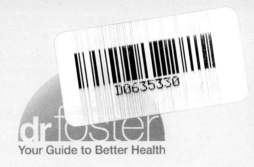

Your Guide to Better Health

GOOD
HOSPITAL
GUIDE

1 3 5 7 9 10 8 6 4 2

Copyright © 2002 by Dr Foster Ltd

First published 2002 by Vermilion,
an imprint of Ebury Press, Random House,
20 Vauxhall Bridge Road, London SW1V 2SA
www.randomhouse.co.uk

Random House Australia (Pty) Limited
20 Alfred Street, Milsons Point, Sydney,
New South Wales 2061, Australia

Random House New Zealand Limited
18 Poland Road, Glenfield, Auckland 10, New Zealand

Random House South Africa (Pty) Limited
Endulini, 5a Jubilee Road, Parktown 2193, South Africa

The Random House Group Limited Reg. No. 954009

Papers used by Vermilion are natural, recyclable products made from wood grown in sustainable forests.

Printed and bound in Great Britain by
Bookmarque Ltd, Croydon, Surrey

A CIP catalogue record for this book is available from the British Library.

ISBN 0091883776

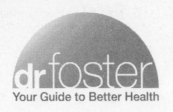

Your Guide to Better Health

GOOD
HOSPITAL
GUIDE

Data Compiled by Dr Foster
Text by Dr Lorna Gold

Vermilion

Who is Dr Foster

Dr Foster provides authoritative information on health services of all kinds in the UK. Our aim is to empower patients with information to help them access the best possible care. We are supervised by an Ethics committee comprising leading figures from the medical profession that has independent legal powers to ensure that guides meet the highest standards.

The ethics committee currently comprises the following membership.

Dr Jack Tinker, dean of the Royal Society of Medicine and chair of the committee

Sir Donald Irvine, president, General Medical Council

Dr Michael Dixon, chair, NHS Alliance

Peter Griffiths, chief executive, Health Quality Service

Dianne Hayter, chief executive, the Pelican Centre, a cancer research charity

Professor Alan Maynard, director health policy unit, York University and chair, York Health Services NHS Trust

Wilma MacPherson, formerly director of nursing and quality, Guy's and Thomas' NHS Trust

Bridget Gill, chair of the Northern and Yorkshire Regional Council of the Institute of Healthcare Management

Kokila Lakhoo, consultant paediatric surgeon, John Radcliffe Hospital

Trevor Campbell Davis, chief executive, Whittington Hospital

Douglas Webb, operations and development director, Friends of the Elderly

Vanessa Bourne, chair, Patients Association

Dr Philip Davies, medical director, Pontypridd and Rhondda NHS Trust

Professor Charles Gillis, formerly director of the West of Scotland Cancer Surveillance Unit.

Further information about Dr Foster and the independent Ethics committee can be found at www.drfoster.co.uk.

Dr Lorna Gold was born in Kilmarnock, Scotland, and studied medicine at the University of Dundee, graduating in 1986. She worked in hospitals until 1992 and for the past eight years has been a full time GP in Handsworth, Birmingham. She is a regular contributor to medical publications and participates in the community-based undergraduate teaching programme for Birmingham University medical students.

Contents

Foreword by Claire Rayner

You hold in your hands a very remarkable document. It is the first ever users' guide to the fifty-year-old National Health Service. Just think about that; fifty years in business and an 'Instructions for Use' manual has never before been provided.

What does that tell you about the NHS and its attitudes to its users? To me it confirms something that I have long suspected about the NHS. As well as being an amazing piece of social engineering, intended from its inception to bring the benefits of modern medicine to the largest number of people, free at the point of use, it has always been somewhat aloof from its users.

Yes, the Service was obviously designed to benefit patients, but the designers regarded patients as merely the raw material of the business of medicine. They were supposed be passive. They were supposed just to lie there waiting to have things done to them and for them and never to question any aspect of their treatment, never to ask questions, never to say anything but a humble 'Thank you' and go away leaving the doctors and nurses and the rest of the staff to go about their mysterious business.

Attitudes have changed over this past half-century. The poorly educated, deferential, grateful, obedient subjects of the 1940s have metamorphosed into the very aware, information-hungry, independent-minded citizens of the 21st Century. Today's patients want doctors and nurses to work with them, to keep them informed, to share their opinions with them and to encourage them to express their own ideas and wishes.

It is no accident that the need to be informed is the top of the list. It has to be. As recently as the 1970s and 80s, when I was writing articles in popular magazines and newspapers explaining the causes, the prevention and the treatment of disease, my mail regularly included bitter complaints (some of them expressed in very pungent terms indeed) from doctors furiously angry about the way I was 'filling their patients' heads with things that 'would only confuse and upset them' and advising me to shut up and leave all matters medical to doctors.

We've come a long way. The Government has responded to the change in popular concern with health matters by insisting that the NHS should be patient-centred in every way. They have decreed it is no longer acceptable for hospitals and GP surgeries to be run for the convenience of the doctors, nurses and other staff but always for that of patients. And this excellent Guide from Dr Foster to provide the sort of information patients need to make the best use for themselves of the NHS is a perfect example of the new thinking.

Is that it, then? Can you now go on your way rejoicing that from here on in all your dealings with the NHS will be idyllic because you are armed with all the facts you need and are therefore in control of what will happen to you? The answer is no. We are here dealing with a huge organisation in which people are more important than the buildings and the equipment in which the work towards health for all is done. A guide to, say, holiday hotels will describe the buildings, the resorts, the local shops and markets and so forth and the likelihood is, if its an honest guide, that you'll set off with a pretty clear idea of what you'll get – and you'll get it.

So in a Guide to, shall we say, hospital A&E services what can you expect? A hotel will tell you in advance if there is room for you. The A&E department is obliged to take all comers even if the demand is so great patients stack up ten deep in waiting room chairs or on trolleys. No Guide in the world could ever foretell accurately the time you might have to wait on any particular evening.

One thing the Guide will make clear is that you sometimes have to make trade-offs in your choices. You may, for example, want to be treated at the most successful orthopaedic unit for your painful knees, but find that they have a much longer waiting list than another which, although not top of the list, is still extremely competent. You may choose that one, only to realise you would have to go to a hospital many miles from home. No visitors. No support system. Suddenly another unit altogether looks an attractive option.

On many occasions you will find you have to weigh the various options and make a choice of the best possible mix – success rates, convenience of access, waiting list – because the ideal or the perfect just can't be achieved (and please note that is as true of the private sector, also included in these pages, as it is of the NHS) But the splendid thing is that such choices are now possible in our newly patient-centred NHS and with this remarkable Guide to hand.

Introduction

Sooner or later all of us will end up in hospital. When we get there we expect to be looked after by doctors and nurses who are competent, working in hospitals that have all the tools necessary to do the job.

How do you know this? The truth is you don't. It is very hard to find out much about the doctor you are going to see or the hospital they work in. What you actually do is rely on the person who sends you – your GP. A GP used to make the decision, choose the hospital and the person to see and you rightly assumed that they would do all these things with your best interests in mind.

This is changing. Patients have found that the level of trust and advice received from their GP can be dependent upon the relationship they have with them, as well as how overworked the GP may be. Increasingly, you, the patient are invited to contribute to the decision about which doctor you are referred to and how your healthcare is managed. This book will help you do just that.

For the first time, we explain in detail how the decisions about your health care are made, who makes them and how you can have your say. We give a detailed guide to every large district general hospital in the country providing you with answers to some of your questions. And we talk you through how to get answers to the rest of your questions.

Do you really have any choice over who treats you in the NHS? In fact there is far more freedom than you realise. The Government favours choice and is currently putting into place measures to tackle long waiting lists. And of course, this guide also covers the private sector, where you are free to seek treatment from whoever you want.

The biggest obstacle to making best use of your options – whether in the NHS or the private sector – is lack of information. This is true both of the public and of GPs. It is remarkable how little official information is provided to GPs about the services that are available in different hospitals and the standards that they meet. This guide will change that. We cover all general acute hospitals plus some smaller hospitals that provide related services such as stroke rehabilitation and give you genuine comparative measures of clinical performance. We have not included community hospitals – i.e. those that do not perform major surgery. We also tell you how the leading specialist hospitals perform in certain areas, for example children's surgery or cancer. Almost all private hospitals have been included. The book has been produced with the guidance of Departmental Health experts, patient organisations, doctors and other health care workers. The issues covered are those raised by patients during focus group research by Dr Foster.

For too long patients have been kept in the dark about the way doctors and hospitals look after their health. This Guide is one in a series of books that will change that. By giving you the facts you need to properly assess the options for your care, it will enable you to get the best service available.

How to use this guide

This guide tells you how health services are provided throughout the country in general and then specifically tells you what each hospital provides in terms of services. The idea is that by combining the two you can get the best care available in your region. For example:

I'm unhappy with the hospital I've been referred to, can my GP refer me to a different one?

On page 15 we explain what you can reasonably expect in this situation. Within the NHS, GPs are in theory free to send patients to any hospital or doctor they choose. The degree to which you and your GP have freedom of choice may be limited by the attitude of your local Health Authority or Primary Care Trust (PCT).

Whatever the degree of choice, the key to making the best of the options available to you is information and a good GP willing to act as your advocate.

I've been waiting for months to see a specialist, how can I speed things up?

Long waiting times are one of the most frustrating aspects of the NHS, but if you have a real medical need, there are several ways you can make sure you are seen by a consultant more quickly. On p17 we explain the options available to you and suggest how to exercise them.

I want to make sure I get the best care possible for my heart condition.

Provision of heart services vary from hospital to hospital, and it may be that you will get better care in one rather than another within your area. For instance, how soon your hospital performs life-saving procedures such as thrombolysis, or whether they have a cardiac rehabilitation unit, could dictate your survival and influence your recovery. On p89 we tell you what measures hospitals should adhere to and which hospitals meet them.

I want to be treated privately, but I don't have health insurance.

Many patients are turning to the private sector for operations rather than wait for one on the NHS. However, these patients may not have insurance schemes and will be paying for their operation out of their life-savings. On p209 we explain why you might choose to be treated privately on a one-off basis, and what schemes are available to finance this.

I don't feel my mother is being treated properly in hospital.

The provision of services for older people in hospital is a major concern. If an older person is admitted as an acute case, say after a fall or a stroke, the kind of care they receive could dictate whether they become long-term inpatients or whether they are up and about as soon as possible and able to return home. On p174 we explain what older people should expect from the NHS and how they can make provision for their care after a hospital stay.

Where to find what you need

The book is divided into three main parts. Section one, *The Patient Pathway*, explains your rights as a patient and talks you through the most common questions that arise about health care. It tells you what you can expect from the system and what you should demand of the system.

Section two, *Focus on Hospital Care*, goes into more specific detail about the issues facing various patient groups. We have chosen heart disease, stroke, cancer, children and older people. Within these sections, we tell you how your hospital measures up against standards of clinical excellence, for example, how long you will have to wait to be seen in A&E, and what lifesaving procedures will be done for you if you are admitted with a heart attack or stroke. We also discuss the pros and cons of the private system, and whether this is a viable alternative to the NHS.

Section three, *Comparing Hospitals*, gives you detailed regional information about hospitals throughout Britain and Ireland.

For each NHS hospital covered in the guide, we tell you what services are available and give you information about staffing levels, waiting times and overall mortality rates. Hospitals are owned by NHS Trusts and most official statistics relate to Trusts not to hospitals. In most cases each Trust owns just one large hospital. However in some cases a Trust may own two or three hospitals – for example, in London, St Bartholomew's Hospital and the Royal London are both run by the Royal London and Barts NHS Trust. Where possible information is given about each hospital. However, official data – such as waiting times – is given for Trusts rather than hospitals because this is how it is collected.

After the NHS hospitals, we list private hospitals by region, again giving extensive detail about the services they provide.

What we tell you about NHS hospital services

Mortality Rates This book includes perhaps the most sophisticated measures currently available. For the first time, you can compare mortality rates for every hospital in the country. We are publishing statistically adjusted mortality rates that allow a genuine comparison of the clinical care provided by hospitals. These figures are based on an analysis of over 100 million patient records held by the Department of Health. The work, conducted by a team under Professor Sir Brian Jarman at Imperial College of Science, Technology and Medicine, has set an important new benchmark for hospital standards. Mortality figures are calculated by looking at all the most seriously ill patients going into hospital – those that account for the vast majority of hospital deaths. The patients have been classified by a range of measures including their age, their sex, their diagnosis and whether they were admitted as an emergency. We have then calculated how many patients should be expected to die on average. We have then compared that with the number of patients who actually died in each hospital. A hospital with a mortality index of 100 is in line with the average. A figure below that indicates a better than expected mortality rate. A higher figure indicates that more people died than would be expected. We also give you mortality rates for heart surgery and the treatment of stroke and broken hip.

It should be stressed that mortality is just one aspect of hospital care and fortunately it is not the principal concern for most people who go into hospital. However it does provide a good first measure of the clinical standards of different hospitals.

The information in the guide indicates a wide variation in the standards of care between hospitals. The facilities and staffing levels in some of the leading teaching hospitals far exceed what is available in many provincial hospitals. Not surprisingly, the large teaching hospitals tend to have much lower death rates.

Staffing Levels The Guide also looks at staffing levels in hospitals and, in particular, the number of doctors and nurses per bed. Staffing is important. The number of doctors per hospital bed is the single most important factor that accounts for the variation in mortality rates.

Waiting times are often the reason a GP may decide to refer a patient to one hospital rather than another. There is often a huge variation in waiting times – the consultant of first choice may have the longest waiting time and it may be better to accept the second or third choice rather than to wait an unacceptable time. The guide gives inpatient and outpatient waiting times for each hospital in the country for a range of specialties.

Waiting times can vary dramatically from one region to another. People in one area can be waiting months for an operation which is available in a matter of weeks at another nearby hospital.

Emergency Services In emergencies, there is no time for making choices. But it is still important for people to know what services their local A&E department offers. How swiftly does it deal with heart attacks? Are there doctors who specialise in children in the hospital at night? How long will you wait in A&E before either being admitted to a hospital bed or discharged? These are important questions to which we provide answers.

Complaints We have looked at how good hospitals are at responding to complaints. It is interesting to note how often hospitals with outstanding achievements in medical care are woefully slow at responding people with a grievance.

What we tell you about private hospital services

Services Private hospitals vary greatly in the types of services offered. Some large city centre hospitals will frequently perform complex heart surgery and will be geared up to cope with the types of emergency that might arise during such an operation. In contrast, smaller rural hospitals will be better prepared for more routine operations such as hip replacements. We tell you what services are offered for cancer and heart disease patients.

Prices We include information about the prices of operations to give you some idea of the variation. However it is important to remember that the price for any individual patient may be different because of their particular circumstances.

Staffing We give details of the number of trained staff in the hospital at any one time and what critical care facilities are available. These are an important part of the hospital's ability to cope with emergencies. Where a hospital has fewer facilities for emergencies it does not mean that the hospital is any less safe – only that it is not equipped to take on higher risk patients or conduct complex operations.

All of us, whether we are patients or doctors, want reassurance that our local medical services will give us adequate care when we need it and in general we get just that. We also want to know how to get the best out of the present service for ourselves and our families, and how to press for that service to become better when they are not as good as the best. This book is a first step to providing patients and GPs with the information they need to make sure that happens.

Section One:
The Patient Pathway

The role of your GP

For most people, 'the doctor' means their general practitioner, or GP. GPs are fully qualified doctors who have spent five years at university followed by at least three years working in hospitals and one year in a training practice. Their job is to look after you when you are sick. If you are unwell, your GP will diagnose your illnesses, treat you when they can, offer support and reassurance when this is appropriate, organise access to other parts of the health service (if for example you need an operation) and monitor you after any treatment in hospital.

Your GP will also play a part in promoting good health, monitoring chronic diseases and liaising with other agencies whose activities can influence the health of individuals or communities. The GP does not work in isolation. Most share a partnership, or group practice, with several other doctors, and all work as part of a Primary Health Care Team, with colleagues as varied as clerical workers, nurses and counsellors. GPs are organised geographically into larger groups called Primary Care Groups or Primary Care Trusts, which are managed jointly by health care workers and lay people and which are able to use NHS funds in a way which is sensitive to the health and social needs of the area. General practice is funded by the government through the Department of Health.

Most GPs are nominally self-employed. They are bound by the regulations set out in their Terms and Conditions of Service, and can be subject to disciplinary proceedings if they breach these regulations. As part of their contract GPs have a financial incentive to attend 30 hours of postgraduate education every year. Until now, this has been left to the individual GP. However, in the near future a process called revalidation will be introduced. This means that every GP who wishes to remain registered with the General Medical Council (a legal requirement for all practising doctors) will be checked at intervals by a team consisting of medical and lay assessors, and GPs who are not performing adequately will have to do extra training or may lose their right to practise.

The way GPs practise medicine is being standardised. Two forces are behind this trend. The first is the move towards evidence-based medicine, which encourages all health care workers to base their care of patients on the results of good quality published research and to be prepared to cast a critical eye over their own practice. The second is a government agency called the National Institute of Clinical Excellence (NICE), which publishes guidelines on important areas of medical treatment, particularly prescribing.

Ninety-eight per cent of us are registered with a GP and often several generations of a family may be under the care of the same one. This means that the GP is better placed than anyone else in the health service to offer holistic care – care which encompasses all aspects of our physical, psychological and social circumstances.

Might I have to wait to see my GP or can I insist on being seen immediately?

The average GP is responsible for around 1,800 patients and most ensure their workload is evenly spread over the week by having an appointment system. The wait for an appointment varies between GPs, and one of the government's targets is that by 2004 everyone should be able to see their GP within 48 hours. Some GPs run open surgeries, where you turn up and wait to be seen. This is useful if you have an urgent problem, but at busy times such as on Monday mornings or during flu epidemics you might have to wait in a long queue. If your problem is a medical emergency such as suspected meningitis or an asthma attack, the receptionist will call a GP away from another patient to see you. There are no other circumstances under which a GP is obliged to see you immediately. If your problem is urgent, even if there are no routine appointments, the receptionist in most practices will arrange for you to be seen that day by a GP. However, there is no guarantee that this will be the GP of your choice.

What is the practice nurse, and what do they do?

The practice nurse is a fully trained nurse. He or she is likely to have had several years of hospital nursing experience after a training—equivalent to a senior staff nurse or ward manager in hospital. Their responsibilities will include most or all of the following:

- Check-ups, contraception, smear tests and education on breast self-examination, ulcer care and removing stitches.
- Health promotion. This includes advice and support for people who are trying to lose weight or stop smoking and advice on sexual health matters.
- Check-ups for patients new to the practice and for people aged over 75.
- Immunisations and advice about keeping healthy when travelling abroad.
- With the health visitor they will offer advice on the health of babies and children and discuss concerns about immunisation with parents. Some practice nurses are also able to advise on other child health issues such as feeding problems and dealing with minor illnesses, but this is more likely to be done by the health visitor. Practice nurses also help the GP with minor surgical procedures and offer ear syringing.
- Help in the management of chronic diseases such as asthma, diabetes and heart disease, and often take blood for tests.
- Some practices operate a system where all emergency consultation requests are handled by a nurse who has received special training and is supported by detailed guidelines – rather like NHS Direct. The nurse can advise on self-care, organise a consultation with a GP, or call an ambulance.

Can I refuse to see the practice nurse and ask to see my GP instead?

You can choose to see your GP instead of the practice nurse for many of the above procedures – immunisation, blood tests and ear syringing, for example. However, the nurse performs these tasks more often than your GP, and is likely to be as skilled at them. If you are having a minor operation or having a contraceptive coil fitted, the GP and nurse both need to be present.

Can I read my medical records if I want to?

Yes, you have had a right to read whatever has been written about you in your medical records since November 1991. If your notes contain information which it would be harmful for you to read, or confidential information about someone else, your GP should remove this first. For example, if it had been recorded in your notes when you were a baby that your older brother was on the at-risk register because your mother had neglected him while suffering from severe postnatal depression, allowing you to read this would breach your brother's and your mother's confidentiality. A recent, well publicised case involved a patient who was distressed on reading in his medical records that he was adopted – a fact which their parents had chosen to conceal from him, and which he would rather not have known. This is only removed from notes when it interferes with the confidentiality of a third party or is of a particularly sensitive nature, and often the GP/hospital/other agency will have sought legal advice before removing it. You can also have access to any information about you that is on your GP's computer system and now nearly half of all GPs make their clinical entries only on computer. Your GP may charge you up to £10 for accessing your records. If your GP prepares a medical report about you for an insurance company, a solicitor or your employer, you can – and should – exercise your right to read the report before it is sent. There will be a charge for such a report. You are entitled to an explanation of anything in your records that you do not understand from your GP. You should not be charged for the time that the GP spends doing this.

What should I look for when choosing a GP?

- Check the surgery building is well maintained, with disabled access, a pleasant waiting room, and evidence of attention to the safety of patients and staff.
- Check the practice leaflet is informative and up to date, and important information is displayed prominently in the waiting room. A well presented practice leaflet suggests care and pride in the way the practice operates.
- Check the staff are cheerful and competent and are happy to deal with any queries you might have.
- Ask whether the practice has a Patient Participation Group which you can join to influence decisions made about the practice and health services in your area.
- Ask your neighbours about the practice, and who they think the best doctors are.

Rather than wait until you are ill to see your GP, it is a good idea to make a brief appointment to see them and make sure that you feel happy with them. This will give you a chance to check:

- That the appointment system is organised to allow you to see that the GP of your choice within 48 hours and that consultations last at least 7 minutes – you may want to choose a surgery that offers 10 minutes or more for each appointment.
- That you are confident that you will be seen within 30 minutes of your appointment time, except in exceptional circumstances such as your GP being called away to deal with a life-threatening emergency.

Then, when consulting your GP you should expect the following:

- You should feel comfortable telling your GP what is troubling you and confident that your symptoms, your beliefs and your anxieties will be respected. They should invite you to participate in decisions about your treatment, explaining the medical issues in a clear and jargon-free manner.
- Further tests or referrals should be organised promptly. Your GP

may even dictate the referral letter while you are in the consulting room.

Your local health authority should be able to supply a list of local GPs. You will probably have to attend the surgery with your NHS card to register. If you have lost your card you may have to complete a special form.

Can I always register with the GP of my choice?

When a GP or a practice has as many patients as they can cope with they have two choices. They can recruit another GP, but this can be very difficult in some parts of the country, or there may not be space for another doctor. Their second choice is to 'close their list' to new registrations. If all the GPs covering your area have closed their lists, then you should apply to the Primary Care Trust who will allocate you to a practice. That practice must accept you, even if their list is closed, but you cannot choose the practice you go to. If you would prefer to see a female doctor, over two-thirds of practices have one so choose a practice that does.

How do I make a complaint about my GP?

Any complaint about GPs or their staff, apart from those where criminal behaviour is involved, should be made to the practice manager in the first instance. Every practice should have a written in-house complaints procedure displayed in the waiting room. Ask for a copy of this. Think carefully about how you express your complaint. Stick to the point and express yourself calmly and rationally. Describe what happened, outline your concerns and suggest how the situation could have been managed better. If you wish to make your complaint in writing, get someone else to go over the letter with you before you send it. Complaints are treated very seriously by GPs, and the vast majority can be resolved to everyone's satisfaction within the practice. If you are not happy with the way the practice handles your complaint, contact your Primary Care

Case history

James Wigg GP Practice

Patients of the James Wigg Practice in North London have access to much more than a GP. Here they will find a wide range of health professionals offering a broad array of services. This means that some patients who would previously have been referred to hospital for specialist treatment can now be treated at their local surgery.

The practice is part of Kentish Town Health Centre and has an unusually large team of staff. There are 13 GPs – one of which focuses on the needs of refugees and homeless people. They are supported by 4 practice nurses, a nurse practitioner and a health visitor. The centre also has 3 counsellors, together with a psycho-sexual counsellor, alcohol counsellor and drugs counsellor. Other services include an antenatal clinic, baby clinic, asthma, diabetes and chronic disease management clinics, and family planning clinics plus an enuresis (bedwetting) service. The centre is also unusual in employing both a welfare rights adviser who gives advice on benefits, and an independent employment adviser.

Usually, patients with mental health problems would require a referral to hospital. However, here they can receive care locally, as a child psychotherapist, a psychotherapist, a psychiatrist and a psychologist all carry out weekly consultations at the centre. There is also a lot of referral between GPs within the practice to those with special interests – in urology or women's health, for example. Referrals are not just confined to GPs – the nurse practitioner and health visitor can also refer patients to the practice's counsellors, psychotherapists or other visiting specialists. The practice nurses can also refer patients with simple injuries to the local casualty department. 'All members of the health team have the same access to patient records on computer, which is almost unheard of,' says Dr Roy Macgregor, one of the GP partners.

The centre is a Beacon Site for its information technology, which means it has been recognised as an example of best practice. It is entirely paperless and all medical records are held on computer. 'The benefit to patients is that all information is summarised on computer screen. Letters from hospital specialists are scanned into the computer and can be called up on screen during the consultation, along with the results of blood tests and blood pressure readings,' says Dr Macgregor. The computer also holds a huge range of patient information leaflets, as well as diagrams that can help patients to understand their condition. This has made consultations longer, but Dr Macgregor says that because they are more detailed and more information is provided, it avoids repeat consultations.

The computer technology has other advantages. The centre is taking part in a pilot to enable GPs to book hospital outpatient appointments via the computer. Dr Macgregor says, 'This allows patients to negotiate an appointment that suits them and take away written confirmation of the time and date there and then.' He adds: 'This has been found to reduce the number of "do not attends" for appointments and since information, including past test results, can be sent to the hospital consultant via the computer, the referrals are also more accurate and more appropriate.'

It will also enable GPs to choose the consultant with the shortest waiting list, instead of relying on printed information. 'By the time waiting lists figures have been collected and printed they are out of date, so having this information electronically will vastly improve things,' says Dr Macgregor.

Trust for advice. If the complaint refers to criminal behaviour such as fraud or sexual assault by your GP, you should take it to the police.

Can I see a GP privately?

Many NHS GPs will see private patients outside their NHS surgery times, such as evenings and weekends. Some GPs choose to do nothing but private work. The advantage of seeing a GP privately is that you are likely to be offered a longer appointment (typically 30 minutes), and if you are at work all day, the appointment times might suit you better. Any GP whom you consult cannot refer you to a consultant on the NHS, arrange tests on the NHS, or give you an NHS prescription, but you can ask your NHS GP to issue an NHS prescription for a drug recommended by your private doctor. If you join a private GP's list, you will normally have to pay a monthly or yearly retainer fee, and you will be charged for individual consultations and prescriptions. Most private medical insurance policies will not pay for you to see a GP privately, although they will pay for consultant referrals recommended by a private GP.

How do I contact a GP when my surgery is closed?

Your GP has a responsibility to make sure that you have access to medical care 24 hours a day. The practice leaflet should explain the arrangements and tell you which telephone number to call if you have an emergency problem at night or at a weekend. Some practices still provide round the clock care for their own patients, but this is rare.

What is NHS Direct?

This is a national telephone network of specially trained nurses who are available 24 hours a day to give telephone advice on health matters to members of the public. At present NHS Direct staff cannot arrange for you to see a doctor, but if necessary they can contact your own GP or your local out of hours service so that you can be offered a consultation. In future, NHS Direct may take on a much wider gatekeeping role in the NHS and within the next two years, all out of hours calls will be handled by NHS Direct. It now covers most of the UK, and can be contacted by telephoning 0845 4647. Further information on NHS Direct is available on its website www.nhsdirect.nhs.uk and the NHS Direct Healthcare Guide is available free from pharmacies.

What are NHS walk-in centres?

In some parts of the country, mainly in city centre areas, it is possible to have a free consultation with a nurse and/or a doctor at a walk-in centre which is run by trained nurses. Some centres, although not all, have doctors on site all of the time. This can be useful if you have an urgent problem but cannot see your own GP – for example, if you are working away from home, or if you work some distance from where you live. (You can, however, see any local GP as a 'temporary resident' and that GP will send the record of your visit to your own GP). Walk-in centres also have longer opening hours and are open seven days a week. If you have a problem which needs to be followed up, the staff at the walk-in centre should contact your own GP. The biggest disadvantage of NHS walk-in centres is that the staff do not have access to your medical records. The development of an NHS-wide computer database of everyone's medical records, or a system of patient-held electronic smart cards, is still many years away. Therefore, NHS walk-in centres are not a realistic alternative to your own GP for anything other than the immediate management of emergency problems. NHS Walk-in centres do not provide travel immunisations.

What is a Medi-Centre?

Medi-Centres are also walk-in clinics staffed by GPs and nurses, but they are run by a private organisation and fees start from £40 for a basic consultation with a doctor and £20 for a telephone consultation. There are five Medi-Centre branches, all in central

London. They offer consultations with a GP or nurse, detailed health screening, blood tests, travel immunisations and simple procedures like ear syringing. All services have to be paid for, including prescriptions. Full details, including the location of the Medi-Centres and a current price list, are on the company website www.medicentre.co.uk.

What will my GP actually do when I consult them?

Your GP will encourage you to tell them about your problem in your own words, then will clarify some of the points by asking questions. This is called 'taking a history'. They may then ask for your consent to examine you. In over 90 per cent of cases, they will be able to make a diagnosis without any further tests.

What if they can't?

Your GP will organise one or more of a range of tests, which may include blood and urine tests, ECGs, X-rays and ultrasound scans. These will either be carried out in the surgery, or in a hospital. Alternatively, they may ask a consultant to see you. The most common reasons for referring to a consultant are :

- Your GP needs an expert second opinion about what might be wrong with you.
- You need an operation or to have tests that only a consultant can arrange, such as an MRI scan.
- You need treatment that only a consultant can prescribe, such as Roaccutane for severe acne.
- Your GP needs help with the management of a complex disease such as rheumatoid arthritis or cancer or for some of your care during pregnancy.

Referrals and waiting lists

Consultants are doctors and surgeons who have a special and usually extensive knowledge of a particular system. This makes them specialists in their particular field. A consultant is the most senior grade of specialist. They will have had extensive training in their specialty, passed a series of postgraduate examinations, and mostly will have performed medical research. Many have ongoing academic, research or managerial commitments. The consultant will also be responsible for a team of doctors who are training in the specialty.

Ultimately, the decision on which consultant to choose and which hospital to visit falls to your GP. However, there is a lot you can do to make sure you have some say in the decision which is reached and it is vital you let your GP know if you are unhappy with any selection. By finding out as much as you can about the hospital you are going to and the procedure you will be undergoing, you can discuss your own findings with your GP, who should in turn respect your choices and preferences.

It is a good idea to make a list of questions about your condition or anything else which worries you and take it with you when you see your GP and later the consultant. Also note down any past and recent medication, past and present medical problems (including those in your family) and any allergies. After you have been referred to a consultant, your GP remains responsible for your care and, even after you have seen the consultant, will often work with them as a team and will continue to look after your other health needs.

There is often a huge variation in waiting times between hospitals to see a consultant. Your GP's first choice of consultant may have the longest waiting time and it may be better to accept the second or third choice rather than wait an unacceptable time. At the back of this guide, we give you the overall outpatient waiting times for each hospital.

Will I always see the consultant to whom my GP referred me?

It would be physically impossible for any consultant to see every patient who has been referred to them, although the majority make a point of seeing the most complicated cases personally. You may be seen by one of the trainee consultants (specialist surgical registrar) or by a clinical nurse consultant, but the consultant should actively supervise your care.

I want to see a consultant. Is my GP obliged to refer me?

If you want to see a consultant and your GP will not refer you, ask them to explain why. It will usually be because you have a condition that can be treated better in general practice. GPs are specialised in the treatment of many common conditions such as minor skin problems, asthma and depression, and many GPs have done extra training in areas like minor surgery and diabetes. Your GP is only obliged to refer you to a consultant if they think that this is an appropriate course of action. They do not have to refer you on demand. If you are unhappy with this decision, ask to see another GP in the practice for a second opinion, or change your GP.

Can I choose which consultant I am referred to?

Yes, provided the consultant of your choice deals with the condition for which you are being referred. There are some limitations. If you are being referred on the NHS, the health authority (or Primary Care Trust) may only fund referrals to local consultants, but you can appeal to the Health Authority (or Primary Care Trust) on this. Under new European Union (EU) directives, you have the right to be referred anywhere in the country if treatment is available for your condition. In some cases, however, there may only be one consultant in your area that specialises in your condition and this will be the person you are referred to. If you are unhappy with this, ask your GP to refer you to a hospital in a different Health Authority.

If you are seeing the consultant privately and your insurance company is paying, check that your chosen consultant is on their approved list.

How does my GP decide which consultant would be best for me? How can I be sure that they have chosen the correct one?

Your GP will base their decision on their existing knowledge of the consultant and the facilities at the hospital in which he or she works. This will include feedback from other patients who have seen that consultant. Your doctor should also be prepared to take your own wishes into account. Ask your GP for the name of the consultant to whom they are referring you, and for their reasons for choosing that consultant. A few hospitals ask GPs not to write to individual consultants, but to let the hospital appointments office allocate each referral to the most suitable consultant, or the one with the shortest waiting list. Tell your GP if you do not wish this type of referral.

I've heard that the hospital I've been referred to is not as good at treating my condition as a different hospital. How can I see a consultant at the hospital of my choice?

Your GP can refer you to the hospital of your choice. If you express a preference for one hospital, or one consultant, over another, most GPs will take this into consideration when referring you. If the hospital of your choice is out of your local area, your GP may need to seek the permission of the Primary Care Trust.

How do I find out more information about the consultant I've been referred to?

Ask your GP to tell you how experienced the consultant is. The Dr Foster website (www.drfoster.co.uk) lists consultants by specialty and areas of expertise. Alternatively, ask your hospital for information about your consultant and a copy of the hospital prospectus (many of these include a potted biography of all the consultants at the hospital).

How does my GP make a referral?

Your GP can make contact with the hospital in one of the following ways:

- By letter. Non-urgent referrals are usually made in this way. The letter is typed and posted to the hospital, where the consultant reads it and decides what level of priority it should be given. The appointments officer then allocates an appointment. Details of the appointment are then sent to you by letter.
- By telephone and fax. If you have an urgent problem, such as suspected cancer, your GP will telephone the hospital to arrange an appointment (most hospitals have a dedicated referral service for cancer) and will send the referral letter by fax. They may be able to tell you the date and time of your appointment there and then. In an emergency, your GP will discuss your case with the duty doctor at the hospital and arrange for you to be seen the same day or admitted. They should give you a referral note to take to the hospital and show to the doctor there. A few consultants allow GPs to put patients straight on to an operating theatre waiting list without the need to see a consultant first (for example for a sterilisation operation).

Do I have a right to see the referral letter and have its contents explained to me?

Yes, and if you feel that your GP has not conveyed the amount of pain you are experiencing, or the effects that the condition is having on your daily life and ability to work, you should ask them to write to the consultant again, stating those points.

What is meant by a waiting list?

There are two sorts of waiting lists – one to see a consultant in outpatients after you have been referred by your GP and then another to be admitted to hospital as an inpatient if you need an operation or procedure. The figures that appear in the newspaper headlines about hospital waiting lists usually refer only to the latter while sick patients wait for an operation. The Patient's Charter introduced a benchmark of a 13-week wait for an outpatient appointment. At the back of this Guide, we tell you which hospitals meet this target.

How long will I have to wait for an outpatient appointment?

There is no guarantee on the maximum length of time you will have to wait between when your GP refers you and when you are actually seen. Instead, there is an 'expectation' that most people should be seen within 13 weeks and everyone should be seen within 26 weeks. Nine out of 10 patients do get seen within these limits and the average waiting time is 7 weeks. But that leaves an unlucky minority who may find themselves waiting up to or even over a year.

If your appointment is cancelled, you should be contacted within 7 days with an offer of a new appointment. You should not have an appointment cancelled more than once.

I think I have been waiting too long to see a consultant. What can I do to speed things up? Does my GP have any influence on waiting times?

If you have a genuinely urgent problem, you will be given priority over people whose condition is less serious. If your condition worsens, tell your GP and ask them to try to speed up your appointment. Most GPs are willing to do this if there is a sound medical or social reason (eg severe pain or inability to work) and if you have a good relationship with your GP, they are more likely to

Case history

Simon Cave, GP

When Simon Cave, a GP in Dorset, refers a patient for hospital treatment, there are a number of factors he must take into account.

'Referral to the hospital sector is common and usually a non-urgent, that is to say non-emergency, situation. So there's time to consider the best treatment for the problem, identify the range of people who could provide that treatment, and find out how available they are. The hospitals in which they work should have the right amount of staff and equipment to deliver that service expertly and safely and there must be confidence in the service to deliver all that is necessary to complete recovery,' he says.

Dr Cave believes that the GP should approach each referral from the perspective of the individual and seek to achieve the very best service available for him or her. Referral to the nearest or most usual hospital should not be automatic (although it may, after consideration, be the most appropriate). Rather, all options should be considered as a matter of course.

Dr Cave suggests that when your GP refers you to a certain hospital, you could ask them that if they or their mother had this condition, would they be making the same decision? After all, a part of the GP's job is to protect the patients, and very few patients have specific knowledge of consultants or hospitals. They depend on their GP to know about the service and Trust, and that the GP will ensure that the service they are sent to is competent and safe.

'When I make a referral it is always with the patient,' says Dr Cave. 'It starts with the condition and the ideal treatment for it. I discuss the risks of treatment and expectations of success with them at the beginning. I then go on to identify the individuals or teams that I know to be competent to provide that ideal service, and the likely waiting time both to be seen and to be operated on – if that is a likely consequence.'

Malignant disease always means that the patient is in for the long haul and often means liaison between many specialists. This means that the choice of initial specialist often determines the ones to whom the patient is later referred.

On the other hand, there is often surprise that 'routine operations' can be less than 100 per cent successful. There can be more than one option to treat a condition and the techniques required for each option are not necessarily within the range of a specific consultant.

With his patients, Dr Cave discusses suitable consultants, their areas of expertise and the waiting time to see them. He also considers their personalities – some are good communicators, some intimidating, some indifferent. 'Patients need personalities who suit them in their different ways', he says. Waiting time is probably the most important factor to the patient and will often override other preferences. Often a patient will choose the consultant with the shortest waiting time. Others, even if uninsured, are prepared to pay private fees to secure the services of a particular Consultant and avoid a long wait.

'The decision as to the final choice of specialist depends on the patient and it is they who weigh up the various factors. Some will opt for the best and disregard all other factors – even the wait. Some will choose the most convenient (often the nearest) and some make a choice based on the experiences of a friend or relative,' says Dr Cave.

However, Dr Cave believes that the GP must ensure that whatever choice the patient makes, it is one that best serves their medical needs.

apply pressure on your behalf. However, the success of this approach varies between hospitals and departments.

You could also try the following:

- Ask your GP to tell you the typical waiting time to see that particular consultant. This should give you an idea of whether you have had to wait longer than normal. All GPs are sent waiting times for consultants in hospitals in their areas and patients can ask for a copy.

- Write to the consultant's secretary, asking if your appointment could be speeded up, and mentioning you are able to accept an appointment that comes up at the last minute because of a cancellation. The secretary may advise you to ask your GP to write and request an early appointment for you.

- Ask your GP or health authority if they have service agreements at hospitals where the lists are shorter than at your local hospital and ask to be referred to any of these.

- Offer to be seen by an NHS consultant privately, who will then, if necessary, refer you back to the NHS for your hospital treatment. Although the cost for this will be around £200, you will have effectively cut up to three months off your total waiting time for treatment.

Can I refer myself directly to a consultant without seeing my GP first?

Even if you are certain that you know what is wrong with you and which consultant you ought to see, you need to be referred by your GP. This applies to both NHS and private referrals in the United Kingdom. Exceptions to this rule are genito-urinary medicine, where you can see a consultant without a referral, and in A&E, if you are admitted as an emergency.

If you are not happy with the consultant you have been referred to, you can ask your GP to refer you to a different one. Your GP will either be able to explain why you are not receiving the treatment you expect or, if appropriate, will be able to put your case to the consultant in a constructive way. They can also refer you to another consultant for a second opinion. If you have a long-term illness and are not confident that your present consultant is doing all they can for you, or if you feel that there is a conflict of agendas which you cannot resolve, ask your GP to refer you to another consultant. When you have a serious chronic illness, it is of paramount importance that you are sure that you are receiving the best possible care.

I don't like hospitals. Can I see a consultant anywhere else?
It may be possible to see the consultant at a community clinic. Ask your GP. However, most consultants work almost exclusively in hospitals. This is because they are responsible for inpatient beds as well as outpatient clinics, and because their time can be used more efficiently if they are based in only one or two sites instead of having to travel around.

If I just turn up at the A&E department will I get to see a consultant more quickly?
The doctors who work in A&E departments cannot arrange outpatient appointments with consultants in other departments but they can ask one of the consultant teams to see you if there is a need to admit you to hospital immediately.

What will happen if my GP thinks I have cancer?
All NHS Trusts are meant to offer patients with suspected cancer an appointment within 2 weeks of referral by their GP. This has made a fundamental difference in the last two years in the treatment of cancer. Most cancer referrals are 'fast tracked' and do not go through the ordinary outpatient system.

Case history

Making a Complaint

When Heather Foster had to call an ambulance for her father, who'd been suffering from shortness of breath for some weeks, she felt he'd been badly let down by his GP. Her father, Ernest, had been to his GP three times in the previous couple of months about breathing problems he'd had, but each time had only been given treatment for a sore throat. Once in hospital, however, doctors realised he had lung cancer, and Ernest died three weeks later.

Heather was upset at how her father had suffered towards the end of his life, and felt that her GP should have realised that he had breathing problems, if not actually diagnose lung cancer. 'I feel that the palliative care should have been started sooner. He could have done without all the pain and suffering he'd had,' Heather said. 'When I told the doctors at the hospital that he had been to the doctor three times, they rolled their eyes, but they didn't say anything.'

Heather first complained verbally to the GP, and then there was an exchange of letters between her and the GP's surgery. But Heather wasn't happy with the GP's explanation. 'The GP kept on saying that my father hadn't ever complained of breathlessness. But you could see that he couldn't even walk about without being out of breath. The GP didn't even look at him. He didn't even listen to his chest. I really wanted to make him sit up and accept that he has to listen to what the patient is saying.'

Heather then contacted Sheffield Community Health Council for advice. They spoke to the surgery on Heather's behalf, but still did not get a satisfactory explanation for why her father's GP had not diagnosed lung cancer. Following the NHS Complaints Procedure, Heather next took her case to the Sheffield Health Authority, and they conducted a review of the case, but concluded that the GP had done nothing wrong and had acted correctly.

Heather was still not happy, and she decided to take her case to the Health Service Ombudsman. The Community Health Council helped her prepare a letter to send to the Ombudsman, explaining what had happened, and the responses she had received so far to her complaint. Sadly, though, the Ombudsman felt it could take no action. Without any other witnesses, or evidence, they said they had to believe what the GP had told them.

There is no guarantee of success if you complain to the Health Service Ombudsman, but a spokesperson for Sheffield County Council offers the following advice to people who are unhappy with treatment they, or a relative, have received. First, you should be clear about what you want. If you want vengeance, you are not going to get it. You can only get an apology, an explanation for what happened, and a promise that it won't happen again. You should also attempt an informal complaint first, for example, with a meeting set up by your Community Health Council with your doctor. Meetings often work better and quicker than letters. Finally, you can try to avoid needing to make a complaint if you are assertive with a doctor or other health professional. If you've got a bad feeling about something, don't just let it go. Ask for an explanation. And if you don't understand something they have told you, tell them.

Where else might my GP refer me to other than a hospital?

- A physiotherapist, for joint and muscle problems.

- A chiropodist or podiatrist, for foot problems.

- A community dietitian, for advice on the management of obesity, diabetes and some digestive problems.

- A community midwife, for care during pregnancy and delivery.

- A district nursing team, if you need nursing care at home. Some areas also have specialised community nursing teams to look after people who would otherwise need to be admitted to hospital, for instance, after suffering a stroke.

- An occupational therapist, for help with rehabilitation after an illness or injury, and to provide aids and appliances to make things easier for you at home.

- A social worker, for example if you need help with benefits, housing (including funding for structural adaptations to your house, such as having stair rails put in), home care services and assessment for a place in a residential or nursing home.

- A community continence advisory team, if you need help with managing bladder or bowel control.

- A family planning clinic, for contraceptive services (although most GPs provide a full range of these).

- A genito-urinary medicine clinic for the management of sexually transmitted infections and other genital problems. If you do not want this referral recorded in your medical records, tell your GP.

- A community paediatrician, for child health and development problems.

- A community mental health team, for a wide range of psychiatric conditions.

- For complementary medicine such as osteopathy or acupuncture. The availability of these services on the NHS varies widely between different areas. If you feel you would benefit from the involvement of any of these agencies in your care, discuss the matter with your GP.

Outpatients

Outpatient departments are non-ward areas where patients meet consultants and their teams for the purpose of diagnosis, deciding on and organising further investigations or treatment and, later, for the continued review of patients who need long-term consultant input into their care. Outpatient examination is limited and appointments times vary from 7 minutes to half an hour, after which you can expect to return home. Make sure that you write down any questions you want to ask during your appointment, or take a friend or relative with you who can take notes for you. It is important that you understand what the consultant says to you, so insist on having your condition explained. At the end of the appointment, make sure that your consultant has given you a treatment plan and that you understand any follow-up procedures you may need to have.

Not everyone needs to be followed up in the outpatient clinic. If you have had a minor operation, or an acute illness from which you have made a complete recovery, you will be discharged back into the care of your GP. If you do need to be seen in outpatients, the consultant will state when they would like to see you (for example, 'in six weeks'), and a member of the clerical staff will be responsible for contacting the consultant's secretary to arrange an appointment for you.

How do I know if I have to go to the outpatient clinic?
You will receive a letter giving the date, time and place of your appointment and advising you whether you need to bring anything with you.

If you need a follow-up appointment, you may be given an appointment card before you leave the ward, or it may be sent to your home address later. If you do not receive an appointment within two weeks of being discharged, contact the consultant's secretary yourself – you may have been overlooked in error.

What should I do if the appointment I've been sent isn't convenient?

Contact the booking office or the consultant's secretary immediately – the number to call should be on your appointment letter. Explain the situation. They may be able to change your appointment to a date and time that suit you better.

What will happen if I accidentally miss my appointment?

Some hospitals and departments will send you another appointment, while others will assume that you have changed your mind about attending and discharge you. As soon as you realise that you have missed your appointment, telephone the booking office or the consultant's secretary. If you are told that your GP needs to refer you again, ask them in person rather than leaving a message with the receptionist.

Why might the hospital cancel or change my appointment?

You should not have your appointment cancelled outright without an explanation. It may be postponed if the doctor you were scheduled to see will be absent and a suitable replacement is not available. If the new date is much later than the original one, you should telephone to ask if alternative arrangements can be made to see you earlier. If it is important on medical or social grounds that you should not have a long wait, ask your GP to write on your behalf.

Can any operations be performed in outpatients?

Procedures which might be performed in outpatients include endoscopies, removal of skin lumps, injection of varicose veins and suction clearance of impacted debris from the ear.

Will there be a crèche or somewhere I can leave my children?

Check with the hospital beforehand. However, very few hospitals provide any sort of organised care for patients' children, so if at all possible you should arrange for friends or relatives to look after children who are too small to cope with coming to outpatients with you. Childcare is a major barrier to good health care for many of the patients who need it most, particularly women and those who are socially disadvantaged. If you feel strongly that your local hospital should provide a childcare facility, you could write to the hospital manager and your Primary Care Trust. If you are unsuccessful, you might want to start a campaign in your community.

In what circumstances might I get my travel expenses paid?
If you are attending an NHS hospital or disablement services centre, you are eligible to have your travel costs reimbursed if your family is receiving Income Support, income-based Jobseeker's Allowance, Family Credit or Disability Working Allowance; if you have a low income; if you are attending a genito-urinary medicine clinic more than 15 miles from your home; if you are a war disablement pensioner being treated for your war injury; if you live in the Scilly Isles or the Scottish Highlands and Islands and are attending a mainland hospital. Should you fall into any of the above categories, you can also claim for accompanying your child. To claim travel costs, you must keep your tickets and receipts and take them to the hospital fares office; if the hospital does not have one, ask reception. If you qualify because you are claiming a social security benefit, you should bring a payment book or letter or HC2 or HC3 certificate to the hospital with you. If you are on a low income and do not receive a qualifying benefit, you should ask the hospital for an HC5 form to claim a refund, or get an HC1 form ('Claim for help with health costs') from the hospital, pharmacy or local Benefits Agency.

What is a one-stop clinic? What sort of conditions are seen in these clinics?
A one-stop clinic is where you can see doctors, nurses and other health care staff who specialise in your condition, and have most

Fiona Robinson

Two weeks after a routine breast scan, Gemma Robinson's mother Fiona received a letter saying there was a query with the results. The letter included details of an appointment at a one-stop clinic in a London hospital for an immediate check-up.

Fiona immediately panicked. On the day, Gemma went along with her for moral support yet secretly thought that it must all be a fuss about nothing. 'She was only 54, after all. Far too young to have breast cancer,' she says. 'We sat in a waiting room which seemed to be full of older women and their husbands. There was even a basket of knitting that you could do if you got bored waiting.' Feeling – and looking – 20 years younger than everyone else, Gemma's mother felt alienated, which made her feel even more nervous.

The one-stop process took all day, during which Fiona was seen by various medical staff and underwent a number of tests, the first of which was a mammogram. At the end of the day, Fiona would see a consultant who would give her the results of the tests.

Two minutes after disappearing into the room for the mammogram Gemma heard her mother 'literally wailing ... I was called in and it turned out the clinician had asked her about "the lump on her breast", presuming Mum already knew that there was something there. This was the first my mum had known that they'd picked up something a few weeks earlier. Obviously it was a terrible mistake, but at the time it felt like a cruel, flippant way to be told you've potentially got something fatally wrong with you. Understandably my mother was very angry and scared. '

However, from that moment on, the one-stop process started to work in Fiona's favour. 'A trained breast cancer nurse immediately appeared and managed to calm Mum down. Then she was seen very quickly by a nurse who took fluid from the lump. This confirmed that the lump was malignant. Ten minutes later we were talking to the consultant who explained Mum's options. On the day I know Mum felt that she was on a roller coaster and that one minute she was feeling great and the next she was told she needed serious surgery and that she was potentially very ill.'

Gemma says that her mother didn't feel she had time to digest the news, although they had to wait another week before being told how large the lump was and what kind of surgery she would need. But Gemma is impressed with the one-stop system. 'From my point of view (ie not the woman who is about to lose a breast) no one wants to hear bad news but at least we were dealt with swiftly. In the space of three hours we'd become part of the whole NHS machine and now my mum was 'in the right hands'. Certainly, the trained breast cancer nurse was an angel that day and she continued to be a huge support all the way through.

Two months later, following surgery, Gemma's mother was given the all clear.

of the tests you need, in one trip to the hospital. One-stop clinics are particularly suited to the management of chest pain, bleeding from the bowel or bladder, breast lumps and some gynaecological problems. You are likely to know the results of any tests the same day.

What if my consultant tells me there's nothing wrong with me but I still feel ill?

The patient's charter stipulates that you have the right to be referred to a second opinion if you and your doctor agree that this is appropriate. You also have a right to see a consultant that is acceptable to you. Ask your GP to refer you a different consultant on the NHS, or consider asking for a referral to a private consultant who you will be able to see more quickly.

If I'm told I need an operation, what questions should I ask the consultant about it?

These might include:
- Who is going to do my operation?
- How experienced is that person?
- How will this operation benefit me compared with not having it done?
- Is there an alternative treatment to surgery?
- What could go wrong and what would be done to remedy this?

How long before I'm admitted to hospital after my outpatient appointment?

There is a guaranteed 18-month maximum on the length of time you will have to wait from seeing the consultant in outpatients to being admitted for your operation and the average waiting time is 3 months. Waiting times vary from one Health Authority to another and at the back of this Guide you can compare hospital waiting times in your area.

I feel as if I have been waiting too long for my operation, is there anything I can do to speed things up?

- If you feel that your condition is worsening or that you are unable to work because of it, tell your GP. They will contact your consultant and you could be reprioritised.
- Remember that some surgeons have shorter waiting times than their colleagues within the same hospital, so ask your GP if you could see one of them instead.
- You could also ask about clinical trials relevant to your condition. These give you the chance to receive cutting-edge treatment for a particular disease from experts in the field.
- If you feel that you have been waiting too long for an appointment, appeal to your GP in the first instance, but then call the hospital direct and tell them that you want to complain to the local Health Authority about how long you have been waiting. If you appointment is not brought forward, call your Health Authority and ask them to act for you.

Can I speed things up by having my treatment abroad?

The Government has recently announced plans to speed up waiting times, and from July 2002 all patients who have been waiting more than 6 months for a heart operation will have the following options:

- Wait for the same hospital and be guaranteed admission within 12 months
- Choose to go to another NHS hospital or a private hospital in the UK
- Travel to Europe, where the treatment will remain free. Foreign treatment will be arranged through a central clearing system and travel costs for both you and a relative or friend will be met.

The European Court of Justice has ruled that patients waiting an unreasonable length of time for treatment on the NHS have a right to seek treatment abroad. Currently the average waiting time for

bypass surgery in other EU countries is 3 months compared to one
year in the UK. The government aims to make these options
available for for hip, knee and cataract patients by 2005.

Can I just go abroad and admit myself to hospital?
If you walk into a hospital in the EU with severe chest pain, you will
be given all the necessary diagnostic and investigative procedures
and receive any necessary treatment under the NHS. However, if you
do this, you run the risk of being seen by a consultant and treated in
a hospital about which you have no information.

**What is a specialist hospital and why might I be referred
to one?**
Most patients who are referred to hospital end up either at a local
district general or a larger treatment site. However, if your
condition cannot be treated in either of these, you will be referred
either by your consultant or the hospital to a specialist hospital.
This is usually because local hospital staff lack the expertise or
facilities to deal with a particular form of treatment. Alternatively,
you may have a rare condition or need a particularly complex
operation that requires a large number of staff. Many specialist
centres are part of large teaching hospitals such as King's College
Hospital, London – a national centre for the treatment of liver
disease.

In the heart disease, cancer and children's section of this Guide,
we name some of the specialist hospitals for these conditions.

Inpatients

If the outcome of your visit to the outpatient clinic is that you
need to be admitted to hospital as an inpatient, it will be for one of
the following reasons:

- You need to have an operation
- You need have tests which can only be carried out in hospital
- You need treatment which can only be given as an inpatient, such as a course of medication through a drip or to stay in hospital for a period of observation.

You can also be admitted to inpatients as an emergency through A&E or directly by your GP if you need immediate treatment.

Any hospital is an alien environment for most people and the idea of being an inpatient can be quite daunting. By finding out as much as possible about what to expect during your admission, you can make the experience less intimidating. It is a very good idea to ask a friend or relative to act as your advocate and make sure they understand your wishes. Should either of you be unsatisfied at any stage with the advice or treatment you are receiving from any member of staff, you should seek a second opinion from someone more senior. You should never feel intimidated to ask questions about your treatment and can insist that they are answered in a way that you can understand.

How can I prepare myself for an operation?

If you know in advance that you are having an operation, take the opportunity to get as fit as possible beforehand. This means stopping smoking; perhaps call the national telephone quitline 0800 169 0169 or visit its website www.giveupsmoking.com. If you are overweight, you should try to lose just a few pounds as this will reduce your risk of problems with the anaesthetic and wound infections. Try to keep to a healthy diet with plenty of fruit, vegetables, wholegrain cereals and protein and take moderate exercise. You can also prepare yourself psychologically by finding out as much as possible about what to expect when you have your operation. Your hospital should send you leaflets on the type of operation you are going to have and how best to prepare yourself for it. Make sure that you receive these. Also, ask the doctor or nurse at outpatients to write down the name

Maureen and Colin Leach

For Maureen and Colin Leach, the infamous NHS waiting lists were more than an inconvenience – for them, they were a matter of life and death, and something that forced them to go thousands of pounds into debt to avoid. Colin, 76, had always been extremely fit and healthy for his age, swimming twice a week. But early last year he suddenly started to get breathless when exercising. His condition deteriorated and soon he got breathless going up the stairs.

Colin went to his GP, who tried to get him an appointment with a consultant cardiologist. Weeks passed and they had received no appointment. Concerned about Colin's worsening condition, they went back to their GP a couple of times, who put them on a 'fast-track'. This meant that Colin was given an electrocardiogram (ECG) and other tests, even though he had yet to see a cardiologist. He eventually saw the cardiologist, who, after yet more tests, discovered that Colin had two badly blocked coronary arteries, for which he would need a bypass operation. Colin was told by the cardiologist that he needed a bypass as soon as possible, but that he would have to wait for at least 12 months for the operation. Colin was also put on the waiting list for a pacemaker, which he would have to have fitted several weeks before the bypass could be done.

Maureen and Colin were horrified that they would have to go on a long waiting list for such urgent treatment. Colin could have had a fatal heart attack at any time. Even if he suffered a heart attack from which he survived, operating on a damaged heart is much more difficult than on a relatively healthy one. Maureen and Colin saw no option but to have the operation done privately. Arranging this was easy and straightforward, and the operation was a success. But the

Leaches had to pay £15,000 for the operation, a sum for which they had to go several thousand pounds into debt.

Colin wrote to his MP and the Minister for Health to complain, and the day before he went into the private hospital he received a letter saying that within five years, the Government hoped to have the waiting list down to three months. However, Colin and Maureen both feel very bitter about this, having paid into the NHS all their working lives. Although Colin has made a good recovery from the operation, the Leaches' fight goes on. They have discovered that, since Colin's pacemaker was fitted privately, it must be routinely checked and maintained privately, too, for which they will have to pay themselves. They are arguing that this should be done on the NHS.

of your condition and the operation that you are going to have so that you can look it up on the internet.

What can I do if my operation is cancelled?

The Trust is obliged to give a new date for your operation within 7 days and Government targets are that your operation should be rescheduled within 30 days. At the back of this Guide, we give you figures for cancelled operations. This will show you which hospitals are more likely to cancel your operation.

What should I do if I have a cold or a sore throat before an operation?

Ring the ward or see your GP that day. He or she will be able to tell you whether your operation will need to be postponed until after you have recovered.

What will happen when I am admitted to hospital?

Hospitals run on such high levels of bed occupancy that you may be asked to telephone on your proposed admission date to confirm that a bed is available for you. When you arrive, you may not be given a bed immediately. A nurse will take your details and put a plastic bracelet giving details of your name, date of birth and hospital reference number on your wrist. Then one of the junior surgical doctors will ask you about your present problem and your general health, examine you and write up a drug chart for any medication you might need. This whole process may be spread over most of a day.

Will I be in a mixed ward?

You might feel distressed at the idea of being in a mixed ward, and an increasing number of hospitals now only have single-sex wards. The Department of Health has made a commitment to eliminate mixed-sex wards in 95 per cent of health authorities by the end of

2002. However, five hospital Trusts have said their schemes for single-sex accommodation will not be completed until after that deadline and for others, pressure on beds and the type of accommodation in some older buildings means the problem is almost impossible to overcome. The department has allocated £40m towards the project but there are fears that the real cost of meeting the target will be much higher. Some consultant wards, including intensive care units, will be able to continue without the need to segregate patients by sex.

The campaign for single-sex wards has been spearheaded by The Patients Association and the Association of Community Health Councils who say that mixed-sex wards make many patients feel uncomfortable and unhappy during their stay. Some hospitals do try to meet requests for single-sex accommodation by making available side rooms on wards but it is not always possible to meet the demand.

Can I stay in my own room?
Private rooms, possibly en-suite, are sometimes available for a small charge to patients who want more privacy whilst staying in hospital. However their availability can never be guaranteed. The rooms cost on average around £40 per night. In some hospitals, they can be pre-booked for planned admissions, particularly on maternity wards and you should call your hospital to ask if amenity rooms can be reserved. However, it is always possible that they will need to be used for another patient at the last moment. It is certainly worth asking for a single room if you cannot sleep on a mixed ward or feel the need for more privacy.

What is day-case surgery, and what operations can be done this way?
If you have day-case surgery, it means that you are admitted to a hospital bed and discharged (sent home) on the same day. Often

you will have attended for a pre-operative check a week or two earlier to make sure you are fit for the operation. Operations typically done as day cases are removal of children's tonsils, male and female sterilisation, varicose vein surgery and hernia repairs.

What is keyhole surgery, and what operations can be done this way?

Keyhole, or laparoscopic, surgery is the term used when an operation is done through two or three tiny cuts around a centimetre long using a fibre-optic camera and special instruments. This means that you have smaller external wounds and can mean that you recover more quickly, although this is not always the case. Keyhole surgery is used for exploratory procedures, female sterilisation, gallbladder removals and an increasing number of other procedures. It can also be used to examine and repair damaged joints – this is called arthroscopic surgery.

I'm being admitted to a teaching hospital. Do I have to agree to being examined by medical students?

Every patient has the right to decide whether to speak to, or be examined by, medical students, and the students should always wear an identity badge clearly displaying their name and status. If you decide not to let students examine you, your wishes will be respected. A medical student will not be given responsibility for prescribing drugs or making decisions about your treatment.

What kind of surgeon will I see?

- **Consultant Surgeon** Your consultant is responsible for managing your care and is assisted by a team of doctors. Whilst you may see your consultant at hospital appointments and on the ward there is no certainty that they will perform your operation. In order to become a consultant in the NHS, their name must be on the General Medical Council (GMC) specialist register.

- **Specialist Surgical Registrar (SpR)** These are senior trainee consultants. Most surgeons spend six years in this post building up their surgical experience and expertise under the supervision of a consultant. After their training is complete and they have become a Fellow of the Royal College of Surgeons (FRCS) they can apply for a position as a fully trained consultant.

- **Senior House Officer (SHO)** Doctors at this level spend between two and four years learning surgery and gaining experience of different surgical procedures. They work under the direct supervision of a consultant. After sitting MRCS (Member of the Royal College of Surgeons) exams, they continue their training under the title of 'Mr', 'Mrs', 'Miss' or 'Ms'.

- **Pre-registration House Officer (PRHO)** All newly qualified doctors spend a year training in a hospital as a House Officer with provision registration with the GMC. Usually six months are spent as a House Surgeon gaining experience in different areas of surgery, and another six months are spent as a House Physician working in general medicine. Each works as a member of a team under the supervision of a consultant. House Officers do most work on the hospital wards and will be your main point of contact as an inpatient.

- **Associate Specialist Surgeon** These surgeons carry out a wide range of surgical care, both on the ward, in the outpatient clinic and in the operating theatre. This might include complex surgery at which they have become expert. They work under the supervision of a consultant.

- **Staff Grade Surgeon** These surgeons have usually had some experience as a registrar, with whom, in many hospitals, they may alternate on the emergency surgical rota. They may perform a range of operations and outpatient consultations under the supervision of a consultant.

What questions should I ask the surgeon before my operation?

- What will be done if complications arise during the operation?
- Where will I be cut, and how big is the cut likely to be?
- How soon can I get up after the operation?
- When will I be able to start eating and drinking?
- When will I be able to have a bath or shower?
- What pain relief am I likely to need?
- Will I get this automatically, or will I have to ask for it?
- Will I have any drips, drains or catheters? What for?
- How long will I be in hospital?
- How long will my stitches or clips need to stay in?
- What restrictions will be placed on my activities when I go home?
- When can I start driving again?
- When can I go back to work?
- When can I start doing sport?
- Will I need to come to the outpatient clinic afterwards?

Why might I be 'nil by mouth'?

It is dangerous to have a general anaesthetic if your stomach is full as you may inhale vomit. Drinking even small amounts of liquid is also dangerous as it causes your stomach to secrete digestive juices. Therefore, before your operation you will be forbidden from eating and drinking for several hours – usually 6–8 hours.

What is an anaesthetic?

An anaesthetic is a substance given to make sure you don't feel anything while the operation is being done. A general anaesthetic means that you are put you to sleep, usually with a relatively painless injection into the back of your hand. A regional anaesthetic is when you are given an injection to make a large part

Consent Forms

This is a form that you sign, in the presence of a doctor (who also signs it), to confirm that you understand fully, and are willing to have, the planned operation or procedure. Do not sign the consent form until you are satisfied that you have been given enough information about your planned operation and that you are sure you want to go ahead with it. Ideally, you should be talked through the procedure by the surgeon performing the operation and if not, another doctor who is qualified to perform it unsupervised. Make sure you understand what you are signing. If the consent form contains a clause that you are not happy about, discuss it with the doctor. For example, for a gynaecological operation there may be something on the form about being examined by medical students while you are under the anaesthetic. Asking for a clause like this to be removed will not prejudice your treatment in any way. Signing a consent form does not take away your rights if problems arise due to the operation being performed negligently. If you are having an operation on one of your arms or legs, make sure that the consent form correctly states whether it is the right or left arm or leg and that the limb is marked with waterproof ink while you are still awake.

of your body, such as a whole limb, numb. A local anaesthetic is when you are given an injection or a cream to make a small area of your body numb. The type of anaesthetic depends upon the type of operation you are having. Most anaesthetics are given by an anaesthetist.

Case history

Caroline Williams

Home comforts and extras, like having her own telephone and television, made all the difference to Caroline Williams, 27, when she spent a week in a London hospital in September 2001.

Caroline's operation, to remove a pituitary tumour, was originally scheduled for the end of August. She went into hospital as planned, but her operation was cancelled the next day because of an emergency. Although she was pleased to be going home, she was disappointed because she had done a lot of mental preparation for the operation.

The operation was rescheduled for the following week. This time, she knew what to expect at the hospital and what to take in, like photos, slippers and other home comforts. She also felt psychologically more in tune with her surroundings. She was put in a single-sex bay in a mixed-sex ward. The three women sharing her bay were all very ill. When she felt ill this didn't affect her, but when she started feeling better and became more aware of her surroundings it became quite upsetting. 'One was in a lot of pain and kept calling out in the night.'

She had a telephone by her bedside. 'Having my own phone made such a huge difference because I could make and receive calls whenever I wanted.' She also paid between £3 and £5 a day for her own television: 'It gave me a direct link to the outside world and brought a feeling of normality to the ward.' The television in the patients' room didn't work and Caroline felt this room needed to be brighter and more stimulating, so that patients would feel inclined to make use of it.

In terms of cleanliness, Caroline says: 'The actual bay was fairly all right, but the bathroom wasn't. There was no soap in the toilets and I had to wear flip-flops in the shower.' But the food and choice of options was a 'pleasant surprise', although Caroline felt there should have been more fibre and fresh fruit. She appreciated little things like being offered hot chocolate in the evenings and iced water each morning.

The nurses and doctors were friendly and caring, but on weekend shifts some could have been more attentive. 'You really have to be proactive about finding things out and getting answers to questions. The older patients seemed to find this harder – one kept worrying that she'd get told off and kept asking if she was allowed to do this and that,' says Caroline.

Caroline's advice to anyone preparing for a hospital stay is to try to make your surroundings homely by displaying photos of loved ones. She also advises taking flip-flops to use in the shower, extra soap, loose change and lots of changes of bed clothing. And she recommends a notebook and pen to jot down questions to ask the doctors. 'The most important thing however is visitors, otherwise the days can seem long and drag by. I was lucky to have so many friends and family around me.'

Will I be conscious when I go into the operating theatre?

If you are having a general anaesthetic, you will be put to sleep in a small room that leads into the operating theatre. If you are having a regional or local anaesthetic, you will be conscious in the operating theatre. Drapes will be arranged so that you will not be able to see the operation being done.

How do I know I won't be mixed up with another patient and have the wrong operation?

When the operating theatre porters collect you from the ward for your operation, the nurse on the ward should confirm who you are and what operation you are having. If this is not done in your presence, tell the porters your name and what you are in for and ask them to check that they are collecting the right person. Again, while you are in the anaesthetic room but before you are given the anaesthetic, ask the anaesthetist to check that the operating theatre staff have the correct information about you.

What if I decide not to have the operation after all?

You can decide not to have the operation at any stage until you are under the anaesthetic, although if the operation is to treat a serious condition you may be asked to sign a form to confirm that you are discharging yourself against medical advice. If you decide in the future that you do want to have the operation, ask your GP to refer you back to the surgeon – but you will need to join the waiting list again.

How will I feel when I come round from the anaesthetic?

Better than you might expect. With modern anaesthetic drugs, it is very unusual to suffer from the sickness or dopiness that used to last for several days after an anaesthetic. One group of people who often do have problems after an anaesthetic are older people. Even apparently fit older people can become quite confused for a few days after a general anaesthetic. Nobody should drive a car on the same day as having a general anaesthetic.

What can I do if I feel I'm not being properly informed about my treatment?

If you are worried about any aspect of your treatment or feel that you don't understand what is happening to you, ask the House Officer to explain. It may help to write your questions down. They should be answered in plain English in a way that you can understand and if they are not, insist that they are. If you feel that your requests are being ignored, ask a friend or relative to act on your behalf and don't be afraid to ask to speak to someone more senior.

Can my relatives visit me in hospital at any time?

Many hospitals now have 'open visiting' rather than the strict visiting hours that were enforced in the past and you should check with the ward if you need to visit outside normal hours. Visiting times in most hospitals are between 2pm and 8pm, although patients are often only allowed visitors for one hour on the first day after a major operation. In certain circumstances, visiting times may be extended: on a maternity unit, the baby's father may be allowed to visit whenever he wants; when a child is in hospital, the parents are encouraged to stay with them at all times; when a patient is seriously ill or dying, their relatives will be allowed to stay with them round the clock if they wish. If your relatives are unable to visit during the set visiting times and need permission to come in the morning or evening instead, tell the ward manager. Special arrangements can usually be made on an individual basis. If you are being tired out by visitors who come too often and stay too long, and you do not feel able to tell them how you feel, ask the ward manager if she can explain to them that you need more rest. Some rules surrounding hospital visiting – for example, limiting the number of visitors each patient can have at any

Case history

David Martin

David Martin, 61, was admitted to hospital in October 2001 to receive chemotherapy treatment for a rare form of leukaemia. He was discharged ten days later. His treatment left him vulnerable to infections, so he was given a lot of medication to take once he got home. But he didn't receive the patient information leaflets that should accompany each drug. All he got was information on when and how often to take his medicines rather than what possible side-effects there might be.

Over the weekend, David vomited and developed a fever. He'd been told to contact the duty haematologist about any concerns. But when his wife, Mary, tried to reach the haematologist on-call on the Saturday evening, she was instead referred to a medical scientist who was unable to help but advised calling the ward. Nurses on the ward advised Mary to give David paracetamol and take him to A&E if he didn't improve. However, David had previously been told by his consultant to avoid A&E because it could put him at risk of picking up an infection. The Martins decided to wait until Monday morning and talk to the team that had cared for him. When they did this David was told to return to the ward immediately, where he was readmitted for a further ten days. He was suffering from a reaction to the antibiotics he'd been taking, and also showed signs of having an infection.

David's advice to anyone caught in a similar situation is: 'If you're told to speak to the duty specialist for your condition and find it difficult to reach them, keep persisting until you do.' He also recommends keeping a notebook where you can record your questions and the specialist's answers.

time, or not permitting small children to visit – are there so that sick people in hospital suffer as little disturbance as possible and to reduce the spread of infection in hospital. These rules are not always enforced properly. If another patient's visitors are disruptive, tell the ward manager.

What is a superbug?

'Superbug' is a popular term for a germ resistant to a large number of antibiotics, the most well-known being the 'methicillin resistant Staphylococcus aureus', or MRSA. This germ is found in many hospital wards and can cause problems with infections, mainly of the skin – including surgical wounds. It cannot be killed by any of the commonly used antibiotics. It can be carried by other patients, or on the skin of hospital staff.

Patients are becoming increasingly concerned about the possibility of getting a hospital acquired infection. Your hospital should be able to give you rates for the number of patients per 1000 admissions who developed an infection while there during the previous 12 months.

What might put me at risk of getting a superbug?

An operation or hospital stay increases your risk. If you have a wound or a skin ulcer, the germ can happily live and multiply in the rich tissue fluids. Lack of hygiene in hospitals almost certainly plays a big part in spreading the infection. Hand washing by staff between seeing patients has been shown to reduce its spread. Most hospitals already run poster campaigns to encourage staff to wash their hands as much as possible and you can always ask a doctor or nurse to wash their hands before they examine or treat you.

What can I do if the ward is dirty?

This has been identified as a real problem in British hospitals, and is starting to be addressed nationally. If you find yourself, as a patient or as a visitor, in a ward with dusty rails and filthy toilets, or if you see staff failing to observe basic hygiene such as washing their hands after treating patients, bring the matter to the attention of the ward manager. If your concerns are dismissed, write a letter to the hospital manager giving a factual description of what you have observed. If the hospital manager's name and contact details are not displayed where you can see them, ask the ward staff or speak to the hospital's information department.

What choices do I have in terms of hospital food?

You should be given three proper balanced meals a day, and a choice of drinks. The quality of hospital food, and the amount of choice available, varies widely between health authorities. Some hospitals prepare food on the premises each day and serve it on the wards – a good arrangement, as it means that portion sizes and special diets can be allocated flexibly, although it means more work for the ward staff. Other hospitals use external caterers, and serve pre-packaged meals rather like airline food. At the very least, you should be able to select a nutritious vegetarian meal from the choices on offer. Hospitals will also offer choices based on the needs of their local community – so, for example, you will get Halal meat dishes in hospitals serving areas with a large Muslim population.

What can I do if I suspect my relative isn't being fed properly in hospital?

Ask for an appointment to discuss the matter with the ward manager and state your concerns. Ask for an assurance that your relative will be given appropriate help to eat each meal. Some families prefer to visit at mealtimes and take personal responsibility for feeding their relatives – you should be allowed to do this if you wish.

Is it possible for a friend or relative to bring in my own food?

Yes, as long as the food that your friend and relative brings you is suitable for any special diet you might be on. For safety reasons, most hospitals will not allow you to heat up your own food on the ward, so ask your friend or relative to bring food that does not need to be heated.

Who decides when I can go home?

A member of the medical team will normally decide when you are fit to go home after discussion with the nurses on the ward. The decision may be made at quite short notice – for example, you may be told during the morning ward round that you can go home at lunchtime on the same day.

Do I get any say? What if I feel I need longer in hospital?

The long hospital stays of the past were not necessarily a good thing. Once active treatment has finished, you will be better off completing your recovery at home, where you can sleep in your own bed and choose your own meals. Hospital departments are under so much pressure that they can only offer you a hospital bed for as long as you have a medical need for one. However, if you do not feel well enough to go home, or you know that your home circumstances will interfere with your recovery, tell the consultant or the ward manager. You may be able to extend your stay if there is a good medical or social reason to delay your return home, or they may arrange a transfer to a nursing home or community hospital. Alternatively, in some areas you may be able to pay for a bed in a convalescent home where you can stay until you feel fully able to care for yourself. As this needs to be booked in advance ask your consultant if they can arrange it for you.

Can I discharge myself from hospital?

You can only be detained in hospital against your wishes if you are being held under the Mental Health Act. Even if your refusal to accept hospital admission or medical treatment for a health problem such as a heart attack or appendicitis appears so irrational that the hospital staff doubt your sanity, the Mental Health Act cannot be used to make you stay in hospital in these circumstances. If you want to discharge yourself, let one of the nurses or doctors attending you know that this is what you want. They will ensure you are seen by someone (usually the duty doctor, or one of the junior doctors on your consultant's team) who will discuss the matter with you, give you the opportunity to explain why you want to discharge yourself, and ensure you understand the possible consequences of doing so. If the doctor thinks it is safe for you to go home, they will discharge you. If not, and you still insist on leaving hospital, you will be asked to sign a form stating that you are discharging yourself against medical advice and take full responsibility for any problems that may arise as a result. When you discharge yourself you are responsible for your own transport, even if you cannot walk, and for organising a supply of your drugs for you to take home. It does not mean that you cannot change your mind and return to the hospital should your circumstances change. You can – but you will have to go through the admissions procedure again.

How will my GP know when I am home and what treatment I received in hospital?

When you are discharged, you should be given a copy of your discharge summary – a handwritten letter stating the dates you were admitted and discharged, the reason for your admission, the diagnosis, what treatment you received and the medication you should continue to take. You should hand this in at your GP's surgery. If you cannot do this, and you will need a visit or a prescription from your GP within the next day or two, ask the ward staff if they will fax or telephone your GP's surgery. A copy of the discharge summary will be posted to your GP, and a more detailed letter will be sent later unless your admission was for something very minor such as removal of a skin lump.

You will also be given a small supply of all your drugs – usually 7 days – to last until you see your GP. A more detailed letter will be sent to your GP by post, but this can take several weeks. If you think you need a visit from your GP, it is better not to rely on the discharge letter to trigger one – you should telephone the surgery and ask for a home visit.

What will happen if I still need painkillers when I am discharged?

You should not be discharged if you still need injectable painkillers. When you go home, a 7-day supply of all the medication you need, including a suitable painkiller if required, will be dispensed from the hospital pharmacy. You do not have to pay for this.

Who can give me advice if I feel I have suffered discrimination while in hospital?

The NHS and the people working in it should not discriminate against you because of your age, sex, race, religion or sexual orientation. If you have suffered discrimination, you must bring it to the attention of the Trust's chief executive in writing.

What should I do if I am unhappy with the way I have been treated in hospital? Who should I complain to?

If you feel there is a problem, then your first point of contact should be the doctors and nurses treating you, as it may be easily solvable. Many hospitals actively encourage patients to report problems, such as dirty toilets or corridors that might otherwise be missed by staff, as it allows them to solve them.

What should I do if I feel my comments are being ignored?

Ask to speak to a more senior member of staff. You can also choose to make a formal complaint to the NHS Trust's chief executive. Complaints about hospital treatment should be made within 6 months of the event. If the issue becomes apparent later, then the complaint should be made within 6 months of you becoming aware of the cause for complaint. When you make a written complaint, the NHS Trust involved should always acknowledge your complaint within 3 days. The complaint is then likely to be sent on to the relevant department or departments in the hospital for investigation. The Department of Health requires that a full response should be provided by the hospital within 20 working days, although this target is not always achieved.

What can I do if I am unhappy with the response?

You can request an independent review within 28 days. You will receive details of how to do this with the Trust's formal response to your complaint. If you are still not satisfied, then you have the option to appeal to the health service Ombudsman, which is independent of both the NHS and the Government. The web address is www.health.ombudsman.co.uk and the website contains a form which you can print out and use if necessary. You can write to the address which is also given on the website or you can telephone on 0845 015 4033. It is not necessary to involve a lawyer.

However, it is not usually possible to involve the Ombudsman unless you have already complained officially and are still not satisfied. At any point in the process you can also contact other organisations for help and advice.

Currently, you can also contact your local Community Health Council, or CHC. These are independent bodies funded by the NHS who act as 'watchdogs' and represent patients within the health service. Under the NHS Plan, the Government intends to abolish the CHCs and replace them with PALS (Patient Advocacy and

Liaison Services), who will perform approximately the same task but will be more closely linked to the local NHS.

If a hospital has actually caused you any form of harm or damage, then you may also be entitled to some form of compensation. Some legal firms will fight cases on a no-win no-fee basis.

Can I get help making a complaint?

The Patients Association is a good source of advice and support. You can speak to a trained volunteer on their helpline between 10am and 4pm Monday to Friday. The telephone number is 0845 608 4455 and all calls are charged at local rate. Their website address is www.patients-association.com. You can e-mail them with details of your experience.

Accident and
Emergency (A&E)

Accident and Emergency (A&E)

The A&E department has a specific role which is the assessment and treatment of trauma, the provision of immediate necessary care for all medical and surgical emergencies and – after assessment and stabilisation – referral to consultant teams if you need to be admitted to a hospital bed.

An emergency admission is any one which is not planned. If you refer yourself to A&E as a result of a 999 call you will be first seen in A&E and then either be sent home or referred to the appropriate consultant team. GP emergency admissions are sometimes sent to A&E but are more usually referred to the consultant team direct.

The best-equipped A&E departments have operating theatres and X-ray and CT scanners available 24 hours a day. These facilities will speed up your diagnosis and treatment. The best-equipped hospitals will also have an intensive care unit (ICU) where patients who cannot breathe for themselves can be ventilated and given one-to-one care. In the data section of this Guide, we tell you which hospitals have these facilities.

Staffing and facilities at different A&E departments can vary and some hospitals are better equipped with dealing with some emergencies than others. Because there is so little scope for choosing which hospital you are admitted to in an emergency, you may feel concern about which hospital you would be taken to and how long you would have to wait to be seen. Government guidelines suggest that the longest you should wait in A&E is 4 hours, after which time you should be admitted to a ward for treatment or discharged with advice as to how to manage your problem. If you are taken to a hospital that meets this target, you are more likely to be found an emergency bed if you need one. In this section, we tell you which hospitals meet these targets.

What sort of problems should I attend A&E with?

Anyone who is unconscious, in severe pain or having difficulty breathing should be taken to A&E. The following is a guide to the problems you should attend with.

- Crushing chest or stomach pain so severe that it stops you from moving or a sudden headache with vomiting.
- Persistent bleeding from any part of the body or head.
- All serious injuries sustained in, for example, a fall.
- Fits or loss of consciousness.
- Any broken bones.
- All bites that puncture the skin need medical attention as they often become infected.
- Any children who have put beads or other small objects into their ears or nostrils (these may be referred to a minor injuries unit).

How do I decide when to call an ambulance?

In most cases, if you can get another form of transport to A&E such as a car with somebody else driving, you should do so. However, there are a few situations in which an ambulance should always be called. These are conditions that are so serious that the patient might collapse and need to be resuscitated on the way to the hospital. This would include any case of suspected meningitis, an asthma attack or a possible heart attack. Never try to transport an unconscious patient to A&E by car or taxi.

How long will I have to wait to be seen and who makes that decision?

Soon after your arrival, a triage nurse or senior house officer will see you and decide how urgently you need to be seen. The waiting time depends on how urgent your problem is and how many people with more urgent problems are ahead of you in the queue. It is common to have to wait several hours if you have a minor injury. Do not eat or drink while you are waiting without asking the triage nurse whether it is all right to do so.

What sort of doctor am I likely to see?

A senior house officer (SHO), the most junior grade of qualified doctor. He or she can take a history, examine you, arrange blood and urine tests and X-rays, suture wounds and organise dressings and plaster casts and prescribe drugs. He or she will then either discharge you, admit you to a short-term observation ward or arrange for a colleague to review you.

In some complex cases the senior house officer may ask a more senior A&E doctor to see you. More commonly, if your problem is serious enough to require admission to hospital, the A&E doctor will refer you to the appropriate consultant team. They will then review you in A&E and, if they agree that your problem is serious, will admit you to a hospital bed. You will then usually be seen by the consultant on the team. The Patient's Charter recommends that all patients who need to be admitted should be found a bed in the hospital within 2 hours.

How does a minor injuries unit differ from A&E?

Some small hospitals have minor injuries units attached. A minor injuries unit is usually staffed by nurses, and medical cover for patients who need to see a doctor is provided either by the patient's own GP or by local GPs on a rota. Some of them will have nurse practitioners who have specialist training and are able to diagnose and treat a wider range of conditions than most nurses. Unlike most A&E departments, minor injuries units may not be open 24 hours a day, and will not usually have X-ray and blood testing facilities on site. They can deal with minor illnesses, soft tissue injuries and suturing uncomplicated cuts, but patients who need tests or more complex treatment have to be referred elsewhere.

What is an intensive care unit?

Intensive care units (ICU) are able to ventilate patients if they are unable to breathe for themselves. The main features of an intensive care unit are the high levels of equipment, mainly for monitoring patients, and the high levels of staffing (one nurse per bed) and staff training.

What is a high dependency unit?

High dependency units (HDU) are able to provide a higher level of care to patients than on normal wards, although not as high as in an intensive care unit and patients generally cannot be kept on ventilators here. As with an intensive care unit though, a high dependency unit is defined by the equipment, the staffing levels (two nurses per bed) and the staff's training.

Focus on A&E

The following tables tell you how well your hospital performs in terms of how quickly you get treated. In England, Wales and Northern Ireland we tell you how many patients were treated and discharged, admitted to hospital or transferred to another hospital within 4 hours. In Scotland, different figures are collected which distinguish between Trolley Cases – people who are put on trolleys and usually admitted to hospital – and Walking Wounded – those who can be treated and discharged home. Trolley Cases should have been seen by a doctor within 30 minutes and treated, discharged or transferred within two hours from arrival. Walking Wounded cases should have been seen by a doctor within 90 minutes and treated, discharged or transferred within two-and-a-half hours from arrival.

In both tables the figure shown is the percentage of patients actually seen within the recommended time.

Scottish A&E

arrival: % within:	TROLLEY CASE		WALKING WOUNDED	
	to Doctor 30 mins	to completion 2 hours	to Doctor 90 mins	to completion 2.5 hours
Aberdeen Royal Infirmary	46.3	45.3	70.5	69.9
Ayr Hospital	75	67.7	89.6	89.3
Balfour Hospital	100	100	100	100
Borders General Hospital	61.6	50.6	89.4	86
Crosshouse Hospital	70.8	83	72.1	77.7
Dr Gray's Hospital	87.9	64.5	92.1	90.2
Dumfries & Galloway Royal Infirmary	87.8	84.1	99.7	94.4
Edinburgh Royal Infirmary	24.7	35.3	53.1	61.1
Falkirk Royal Infirmary	43.5	46.8	62.2	66.2
Gilbert Bain Hospital	87.5	50	100	96.8
Glasgow Royal Infirmary	23.3	51.9	64.7	81.1
Hairmyres Hospital	61.2	60	68.2	72.4
Inverclyde Royal Hospital	66.4	76.3	84.6	87.5
Law Hospital	91	77.1	84.9	88.7
Monklands District General Hospital	38.6	62.2	74.6	78.2
Ninewells Hospital	63.7	67.5	89.4	91.1
Perth Royal Infirmary	88.7	91.5	98	96.9
Queen Margaret Hospital	74.3	56.5	95.7	94.3
Raigmore Hospital	65.7	53	79.4	81.5
Royal Alexandra Hospital	45.6	69.9	78.3	85.6
Southern General Hospital	45.1	53.8	72.3	66.8
St John's Hospital at Howden	83.3	43.8	66.1	76.1
Stirling Royal Infirmary	74.2	83.8	91.7	91.1
Stobhill Hospital	49.4	65.1	75.6	77.5
Vale of Leven District General Hospital	79.7	82	83.6	88.2
Victoria Hospital, Kirkcaldy	75.5	82.7	95.7	97.3
Victoria Infirmary, Glasgow	87.3	95.6	91.1	96.8
Western Infirmary, Glasgow	48.2	61.8	75.3	78.6
Western Isles Hospital	84.2	77.8	97.9	93.

Wishaw Hospital is not included in this table. This hospital opened in 2001 and consequently no data has been collated for it as yet.

A&E waiting England NI and Wales

If the hospital has not provided us with information, a dash appears instead of a figure.

	% treated within 4 hours
Eastern	
Stamford & Rutland Hospital	100
Bedford Hospital	99
James Paget Hospital	98
Queen Elizabeth Hospital	94
West Suffolk Hospital	89
Hinchingbrooke Hospital	87
Southend Hospital	86
Addenbrooke's Hospital	80.4
Norfolk & Norwich University Hospital	80
Colchester General Hospital	75
Queen Elizabeth II Hospital	69.6
Lister Hospital	69.6
Princess Alexandra Hospital	69
Basildon Hospital	66.2
Broomfield Hospital	63
Luton & Dunstable Hospital	62.2
Watford General Hospital	60
Hemel Hempstead General Hospital	60
Edith Cavell Hospital	-
Orsett Hospital	-
Peterborough District Hospital	-
Ipswich Hospital	-

	% treated within 4 hours
London	
King's College Hospital	92
Homerton Hospital	92
Queen Mary's Hospital	87
University Hospital Lewisham	79
Whittington Hospital	75
Hammersmith Hospital	72
Kingston Hospital	69
King George Hospital	69
Hillingdon Hospital	68
Queen Mary's Hospital (Sidcup)	67
Royal Free Hospital	67
North Middlesex University Hospital	66
Ealing Hospital	65

	% treated within 4 hours
Bromley Hospital	64.1
Mayday Hospital	64
Charing Cross Hospital	64
St Thomas' Hospital	58
Epsom General Hospital	55
St Helier Hospital	55
Newham General Hospital	54
St George's Hospital (London)	50
Oldchurch Hospital	49
Northwick Park Hospital	49
Central Middlesex Hospital	49
Middlesex & University College Hospitals	47.4
West Middlesex University Hospital	45
St Bartholomew's Hospital	41
Royal London Hospital	41
Whipps Cross University Hospital	33
Barnet Hospital	-
Chase Farm Hospital	-
St Andrew's Hospital	-
Queen Elizabeth Hospital	-
St Mary's Hospital	-

	% treated within 4 hours
North West	
Royal Lancaster Infirmary	97.7
St Helens Hospital (Merseyside)	97
Furness General Hospital	95.75
Burnley General Hospital	94
Blackburn Royal Infirmary	94
Leighton Hospital	94
Countess of Chester Hospital	93
Royal Bolton Hospital	90
Macclesfield District General Hospital	87
Tameside General Hospital	82.5
Southport & Formby District General Hospital	82
Wirral Hospital (Arrowe Park & Clatterbridge)	80
Chorley & South Ribble District General Hospital	79.4

A&E waiting England NI and Wales

	% treated within 4 hours		% treated within 4 hours
Royal Preston Hospital	79.4	Middlesbrough General Hospital	89
Royal Oldham Hospital	78.91	Wansbeck General Hospital	85
Fairfield General Hospital	78.3	Bradford Royal Infirmary	84
Hope Hospital	77.6	Sunderland Royal Hospital	82
Ormskirk and District General Hospital	76	University Hospital of North Durham	70
Halton General Hospital	75	West Cumberland Hospital	99.3
Wythenshawe Hospital	75	St James's University Hospital	-
Warrington Hospital	75	Leeds General Infirmary	-
North Manchester General Hospital	70	Wharfdale General Hospital	-
Rochdale Infirmary	68	Seacroft Hospital	-
Stepping Hill Hospital	58	Chapel Allerton Hospital	-
University Hospital Aintree	53.5	Huddersfield Royal Infirmary	-
Whiston Hospital	47	Royal Victoria Infirmary	-
Royal Liverpool University Hospital	44.4	Bridlington & District Hospital	-
Bury General Hospital	-	Scarborough General Hospital	-
Leigh Infirmary	-	Whitby Hospital	-
Royal Albert Edward Infirmary	-	Ryhope Hospital	-
Manchester Royal Infirmary	-	University Hospital of North Tees	-
Blackpool Victoria Hospital	-	Hull Royal Infirmary	-
Trafford General Hospital	-	University Hospital of Hartlepool	-

Northern and Yorks		**South East**	
Queen Elizabeth Hospital	100	Radcliffe Infirmary	100
Bishop Auckland General Hospital	100	North Hampshire Hospital	98.5
Darlington Memorial Hospital	100	Royal Hampshire County Hospital	97.7
Airedale General Hospital	99.94	Worthing Hospital	92
Calderdale Royal Hospital	99	Eastbourne District General Hospital	86.5
Harrogate District Hospital	99	St Mary's Hospital (Newport)	86.33
Friarage Hospital	98	Princess Royal Hospital	85.9
Cumberland Infirmary	97.9	Medway Maritime Hospital	84
Hexham General Hospital	96	Heatherwood Hospital	83
York District Hospital	95	Wexham Park Hospital	83
South Tyneside District Hospital	94.2	St Peter's Hospital	82
Pinderfields General Hospital	94	Queen Elizabeth The Queen Mother Hospital	80
Pontefract General Infirmary	94	William Harvey Hospital	79
Dewsbury and District Hospital	93.3	Conquest Hospital	76.2
North Tyneside General Hospital	91	Horton Hospital	76
Newcastle Hospitals*	90	Kent and Sussex Hospital	76

* Newcastle Hospitals comprises: Freeman Hospital, Royal Victoria Infirmary and Newcastle General Hospital.

A&E waiting England NI and Wales

	% treated within 4 hours
Northampton General Hospital	76
Kent & Canterbury Hospital	76
St Richard's Hospital	74.4
Stoke Mandeville Hospital	70
Royal Berkshire & Battle Hospitals	70
Maidstone Hospital	69
Kettering General Hospital	67
East Surrey and Crawley Hospitals	63.1
Crawley Hospital	63.1
John Radcliffe Hospital	57
Milton Keynes General NHS Hospital	49
Royal Sussex County Hospital	46
Frimley Park Hospital	40
Royal Surrey County Hospital	33
Southlands Hospital	-
Wycombe Hospital	-
Battle Hospital	-
Royal South Hants Hospital	-
Pembury Hospital	-
Darent Valley Hospital	-
Queen Alexandra Hospital	-
St Mary's Hospital (Portsmouth)	-
Southampton General Hospital	-

South West

	% treated within 4 hours
Taunton & Somerset Hospital	99.87
Yeovil District Hospital	95
North Devon District Hospital	95
Royal Devon & Exeter Hospital	92.8
Cheltenham General Hospital	92
Gloucestershire Royal Hospital	90
Weston General Hospital	90
Torbay District General Hospital	89
Southmead Hospital	85
Frenchay Hospital	83
Derriford Hospital	77
Royal Bournemouth Hospital	75
Salisbury District Hospital	74.8
Poole Hospital	71

	% treated within 4 hours
Royal Cornwall Hospital	70
Bristol Royal Infirmary	63
Royal United Hospital	55
St Michael's Hospital	-
Standish Hospital	-
Stroud General Hospital	-
Princess Margaret Hospital	-
Cirencester Hospital	-
Bristol General Hospital	-
Dorset County Hospital	-

Trent

	% treated within 4 hours
Doncaster Royal Infirmary & Montagu Hospital	97.5
Diana, Princess of Wales Hospital	100
Grantham & District Hospital	97.2
Scunthorpe General Hospital	95.9
Bassetlaw District General Hospital	95.9
Pilgrim Hospital	92.1
Barnsley District General Hospital	89
Lincoln County Hospital	88.7
King's Mill Hospital	88
Derbyshire Royal Infirmary	74
Northern General Hospital	73.7
Queen's Medical Centre	72
Chesterfield & North Derbyshire Royal Hospital	64.2
Leicester Royal Infirmary	59
Rotherham District General Hospital	-
Skegness & District Hospital	-
Louth County Hospital	-

West Midlands

	% treated within 4 hours
Princess Royal Hospital	100
George Eliot Hospital	100
Hospital of St Cross	98
Coventry and Warwickshire Hospital	97
County Hospital (Hereford)	96
Manor Hospital (Walsall)	95.2
Worcester Royal Infirmary	95

A&E waiting England NI and Wales

	% treated within 4 hours
Alexandra Hospital	95
Kidderminster Hospital	95
Solihull Hospital	94.2
New Cross Hospital	92
Selly Oak Hospital	92
Royal Shrewsbury Hospital	90
Staffordshire General Hospital	83
Sandwell General Hospital	80
Good Hope District General Hospital	74.5
Birmingham Heartlands Hospital	74.3
City Hospital	58
Dudley Group of Hospitals*	51.6
General Hospital (Hereford)	-
North Staffordshire Royal Infirmary	-
Warwick Hospital	-
Queen's Hospital (Burton)	-
North Staffordshire Hospital	-

N. Ireland	% treated within 4 hours
Antrim Hospital	97.2
Whiteabbey Hospital	96
Belfast City Hospital	93
Mater Hospital	92
Ulster Hospital	14.6
Daisy Hill Hospital	-
Altnagelvin Area Hospital	-
Causeway	-
Craigavon Area Hospital	-
Erne Hospital	-
Lagan Valley Hospital	-
Mid-Ulster Hospital	-
The Royal Hospitals	-
Tyrone and Fermanagh Hospital	-
Tyrone County Hospital	-
Downe Hospital	-

Wales	% treated within 4 hours
Singleton Hospital	100
Llandudno General Hospital	100
Withybush General Hospital	99.3
West Wales General Hospital	99
Bronglais General Hospital	98.4
Ysbyty Gwynedd	98
Prince Charles Hospital	96.8
Glan Clwyd District General Hospital	94.7
Royal Glamorgan Hospital	92.6
Prince Philip Hospital	92
Caerphilly District Miners' Hospital	90
Princess of Wales Hospital	88
University Hospital of Wales	85.56
Morriston Hospital	85
Llandough Hospital	-
Wrexham Maelor Hospital	-
Nevill Hall Hospital	-
Royal Gwent Hospital	-
Neath General Hospital	-

* Dudley Group of Hospitals comprises: Russells Hall, Wordsley, Corbett and Guest Hospitals.

Section Two:

Focus on Hospital Care

Heart Disease

Heart disease

One of the areas of the NHS on which the most demand is placed is its heart services. More people die from coronary artery disease than from any other disease in the UK and there are 270,000 heart attacks in the UK each year.

Standards of care provided to heart patients vary between hospitals. If you have a known heart problem, you, together with your GP, may want to take several factors into account when choosing the hospital at which you receive treatment. In this Guide we describe some of the more important differences between hospitals, for example which hospitals have coronary care units – special wards set up to provide a high level of care for patients that have suffered heart attacks, undergone heart surgery or are particularly weak. We also tell you which hospitals perform coronary angiography – currently the gold standard test for coronary artery (ischaemic heart) disease – but one that requires skill to perform. The Government has suggested that hospitals that do this test should perform at least 500 per year. This aims to ensure that the practitioners have enough experience. In this section, we list those hospitals which meet this target.

Your chances of surviving a heart attack depend to a great extent on how fast you get to hospital and how quickly you are treated. Thrombolysis, which involves giving patients clot-busting drugs, is one of the most important ways of treating a heart attack but its effectiveness depends on it being done quickly. Hospitals aim to perform thrombolysis within 30 minutes of a heart-attack patient entering the hospital. In this section we list those hospitals which currently meet that target.

One of the most effective treatments for coronary artery (ischaemic heart) disease is heart bypass surgery. Heart bypass surgery – or coronary artery bypass grafting – has been one of the great success stories of modern medicine. It has gone, in just a few decades, from being a new experimental treatment to being a relatively safe routine procedure that can add years and even decades to people's lives. In this section, we look at the relative success rate of different hospitals at performing this treatment.

The aims of the National Service Frameworks for heart disease include:

- A 40 per cent reduction in deaths from heart disease by 2010.
- Provision of rapid-access chest pain clinics to speed up the assessment of people who are referred by their GP with suspected heart disease and to speed up the emergency treatment of heart attacks.
- An increase in the number of coronary angiographies and coronary angioplasties.
- An increase in the number of coronary artery bypass graft procedures.
- A reduction in the waiting times for surgical procedures to treat heart disease.
- An increase in the number of people who receive cardiac rehabilitation after a heart attack or heart bypass surgery.
- Those discharged after a heart attack should be given beta-blockers.

What is heart disease?

There are many types of heart disease. They include problems with the muscles, the valves or the rhythm of the heart (arrhythmias) and congenital heart disease, which is the result of being born with an abnormality in the structure of the heart. However, the commonest type of heart disease is **ischaemic heart disease**, or coronary artery disease, which develops when the coronary artery becomes narrowed and blood supply to the heart becomes insufficient.

Heart disease can vary in severity from an insignificant hole between the walls of the heart which closes by itself, to major structural abnormalities which prevent the baby from surviving more than a few hours after birth. About one baby in 100 is born with some form of congenital heart disease. This section will use the term 'heart disease' to mean ischaemic heart disease, which is one of the biggest health problems in the UK.

What causes heart disease?

Family History If several close relatives – parents and siblings – had a heart attack before age 60, your risk of heart disease is higher.

Sex Heart disease is rare in men before the age of 40 and in women before the menopause, but increases rapidly thereafter. On average, men tend to develop heart disease around 10 years earlier than women. However, women's risk increases after the menopause but is reduced by having previously used hormone replacement therapy (HRT).

Smoking has been directly linked to heart disease and if you stop smoking, your risk is significantly reduced.

Diabetics also have a greater risk of heart disease and are advised to control their illness to the best of their ability.

High Blood Pressure if linked with other contributory factors, such as high cholesterol.

Cholesterol If your cholesterol is very high you may need drugs to help control it.

Diet The UK and Scotland are near the top of the European heart disease league. Being overweight puts extra strain on the heart. Eating a diet high in fats (especially saturated fats – animal and dairy fats), sugar, salt and heavily processed 'convenience' foods, and low in fruit, vegetables, fibre and known protective foods such as oily fish, is bad for your heart.

Moderate alcohol consumption – 14 units a week for women and 21 for men – has been shown to protect against heart disease, but if you drink a lot more than this then you are increasing your risk of heart disease.

How does my GP assess my risk of heart disease?

Your GP assesses your risk of developing heart disease by a process called 'risk profiling'. They will take various factors into account including your family history, age and sex, whether you smoke, have diabetes or whether your blood pressure and cholesterol levels are high. When they have assessed your level of risk they may advise you on lifestyle changes to reduce it. They may also recommend medication to reduce your risk further and if your risk is very high you may be referred to heart specialist (cardiologist).

What causes high blood pressure?

In around 95 per cent of cases of high blood pressure, or hypertension, no cause can be found. This type is called essential hypertension. The other 5 per cent of cases are caused by a range of uncommon diseases of the heart, kidneys and hormones. This is called secondary hypertension.

How often should I have my blood pressure measured?

The British Hypertension Society recommends that all adults should have their blood pressure measured every 5 years until the age of 80. If your blood pressure has ever been high, or is at the high end of normal, it should be measured once a year. If you are having treatment for high blood pressure, you may need more frequent measurements.

Do I need to have any other tests if my blood pressure is high?

You should have tests to check for other heart disease risk factors and to ensure that your high blood pressure has not damaged any important organs. These include: a urine dipstick test for sugar and protein, tests for kidney function, blood glucose and cholesterol and an electrocardiogram (ECG – see p82). These tests should be repeated annually.

Can I reduce my blood pressure without drugs?

Yes, though you may also need drug treatment if it is very high. The measures that are shown to work are losing weight if you are overweight, eating less salt in your diet, exercising until you are slightly breathless for at least 20 minutes 3 times a week, and keeping your alcohol intake below the recommended maximum level of 14 units a week for women and 21 units a week for men.

What sort of drugs might I be given to reduce my blood pressure?

There are about ten different classes of blood pressure-lowering drugs, with several individual drugs in each class. Experts currently believe that tailored therapy – planning a medication regime to suit each patient – is the best way to treat high blood pressure. The choice of drugs is often dictated by how well the patient tolerates any side-effects. Most drugs for high blood pressure can be taken once a day.

What is cholesterol?

This is a fatty substance which our bodies need to survive – there is cholesterol in every human cell, and as well as getting cholesterol from animal products in our diets we manufacture it in our livers. Problems arise when cholesterol carried in our bloodstream sticks to the walls of major blood vessels to form fatty plaques called atheroma. These plaques narrow the bore of the blood vessels and if they burst and become ragged, their surface is a perfect site for a blood clot to form and block the blood vessel completely. This is how most heart attacks and strokes (blockages of arteries in the brain) happen.

Blood cholesterol can be lowered by drugs more effectively than by diet alone. **Statins** (the commonest group of cholesterol-lowering agents) are recommended for those at moderate or high risk of having a heart attack or stroke within the next ten years.

What causes high cholesterol?

A combination of your family history and lifestyle factors. Some families are affected by a range of genetic conditions called the familial hyperlipidaemias, which cause extremely high blood cholesterol levels and lead to heart disease at an unusually early age – sometimes in the teens. People with these conditions need very aggressive treatment with diet and a combination of cholesterol-lowering drugs. An underactive thyroid gland can cause high cholesterol, and the cholesterol level falls when the thyroid problem is treated. For most people, however, the main factor causing high cholesterol is a diet high in saturated fat.

How can I reduce my blood cholesterol?

Keep your weight within the normal range for your age and height, eat healthily and exercise regularly. This will not only lower your blood cholesterol, but will also ensure that a high proportion of your cholesterol is transported in a form that will not harm your arteries. It is also important to stop smoking to reduce your risk of coronary artery disease overall. If your cholesterol is very high, diet alone is unlikely to reduce it sufficiently to make a difference to your risk of heart disease.

How often should I have my cholesterol measured?

Every 5 years if you are a man, or if you are a woman who has gone through the menopause. A younger woman with a normal cholesterol level would not need to have another measurement until after the menopause. If you are on treatment for high cholesterol you should have your cholesterol measured annually.

Heart Attack

The heart does not take oxygen from the blood that it pumps around the body. It has its own blood supply, the coronary arteries (so-called because they surround the heart muscle like a crown). The coronary arteries are particularly vulnerable to fatty deposits called atheroma. A heart attack, usually called a myocardial infarction, or MI, by health professionals, occurs when a smooth plaque of atheroma bursts open, leaving a rough surface on which a blood clot can form. This clot, or thrombus, cuts off the supply of blood to part of the heart muscle and the muscle cells quickly die. The consequences of this depend on which part, and how much, of the heart is damaged. Some heart attacks only involve part of the thickness of the heart muscle and cause no symptoms; others prevent the heart from beating and cause sudden death.

What symptoms might I expect if I have a heart attack?

An uncomfortable feeling, usually in the centre of your chest or like a tight metal band around your chest, and heavy or crushing in nature. Sometimes it will be in your left shoulder, arm and hand, your neck and your jaw, or any combination of these. Sometimes pain is felt in both arms. Other symptoms are hortness of breath, clamminess and sweating, sometimes with vomiting. Heart attacks tend to occur in people who are known to have risk factors for heart disease.

What should I do if I suspect I'm having a heart attack?

Swallow an aspirin – which helps prevent further clot formation – and dial 999. If you are having a heart attack, it is important to get the diagnosis confirmed and treatment started as quickly as possible. Don't wait for a visit from your GP or try to make your own way to hospital.

What will the ambulance crew do?

Anyone with chest pain is given priority by ambulance control. When they arrive, the crew will record an ECG trace (see p82) and measure your pulse and blood pressure, put a cannula into one of your arm veins in case you need emergency drugs, give you oxygen and a morphine-based painkilling injection, and transport you to A&E as quickly as possible. They will also alert the A&E staff that they are bringing in someone with a suspected heart attack.

What will happen in A&E?

Your pulse, blood pressure, breathing rate and another ECG (see p82-3) will be recorded and if you have developed an irregular heartbeat or a very low blood pressure you will be given treatment for this. Once you are stable, a junior doctor will take your history, examine you, take blood tests, and arrange for you to be admitted to the Coronary Care Unit (CCU). There, you will be under the care of the on-call medical team, or the cardiology team if the hospital has one.

What are thrombolytic ('clot-busting') drugs, and how are they used?

The standard treatment for most heart attacks is **thrombolysis** – an intravenous infusion of a drug that dissolves the clot blocking the artery and, if given early enough, allows the damaged heart muscle to recover. This should ideally be given within an hour of the heart attack occurring, although they may still be of some benefit up to 12 hours later.

In its National Service Framework for heart disease, the Government has set a target of 75 per cent of patients receiving thrombolysis within 30 minutes of reaching hospital. On p90, we tell you which hospitals achieve this.

In rural areas, where there might be a significant delay in the patient reaching hospital from home, this target is not particularly helpful. A study in rural Scotland showed that administration of thrombolysis by GPs prior to admission reduced the number of deaths in patients who had had heart attacks.

In future, ambulance crews may be trained to administer these drugs.

Are they dangerous?

They will cause clots elsewhere in the body to dissolve too, so they can be risky in patients who have recently had bleeding from a stomach ulcer or had major surgery or a bleed in the brain. In most patients, the risks of treatment are greatly outweighed by the risks of not giving these drugs.

What is a Coronary Care Unit?

This is where people who have had heart attacks or other acute cardiac events are nursed. The Coronary Care Unit (CCU) is equipped with sophisticated monitoring equipment, and the nurses are specially trained to deal with emergencies such as irregular heartbeats and cardiac arrest (when the heart stops beating).

In the CCU, you will have continuous monitoring of your heart rhythm and regular ECGs and blood tests. After an uncomplicated heart attack, you can expect to spend around three days in the CCU before being transferred to the main medical ward for a few days.

What is cardiac rehabilitation?

This is an exercise and lifestyle management programme for people who have had a heart attack or heart bypass surgery. The aim of the programme is to reduce the risk of subsequent cardiac problems and to promote a return to a full a normal life.

Cardiac rehabilitation programmes are run by specially trained nurses, often with the support of physiotherapists and dietitians. Most people are offered 6–8 sessions at weekly intervals. These programmes are shown to improve life expectancy and should be offered to all suitable patients, though not all hospitals currently do so.

Angina Pectoris

Angina pectoris is chest pain which may be associated with shortness of breath caused by coronary artery (ischaemic heart) disease. It occurs when the heart muscle is temporarily starved of oxygen and the stressed muscle cells release a substance that causes pain. It is typically brought on by exercise, and many sufferers know exactly how far, and how fast, they can walk before the pain starts. Similarly, it typically goes away after resting for a short time. If you have angina that comes on at rest, or is getting worse quickly, see your GP as a matter of urgency – you are at extremely high risk of having a heart attack in the near future and may need to be admitted to hospital for emergency treatment.

What will be done to find out whether I have heart disease?
If you or your doctor suspect that you might have heart disease, these are the ways used to confirm or rule out the diagnosis.
Taking a history Your doctor will ask you to describe your symptoms in your own words, and will then ask questions to get more details. They will also want to know what illnesses run in your family and whether you smoke. This information helps your doctor to decide whether heart disease is a likely explanation for your symptoms.
Examination Your doctor will weigh you, check your pulse and blood pressure and examine your chest thoroughly. They may also examine your abdomen and check the blood supply to your legs. They may also give you aspirin.

Case history

John Carter

John Carter, 48, had no indication there was anything wrong with him before he suffered heart failure. He had done a six-hour shift at his transport company office and come home as normal. He was due to be going on a four-day residential course the next day. Suddenly, when he got home, John experienced all the symptoms of a heart attack: crushing chest pain, clammy hands, pins and needles, grey skin. His wife immediately called the local health call centre and asked for advice over the phone. The call centre was staffed by medical staff and doctors who were trained to respond to emergencies.

Over the phone John's wife was told that they would order an ambulance immediately. In the ambulance, John was wired up to an ECG machine, but it wasn't until they got to the hospital that any irregularity on the monitor really showed up. The doctors also discovered that there was a blood clot in one of the major arteries of John's heart; they tried to thin it out and wash it away with warfarin, but it didn't respond. They flooded the vein with dye to find the blockage and began inserting a wire in order to prepare for an angioplasty. Meanwhile, John was wheeled into theatre, at this stage only half-awake. His consultant visited him at his bedside just before the heart operation. 'My consultant understood how frightened I was, so did the surgeon. Because it was done by local anaesthetic, the surgeon explained things while he was doing it – but in a very positive way. I had the stent op, where a surgical spring is inserted into an artery and remains there permanently.' John describes it as being like a 'pit prop'– because the artery tends to lose its elasticity after being widened. John was also given medication to prevent plaque from building up around the stent, after which tissue can grow around it.

John was in the theatre about an hour and a half and when he came round the consultant's understudy was there to explain the method of the operation and what drugs he had been given. At all times John says, he felt well informed and 'impressed by the care they took'. A few days later John met the cardiac rehabilitation counsellor who was responsible for his aftercare. Once a patient is discharged, the counsellor will visit them in their own home and give advice on diet and exercise. The consultant had advised a change of diet: he now has a curry once a month rather than twice a week, plus more fruit and vegetables but finds the diet sometimes hard to stick to.

John also takes soluble aspirin and a cholesterol-reducing medication every day. Initially, John had an appointment with the hospital gym once a week to do cardiac exercises, stepping, stretching and light weights. This carried on for three months until John felt fully recovered. He also contacted the British Heart Foundation for advice and literature.

'I have a very good cardiac nurse I can phone at any time. The consultant seemed to take a very close interest in my case, which was a great help. I feel I have been very fortunate.'

The following tests may then be organised:

An electrocardiogram (ECG). Wires clipped to sticky pads on your chest, wrists and ankles measure the natural electrical currents generated by your heart. This is one of the more important test for diagnosing heart disease and the critical test for diagnosing a heart attack.

A chest X-ray to look at the size and shape of your heart and the condition of your lungs.

Blood tests to look for anaemia, infection and thyroid problems – all of which can unmask heart disease – and for diabetes, kidney disease and raised cholesterol, which often accompany heart disease.

Most angina is stable. However, a handful of patients will have unstable angina, and if it is getting worse or you have enough risk-factors to suggest heart disease, your GP will then refer you to a consultant for further tests. You may be able to have all your tests done in a **rapid-access pain clinic**. These are NHS outpatient clinics which aim to ensure that patients with suspected heart disease are seen by a consultant within two weeks of referral and have the appropriate tests done quickly, usually at a 'one-stop' clinic. Not all areas have rapid-access chest pain clinics yet, but they form part of the Government's National Service Framework for heart disease and will become available nationwide over the next few years.

What tests might the consultant do?

Exercise tolerance test in which the strain on your heart is monitored by a continuous ECG while you walk at various speeds on a treadmill. This shows how your heart copes with exercise and is one of the crucial tests for diagnosing coronary artery disease. If it is positive (abnormal), then you will often need to go on to have a coronary angiogram to establish the pattern of disease (see below).

24 hour ECG where you wear a small portable ECG machine which monitors your heart rhythm as you go about your normal activities. This is very useful if you have occasional bouts of an irregular heartbeat but is not routinely performed in the diagnosis of coronary artery (ischaemic heart) disease.

Echocardiogram a non-invasive ultrasound scan of your heart. This shows how well heart your is pumping blood.

Thallium scan which shows how well different parts of your heart are supplied with blood.

Cardiac Catheterisation in which a thin tube is inserted into a blood vessel under local anaesthetic and threaded through to the chambers of the heart to monitor blood flow, blood pressure, blood chemistry, and the output of the heart, and to take a sample of heart tissue. This test is used to diagnose congenital heart disease and coronary artery (ischaemic heart) disease.

Coronary angiography in which a thin plastic tube is threaded through a groin or arm artery to the coronary arteries, and a dye is injected directly into the coronary arteries. The blood supply to your heart is then shown up on a moving X-ray film. This test shows whether any of the important arteries around your heart are narrowed or blocked, and helps your consultant decide whether a heart bypass operation or coronary angioplasty (see below) would help you. It is the gold standard test for coronary artery (ischaemic heart) disease, but it carries a small risk of serious complications. In this section, we tell you which hospitals perform coronary angiography.

Coronary Angioplasty in which a fine flexible wire with a balloon on its tip is passed into an artery in the groin and up to the heart. Using X-rays to monitor its position, the balloon is slipped into the blocked segment of the artery and inflated so that the blockage is crushed against the wall of the artery, leaving space for the blood to flow through. The balloon is then removed. Sometimes a short mesh tube called a **stent** is left in place to hold the artery open.

Coronary angioplasty avoids the need to open the chest and use cardiopulmonary bypass (see below), but it carries a small risk of serious complications. There is roughly a 1 to 2 per cent risk of a serious complication – these include a heart attack, a stroke, requiring an emergency heart bypass operation and death. This risk varies according to how unwell you are prior to the procedure and the skill of the team carrying out the procedure.

If the outcome of these tests are that you have coronary artery (ischaemic heart) disease you will then assessed for your risk factor of having a heart attack. The majority of patients with coronary artery disease are not referred for an operation. You may be treated with drugs alone, or by a combination of medication (aspirin plus drugs to control your cholesterol) and angioplasty. However, if you need an operation, you will be given drugs to control high blood pressure plus aspirin or other drugs to prevent blood clots.

Why might someone with heart disease be offered an operation?

Heart operations are done for several reasons. All of these operations are complex, and are done by highly trained teams of specialists. Most require cardiopulmonary bypass, in which a machine temporarily takes over the function of the heart and lungs so that the heart can be stopped while it is operated on. For adults, there are two common types of heart operation.

Coronary Artery Bypass Grafting (Heart Bypass Operation).
This operation is done if the pattern of narrowings in the arteries is not suitable for angioplasty. To know if it is needed, you first need to have coronary angiography.

If lengths of the arteries which carry blood to the heart muscle are severely narrowed, this operation can be used to bypass the damaged areas using lengths of the patient's own leg veins or chest wall or forearm arteries. It is a major operation which takes several hours, leaves a long scar down the middle of the chest and usually needs cardiopulmonary bypass. However, these days it is a surprisingly safe operation – in those whose heart is relatively healthy before having it the mortality rate for all patients overall is about 2–3 per cent. It improves the symptoms of angina but also improves life expectancy in many patients. If you have this operation, you will generally spend 24–48 hours being closely monitored in the intensive care or coronary care unit, and 5 to 10 days in hospital altogether. In this section, we give you the mortality rate for each hospital performing this operation and what percentage of patients are operated on within 6 months of referral.

Heart valve replacement. Sometimes the one-way valves that regulate blood flow in and out of the heart become blocked or leaky. In the past this was often due to the effects of a disease called rheumatic fever, but now it is more often the result of wear and tear due to age. If the valve needs to be replaced, a general anaesthetic and cardiopulmonary bypass are used. The surgeon cuts out the damaged valve and replaces it with a valve made either from bovine tissues or from artificial materials, often metal and plastic. As with coronary artery bypass grafting, you will be closely monitored for a few days after the operation and will be in hospital for 5 to10 days. In this section, we give you the mortality rate for each hospital performing this operation, and tell you how long you will have to wait to receive it.

Although the prospect of heart surgery can be alarming, it is important to remember that most people who have these operations make an uneventful recovery, notice big improvements in their quality of life and can often stop taking some of their heart drugs. Coronary artery bypass grafting and heart valve replacement can also lengthen the life expectancy of someone with heart disease.

Case history

John Denny

John Denny of Birmingham found that the exercise group he joined after his triple heart bypass was 'far more useful than any GP's advice'. He feels that the NHS exercise therapy groups for heart patients are a superb clearing house of information and that 'like any user group, they know what they are talking about'.

Now 50, Denny used to cycle 100 miles in a day. However, he was overweight and began to suffer from attacks of breathlessness. 'It took a long time for my angina to get diagnosed – the early symptoms are easy to confuse with flu' he says. He knew that it could only be diagnosed if he had an exercise ECG and he waited six months for an appointment. A year after that, he was given a triple bypass operation.

Denny collected his own information about his condition. He found his GP helpful but busy, and thinks that 'unless they have had angina, no doctor will really understand the symptoms. For example, they always ask about pains in the chest – in fact it's just a dull ache and not pains'. Though he didn't see the consultant before his operation, he was very well briefed by the anaesthetist, who took time to explain everything.

Later his GP discussed diet with him. 'I chose to eat more fruit, less butter and less margarine, and take more exercise.' He still gets angina in cold weather – something for which his GP had not prepared him.

'On the whole I was in the hands of the hospital system and had little useful information from doctors, none from a consultant. The best advice was from the people in the therapy group – there's no shortage of people with a heart condition and they are very willing to share useful advice.'

Heart Failure

Heart failure is not the same thing as a heart attack, although a heart attack can cause heart failure. Heart failure can result from anything that weakens the heart muscle fibres, such as high blood pressure and heart attacks, or anything that causes the heartbeat to become irregular or which forces the heart to do extra work, such as anaemia, fever, or an overactive thyroid gland. The most serious form of heart failure is called left ventricular failure and involves the main pumping chamber of the heart. Symptoms are shortness of breath on exercise and on lying flat in bed. People with heart failure often report waking up gasping for breath at the same time each night and having to prop themselves up on pillows or sleep in a chair to prevent this from happening. It is a serious condition – people with severe heart failure are less likely to survive twelve months than people with most cancers.

How is heart failure treated?

The treatment of heart failure has been transformed by the availability of very effective drugs called ACE inhibitors. These, together wtih water tablets, reduce the load on the heart and make the heart muscle beat more efficiently. Most people will also be given low dose aspirin to thin the blood.

Can Complementary Therapy help with heart disease?

Complementary therapies cannot cure heart disease, but conventional doctors are now recommending diet and lifestyle changes that have long been the staple of complementary medicine. However, some alternative medicines may interfere with conventional drugs and you should always consult with your GP or consultant before taking them.

Exercise, group therapy and stress management may play a part in reducing symptoms or heart disease and acupuncture is popular in the treatment of high blood pressure. Recent studies suggest that folic acid and vitamin B supplements my reduce homocysteine, which damages artery walls, and a 1996 study by Cambridge University found that daily vitamin E supplements could reduce the risk of heart attack in patients with atherosclerosis by 77 per cent.

Although there is no clinical evidence to suggest that it works, arnica, the homeopathic standby for shock and bruising, is routinely recommended before and after heart surgery to help healing and minimise physical trauma. Antioxidant nutrients, particularly vitamin C, are also believed to have a role in wound healing.

Focus on heart disease

In the following table, we tell you which hospitals perform heart bypass operations (coronay artery bypass graft) and how they perform in terms of waiting times and mortality rates for heart bypass operations.

The following table compares heart surgery services in English hospitals. The first column is the standardised mortality ratio for heart bypass operations. A rate of 100 is in line with the average, a figure above 100 indicates a higher than average mortality rate, a figure less than 100, a lower rate. The hospitals are banded according to whether the figure is significantly higher or lower than average (using 99 per cent confidence intervals). There are four hospitals with significantly low rates and two with significantly high rates. Hospitals with a very high or low number may not necessarily be significantly above or below average if, for example, they treat relatively few patients.

The second column gives an indication of waiting times for different hospitals. The figure is the percentage of patients who have been operated on by a cardiothoracic surgeon within six months.

Coronary Artery Bypass Graft (CABG)

	heart bypass mortality rate	% of patients seen within 6 months
LOW		
Bristol Royal Infirmary	48	73%
Derriford Hospital	51	64%
Leeds General Infirmary	54	55%
Southampton General Hospital	62	68%
AVERAGE		
Royal Free Hospital	38	100%
Nottingham City Hospital	55	71%
Royal Sussex County Hospital	76	72%
Blackpool Victoria Hospital	79	52%
Manchester Royal Infirmary	79	70%
Northern General Hospital	88	73%
Newcastle Hospitals*	89	74%
Royal London Hospital	92	51%
St Bartholomew's Hospital	92	51%
Queen Elizabeth Hospital (Birmingham)	98	42%
Glenfield Hospital	102	57%
St Mary's Hospital (London)	103	83%
King's College Hospital	105	78%
James Cook University Hospital	107	74%
North Staffordshire Hospital	111	60%
Guy's Hospital	112	71%
St Thomas' Hospital	112	71%
John Radcliffe Hospital	115	61%
Castle Hill Hospital	116	64%
St George's Hospital (London)	116	77%
Hammersmith Hospital	155	100%
HIGH		
Middlesex & University College Hospitals	170	68%
Walsgrave Hospital	182	50%
Wythenshawe Hospital*	-	59%

* Newcastle Hospitals comprises: Freeman Hospital, Royal Victoria Infirmary and Newcastle General Hospital.

* Wythenshawe Hospital is currently querying their mortality fiqure, which in the last analysis was significantly higher than avearage.

Focus on heart disease

In the following tables, we give you statistics on how your hospital performs in standards of coronary care. We tell you whether your hospital performs the following:

Thrombolysis in 30 minutes: This potentially life-saving procedure is shown to be more effective if performed within 30 minutes of admission to A&E.

Angiography: Although your hospital may have a coronary care unit, they might not provide angiography (see p83) – this means that you may have to be referred to a different hospital for this test.

Meets NSF guidelines for catheterisations: The National Service Framework for heart disease suggests that a unit should perform 500 cardiac catheterisations a year. Trusts that perform a high level of operations are likely to more experienced at this procedure.

Coronary care

If the hospital has not provided information, a dash appears instead of yes or no.

	Thrombolysis in 30 mins	Coronary angiography	NSF for catheterisations
Eastern			
Addenbrooke's Hospital	Yes	No	No
Basildon Hospital	Yes	No	No
Bedford Hospital	Yes	No	No
Broomfield Hospital	Yes	No	No
Colchester General Hospital	No	Yes	No
Hemel Hempstead General Hospital	No	No	No
Hinchingbrooke Hospital	No	No	No
Ipswich Hospital	Yes	No	No
James Paget Hospital	No	No	No
Lister Hospital	No	Yes	Yes
Luton & Dunstable Hospital	-	No	No
Mount Vernon Hospital	-	No	No
Norfolk & Norwich University Hospital	No	Yes	Yes
Orsett Hospital	-	-	-
Peterborough District Hospital	Yes	No	No

Coronary care

	Thrombolysis in 30 mins	Coronary angiography	NSF for catheterisations
Princess Alexandra Hospital	No	No	No
Queen Elizabeth Hospital	No	No	No
Queen Elizabeth II Hospital	No	No	No
Southend Hospital	No	Yes	Yes
St Albans City Hospital	-	Yes	Yes
St John's Hospital	-	No	-
Stamford & Rutland Hospital	-	No	-
Watford General Hospital	-	No	No
West Suffolk Hospital	No	No	-

London

Barking Hospital	-	No	-
Barnet Hospital	-	No	No
Bromley Hospital	Yes	No	No
Central Middlesex Hospital	Yes	No	No
Charing Cross Hospital	No	No	No
Chase Farm Hospital	-	No	No
Chelsea and Westminster Hospital	No	No	No
Ealing Hospital	Yes	No	-
Epsom General Hospital	-	No	No
Farnborough Hospital	-	No	No
Guy's Hospital	No	No	No
Hammersmith Hospital	No	Yes	Yes
Harold Wood Hospital	-	No	No
Hillingdon Hospital	Yes	No	No
Homerton Hospital	No	No	No
King George Hospital	No	No	No
King's College Hospital	No	Yes	Yes
Kingston Hospital	Yes	No	No
Mayday Hospital	Yes	Yes	Yes
Middlesex & University College Hospitals	No	Yes	Yes
Newham General Hospital	No	No	No
North Middlesex University Hospital	Yes	Yes	Yes
Northwick Park Hospital	Yes	Yes	Yes
Oldchurch Hospital	-	No	No
Orpington Hospital	-	No	No
Queen Elizabeth Hospital	Yes	Yes	Yes
Queen Mary's Hospital (Sidcup)	Yes	No	No
Queen Mary's Hospital (Hampstead)	-	No	No

Coronary care

	Thrombolysis in 30 mins	Coronary angiography	NSF for catheterisations
Royal Free Hospital	-	Yes	Yes
Royal London Hospital	Yes	No	-
St Andrew's Hospital	-	-	-
St Bartholomew's Hospital	Yes	Yes	Yes
St George's Hospital (London)	Yes	Yes	Yes
St Helier Hospital	Yes	No	No
St Mary's Hospital	Yes	Yes	Yes
St Thomas' Hospital	Yes	Yes	Yes
University Hospital Lewisham	No	No	No
West Middlesex University Hospital	Yes	No	No
Whipps Cross University Hospital	No	No	No
Whittington Hospital	No	No	No

North West

	Thrombolysis in 30 mins	Coronary angiography	NSF for catheterisations
Blackburn Royal Infirmary	Yes	No	No
Blackpool Victoria Hospital	No	Yes	Yes
Broadgreen Hospital	Yes	Yes	Yes
Burnley General Hospital	Yes	No	No
Bury General Hospital	-	No	No
Chorley & South Ribble District General Hospital	No	No	No
Countess of Chester Hospital	-	Yes	No
Fairfield General Hospital	No	No	No
Furness General Hospital	No	No	No
Halton General Hospital	Yes	No	No
Hope Hospital	Yes	No	No
Leigh Infirmary	-	No	No
Leighton Hospital	No	No	No
Macclesfield District General Hospital	No	No	No
Manchester Royal Infirmary	Yes	Yes	Yes
North Manchester General Hospital	Yes	No	No
Ormskirk and District General Hospital	Yes	No	No
Queens Park Hospital	No	No	No
Rochdale Infirmary	No	Yes	Yes
Rossendale General Hospital	-	No	No
Royal Albert Edward Infirmary	Yes	No	No
Royal Bolton Hospital	Yes	No	No
Royal Lancaster Infirmary	Yes	No	No
Royal Liverpool University Hospital	Yes	Yes	No
Royal Oldham Hospital	Yes	No	No

Coronary care

	Thrombolysis in 30 mins	Coronary angiography	NSF for catheterisations
Royal Preston Hospital	No	No	No
Southport & Formby District General Hospital	Yes	No	No
St Helens Hospital (Merseyside)	-	-	-
Stepping Hill Hospital	Yes	No	No
Tameside General Hospital	No	No	No
Trafford General Hospital	No	No	No
University Hospital Aintree	Yes	No	No
Warrington Hospital	Yes	No	No
Westmorland General Hospital	No	No	No
Whiston Hospital	No	No	-
Wirral Hospital (Arrowe Park & Clatterbridge)	Yes	Yes	Yes
Withington Hospital	No	No	No
Wythenshawe Hospital	No	Yes	Yes

Northern and Yorks

	Thrombolysis in 30 mins	Coronary angiography	NSF for catheterisations
Airedale General Hospital	Yes	Yes	Yes
Bishop Auckland General Hospital	No	No	No
Bradford Royal Infirmary	Yes	Yes	Yes
Bridlington & District Hospital	-	No	No
Calderdale Royal Hospital	No	Yes	No
Castle Hill Hospital	No	Yes	-
Chapel Allerton Hospital	-	-	-
Cumberland Infirmary	Yes	Yes	No
Darlington Memorial Hospital	No	No	No
Dewsbury and District Hospital	Yes	Yes	Yes
Newcastle Hospitals*	Yes	Yes	Yes
Friarage Hospital	Yes	No	No
Harrogate District Hospital	-	No	No
Hexham General Hospital	No	No	No
Huddersfield Royal Infirmary	-	No	No
Hull Royal Infirmary	No	Yes	Yes
James Cook University Hospital	Yes	Yes	Yes
Leeds General Infirmary	Yes	Yes	Yes
Middlesbrough General Hospital	-	No	No
North Tyneside General Hospital	No	Yes	No
Pinderfields General Hospital	No	Yes	Yes
Pontefract General Infirmary	No	Yes	Yes
Princess Royal Hospital	-	-	-

* Newcastle Hospitals comprises: Freeman Hospital, Royal Victoria Infirmary and Newcastle General Hospital.

Coronary care

	Thrombolysis in 30 mins	Coronary angiography	NSF for catheterisations
Queen Elizabeth Hospital	Yes	Yes	Yes
Royal Victoria Infirmary	-	No	No
Ryhope Hospital	-	-	-
Scarborough General Hospital	Yes	No	No
Seacroft Hospital	-	-	-
South Tyneside District Hospital	Yes	No	No
St James's University Hospital	Yes	No	No
St Luke's Hospital (Bradford)	Yes	No	No
St Luke's Hospital (Huddersfield)	-	-	-
Sunderland Royal Hospital	No	Yes	Yes
University Hospital of Hartlepool	Yes	No	No
University Hospital of North Durham	Yes	No	No
University Hospital of North Tees	No	No	No
Wansbeck General Hospital	No	Yes	No
West Cumberland Hospital	Yes	Yes	Yes
Wharfdale General Hospital	-	No	No
Whitby Hospital	-	-	-
York District Hospital	-	Yes	Yes

South East

	Thrombolysis in 30 mins	Coronary angiography	NSF for catheterisations
Amersham Hospital	-	No	-
Ashford Hospital	No	No	No
Buckland Hospital	-	No	No
Churchill Hospital	-	No	-
Conquest Hospital	Yes	Yes	Yes
Crawley Hospital	Yes	No	No
Darent Valley Hospital	No	No	No
East Surrey and Crawley Hospitals	Yes	No	No
Eastbourne District General Hospital	Yes	Yes	Yes
Frimley Park Hospital	Yes	No	No
Heatherwood Hospital	No	No	No
Horton Hospital	No	No	No
John Radcliffe Hospital	No	Yes	Yes
Kent & Canterbury Hospital	No	No	No
Kent and Sussex Hospital	Yes	No	No
Kettering General Hospital	No	No	No
Maidstone Hospital	Yes	No	No
Medway Maritime Hospital	Yes	No	No
Milton Keynes General NHS Hospital	Yes	No	No

Coronary care

	Thrombolysis in 30 mins	Coronary angiography	NSF for catheterisations
North Hampshire Hospital	Yes	Yes	Yes
Northampton General Hospital	No	Yes	No
Pembury Hospital	-	-	-
Princess Royal Hospital	No	No	No
Queen Alexandra Hospital	No	No	No
Queen Elizabeth The Queen Mother Hospital	Yes	No	No
Queen Victoria Hospital	-	No	-
Radcliffe Infirmary	-	No	No
Royal Berkshire & Battle Hospitals	Yes	Yes	Yes
Royal Hampshire County Hospital	No	No	No
Royal South Hants Hospital	-	-	-
Royal Surrey County Hospital	Yes	Yes	Yes
Royal Sussex County Hospital	Yes	Yes	Yes
Southampton General Hospital	-	Yes	Yes
Southlands Hospital	-	-	-
St Mary's Hospital (Portsmouth)	No	Yes	Yes
St Mary's Hospital (Newport)	Yes	No	No
St Peter's Hospital	No	Yes	No
St Richard's Hospital	Yes	No	No
Stoke Mandeville Hospital	Yes	No	No
Wexham Park Hospital	No	No	No
William Harvey Hospital	Yes	No	No
Worthing Hospital	No	No	No
Wycombe Hospital	No	No	No
South West			
Bristol General Hospital	-	No	No
Bristol Royal Infirmary	Yes	Yes	Yes
Cheltenham General Hospital	Yes	Yes	Yes
Cirencester Hospital	-	-	-
Derriford Hospital	No	Yes	Yes
Dorset County Hospital	No	Yes	-
Frenchay Hospital	No	Yes	No
Gloucestershire Royal Hospital	No	No	No
North Devon District Hospital	No	No	No
Poole Hospital	No	No	-
Princess Margaret Hospital	-	Yes	No
Royal Bournemouth Hospital	No	Yes	Yes
Royal Cornwall Hospital	No	Yes	Yes

Coronary care

	Thrombolysis in 30 mins	Coronary angiography	NSF for catheterisations
Royal Devon & Exeter Hospital	No	Yes	No
Royal United Hospital	Yes	Yes	Yes
Salisbury District Hospital	No	No	No
Southmead Hospital	No	Yes	No
St Michael's Hospital	-	-	-
Standish Hospital	-	-	-
Stroud General Hospital	-	No	No
Taunton & Somerset Hospital	Yes	Yes	Yes
Torbay District General Hospital	Yes	Yes	Yes
West Cornwall Hospital	-	No	No
Weston General Hospital	Yes	No	No
Yeovil District Hospital	Yes	No	No

Trent

	Thrombolysis in 30 mins	Coronary angiography	NSF for catheterisations
Barnsley District General Hospital	Yes	No	-
Bassetlaw District General Hospital	No	No	No
Chesterfield & North Derbyshire Royal Hospital	Yes	No	No
Derby City General Hospital	Yes	No	-
Derbyshire Royal Infirmary	Yes	Yes	Yes
Diana, Princess of Wales Hospital	No	Yes	Yes
Doncaster Royal Infirmary & Montagu Hospital	No	Yes	No
Glenfield Hospital	Yes	Yes	-
Grantham & District Hospital	Yes	No	-
King's Mill Hospital	Yes	No	No
Leicester General Hospital	Yes	No	No
Leicester Royal Infirmary	Yes	No	No
Lincoln County Hospital	Yes	Yes	Yes
Louth County Hospital	Yes	No	-
Northern General Hospital	Yes	Yes	Yes
Nottingham City Hospital	Yes	Yes	Yes
Pilgrim Hospital	Yes	No	No
Queen's Medical Centre	No	Yes	Yes
Rotherham District General Hospital	No	No	No
Royal Hallamshire Hospital	Yes	No	No
Scunthorpe General Hospital	-	No	No
Skegness & District Hospital	-	No	No

Coronary care

	Thrombolysis in 30 mins	Coronary angiography	NSF for catheterisations
West Midlands			
Alexandra Hospital	Yes	Yes	No
Birmingham Heartlands Hospital	Yes	Yes	Yes
City Hospital	Yes	Yes	Yes
County Hospital (Hereford)	No	Yes	No
Coventry and Warwickshire Hospital	Yes	No	No
Dudley Group of Hospitals*	Yes	Yes	Yes
General Hospital (Hereford)	-	No	No
George Eliot Hospital	Yes	No	No
Good Hope District General Hospital	Yes	Yes	No
Hospital of St Cross	Yes	No	No
Kidderminster Hospital	-	No	No
Manor Hospital (Walsall)	Yes	Yes	Yes
New Cross Hospital	Yes	No	No
North Staffordshire Hospital	No	Yes	Yes
North Staffordshire Royal Infirmary	Yes	No	No
Princess Royal Hospital	Yes	Yes	No
Queen Elizabeth Hospital (Birmingham)	Yes	Yes	Yes
Queen's Hospital (Burton)	Yes	No	-
Royal Shrewsbury Hospital	Yes	Yes	No
Sandwell General Hospital	Yes	Yes	Yes
Selly Oak Hospital	Yes	Yes	Yes
Solihull Hospital	Yes	No	No
Staffordshire General Hospital	Yes	No	No
Walsgrave Hospital	Yes	Yes	Yes
Warwick Hospital	Yes	No	No
Worcester Royal Infirmary	Yes	Yes	No
N. Ireland			
Altnagelvin Area Hospital	Yes	Yes	No
Antrim Hospital	Yes	No	No
Belfast City Hospital	Yes	Yes	Yes
Causeway	Yes	No	-
Craigavon Area Hospital	No	Yes	No
Daisy Hill Hospital	Yes	No	No
Downe Hospital	Yes	No	No
Erne Hospital	-	No	No
Lagan Valley Hospital	-	-	-

* Dudley Group of Hospitals comprises: Russells Hall, Wordsley, Corbett and Guest Hospitals.

Coronary care

	Thrombolysis in 30 mins	Coronary angiography	NSF for catheterisations
Mater Hospital	Yes	No	No
Mid-Ulster Hospital	-	No	No
The Royal Hospitals	-	Yes	Yes
Tyrone County Hospital	-	-	-
Ulster Hospital	Yes	Yes	No
Whiteabbey Hospital	-	No	-
Scotland			
Aberdeen Royal Infirmary	-	Yes	No
Ayr Hospital	Yes	Yes	Yes
Balfour Hospital	-	No	No
Borders General Hospital	-	No	No
Crosshouse Hospital	Yes	No	No
Dr Gray's Hospital	No	No	No
Dumfries and Galloway Royal Infirmary	Yes	Yes	No
Falkirk Royal Infirmary	No	No	No
Gartnavel General Hospital	-	No	No
Gilbert Bain Hospital	-	-	-
Glasgow Royal Infirmary	-	Yes	No
Hairmyres Hospital	Yes	Yes	Yes
Inverclyde Royal Hospital	Yes	Yes	No
Lorn and Islands District General Hospital	-	No	-
Monklands Hospital	Yes	No	No
Ninewells Hospital	-	Yes	Yes
Perth Royal Infirmary	-	No	No
Queen Margaret Hospital	No	No	No
Raigmore Hospital	Yes	Yes	No
Royal Alexandra Hospital	Yes	No	No
Royal Infirmary of Edinburgh	Yes	Yes	Yes
Southern General Hospital	-	-	-
St John's Hospital at Howden	-	No	No
Stirling Royal Infirmary	No	No	No
Stobhill Hospital	-	No	No
Stracathro Hospital	-	No	No
Vale of Leven District General Hospital	Yes	No	No
Victoria Hospital	-	No	No
Victoria Infirmary	-	No	No
Western General Hospital	Yes	Yes	Yes
Western Infirmary	-	Yes	No

Coronary care

	Thrombolysis in 30 mins	Coronary angiography	NSF for catheterisations
Western Isles Hospital	-	-	-
Woodend Hospital	-	No	No

Wishaw Hospital is not included in this table. This hospital opened in 2001 and consequently no data has been collated for it as yet.

Wales

	Thrombolysis in 30 mins	Coronary angiography	NSF for catheterisations
Bronglais General Hospital	No	No	-
Caerphilly District Miners' Hospital	No	-	-
Glan Clwyd District General Hospital	No	No	No
Llandough Hospital	No	No	No
Llandudno General Hospital	No	No	-
Morriston Hospital	Yes	Yes	Yes
Neath General Hospital	No	No	-
Nevill Hall Hospital	Yes	Yes	No
Prince Charles Hospital	Yes	No	No
Prince Philip Hospital	No	No	No
Princess of Wales Hospital	No	Yes	Yes
Royal Glamorgan Hospital	Yes	No	No
Royal Gwent Hospital	Yes	Yes	No
Singleton Hospital	-	No	No
St Woolos Hospital	-	No	No
University Hospital of Wales	No	Yes	Yes
West Wales General Hospital	No	No	No
Withybush General Hospital	Yes	No	No
Wrexham Maelor Hospital	No	No	No
Ysbyty Gwynedd	Yes	No	No

HEART SPECIALIST HOSPITALS

Eastern

	Thrombolysis in 30 mins	Coronary angiography	NSF for catheterisations
Papworth Hospital	-	Yes	Yes

London

	Thrombolysis in 30 mins	Coronary angiography	NSF for catheterisations
London Chest Hospital	-	Yes	Yes
Harefield Hospital	-	Yes	Yes
Royal Brompton Hospital	-	Yes	Yes

North West

	Thrombolysis in 30 mins	Coronary angiography	NSF for catheterisations
Cardiothoracic Centre Liverpool	-	-	-

Stroke

Stroke

Stroke kills 60,000 people a year in Britain, making it the biggest cause of death after heart disease and cancer. Stokes account for between 10 and 15 per cent of emergency hospital admissions to medical wards. The key to a good recovery from stroke is access to good treatment and care as soon as you are admitted. This includes quick access to CT and MRI scans and prompt treatment with physiotherapy. Some hospitals have a policy on this – others don't. However, stroke patients often have little choice other than to go to the nearest hospital as an emergency admission. There is a huge variation in hospital standards, and you may be 70 per cent more likely to die in one hospital than another if admitted for stroke.

If one of the arteries that carry blood to the brain becomes blocked, cutting off the blood supply to part of the brain, or bursts and causes bleeding into the lining of the brain, the functions controlled by the affected part of the brain stop working. This is called a stroke. The actual symptoms and signs of a stroke depend on which artery is blocked. The most common effects are loss of speech, drooping of the lower half of the face on one side, weakness of the limbs of one side of the body, or partial loss of vision. Strokes can also affect vital functions like breathing and cause sudden death. It is one of the biggest causes of death and disability in the UK, and costs the NHS more than any other single condition. Every year about one person in 400 will have a stroke, and half of those affected will be over 75. The following will be critical in their survival and recovery:

- Whether the A&E staff rapidly identify the nature of the problem and arrange admission to a specialist ward.
- Whether the hospital has a dedicated stroke unit with separate wards and teams of doctors and nurses who are focused entirely on the treatment of strokes.

- Whether you are seen by a physiotherapist within 72 hours of admission.
- If your hospital has a consultant stroke unit, there will be dedicated beds and staff who have received extra training in the management of strokes. We tell you where these hospitals are. Critical in quantifying whether a hospital is good at treating stroke patients is the number of suspected stroke victims given a CT scan within 24 and 48 hours and whether there is a stroke rehabilitation team. As stroke mainly affects older people, these patients have a right to be concerned whether there is an age bar on access to rehabilitation services.

The National Service Framework suggests that older people thought to have had a stroke should have access to diagnostic services, be treated appropriately by a specialist stroke service, and subsequently, with their carers, participate in a multidisciplinary programme of secondary prevention and rehabilitation.

What causes strokes?

There are three main causes of strokes. The first is age-related narrowing of the blood vessels in the brain or the blood vessels in the neck that lead to the brain. This is due to thickening of the muscle wall and fatty deposits (atheroma) sticking to the internal surface.

Another cause is blood clots from other parts of the body, for instance from the heart, travelling to the brain and getting stuck so that they block the flow of blood. These first two causes account for about three-quarters of strokes.

The other major cause of stroke is bleeding into the brain (intracranial haemorrhage or subarachnoid haemorrhage). This occurs due to weakness of the blood vessel walls, either inherited or caused by high blood pressure.

High blood pressure is an important risk factor for all three types of stroke.

What procedures might I be offered to prevent a stroke?

There are different procedures to try to prevent strokes caused by blocked arteries in the neck:

- Carotid angioplasty, in which a fine flexible wire with a balloon on its tip is passed into one of the arteries in your neck. The balloon is inflated to compress the plaques of atheroma and widen the artery. The whole procedure is controlled using a continuous X-ray film.

- Carotid Endarterectomy, which is a major operation usually performed under general anaesthetic to remove the blockage in the artery. Other procedures are equally effective, but the evidence suggests that they only bring significant benefit in people who have had transient ischaemic attack (TIA) within the past six months, have one or both neck arteries narrowed by at least 70 per cent and who are in good general health, with no uncontrolled angina or high blood pressure and no other serious diseases. It is important to have procedures like these performed in a consultant unit which does them regularly, as such units have the lowest rate of serious complications. There is a relatively low risk of the procedure causing a stroke, but the operation reduces the risk of a stroke in the long run.

What is a transient ischaemic attack?

A transient ischaemic attack, or TIA, is the name given to a condition in which someone shows signs of having had a stroke, but recovers fully in less than 24 hours. If you have a TIA, however minor, there is a one in eight chance that you will have a stroke within twelve months.

What can be done to prevent this from happening?

Anyone who has a TIA should inform their GP. Even if the symptoms have completely gone, the diagnosis can often be made from the history. The GP will usually prescribe aspirin, or an alternative if you cannot take aspirin, and arrange an urgent referral to a neurologist, a vascular surgeon or a dedicated rapid access TIA clinic, depending on local arrangements. At the clinic, you can expect to have a test called a duplex scan, which is a painless ultrasound scan to measure the internal diameter of the main arteries in your neck and see if they are blocked. You may also be referred for a CT scan to rule out other, rarer, problems such as blood clots and brain tumours. The doctors may to want to do an ECG of the heart and take some blood tests.

What can be done to reduce my risk of a stroke?

If you smoke, stop. If you have high blood pressure, it is critical that it is brought under control with medication. You should be prescribed an antiplatelet drug such as aspirin, ticlopidine or a combination of aspirin and dipyridamole. If you have diabetes or high cholesterol, there is some evidence that bringing these under control with medication will reduce the risk of stroke. The strongest evidence for the effect of cholesterol-lowering drugs is with one called pravastatin. If you have a condition called atrial fibrillation, a common disturbance of the heart rhythm which is strongly associated with stroke, you may be put on warfarin to prevent blood clots. Moderate exercise and drinking a small amount of alcohol every day (e.g. a glass of wine, but not more than this) are also shown to reduce the risk of stroke.

What should happen if I have a stroke?

You should go to A&E as quickly as possible, normally by ambulance. Once the doctor has examined you and is confident that you have not had a haemorrhage, you will be given aspirin and admitted to hospital. You should have a CT scan of the brain during your admission. Sometimes the doctors will wait for the CT scan before giving aspirin if they think there is a high risk that the stroke was caused by a haemorrhage (aspirin would make this worse).

Case history

Amanda Pitt-Brown

A little over a month after having her fourth child, Amanda Pitt-Brown had a stroke, which left her right side completely paralysed and her speech distorted. Tests revealed that it may have been the Pill – which Amanda had been on for no more than a week before she became ill – that caused it. She had been suffering a headache for two days before her stroke, but had put it down to the strain of now having four children. Then she suddenly felt 'very peculiar'. She went into the bathroom and sat on the side of the bath. When she collapsed, her husband managed to catch her before she hit the floor.

In the ambulance on the way to the hospital, Amanda still felt alert and aware of what was going on around her; she was also convinced that she was still talking coherently, but to everyone else what was coming out of her mouth was nonsense. When she reached the hospital, Amanda was unconscious and remained in a deep sleep for the following three days, waking intermittently. When she finally woke up, she was surrounded by books on stroke. Amanda thought they were for somebody else on the ward: 'I thought that stroke was something that only happened to old people.' From time to time nurses came around to ask her questions, such as 'who was the Prime Minister, when was my birthday … It was pointless; I knew the answers, but I couldn't speak.' No one told her what had happened; that task fell to her husband. Although she could think quite clearly, her thought processes were slower and she could not express herself properly. Her entire right side felt 'dead' and the doctors told her she might never walk again.

Each time her consultant came to check on her, he spoke over her – to the nurses, her husband – as if she wasn't there.

'He said negative things about my prognosis, and his attitude was patronising and arrogant – he never once introduced himself to me or sat down by my bed. Even though I couldn't speak, I could understand; my family and friends were well aware of this.' After six weeks, and having only ever seen her consultant three or four times, Amanda discharged herself. 'I wanted to be with my family, and I wanted to be at home: my own bed, my own bathroom, my own food.'

Amanda still visited the hospital every morning for intensive speech and physiotherapy, and her parents paid for her to see a private physiotherapist and a private stroke specialist. After this, her hand – which hadn't moved for 18 months – started to respond to treatment. Amanda believes that the idea that stroke patients make all their progress in the first year is 'ludicrous'. 'I made all my progress after the first year. People are too ready to believe everything they are told, just because it comes from someone in a white coat,' she says.

Two years later, Amanda was finally discharged from hospital; her speech therapist said the best treatment for her speech was practice: just talking to other people. She doesn't see her private consultant any more. She has also changed her GP, as she feels that her former doctor did not outline the risks associated with the Pill. 'My new GP treats me with respect and has an amazing ability to listen.'

Six years on, Amanda's speech is almost back to normal, but she still has problems with her right arm. She says 'I still get very frustrated, but I am a survivor.'

How long will it take me to recover from a stroke?

If you have a stroke, relatively few people make a full recovery and regain the ability to do everything as well as before. You can go on improving for a year or more after a stroke, although most of your recovery will take place within the first three months. One in two stroke sufferers will become depressed in the months following the stroke. This can interfere with recovery, so it is important that it is recognised and treated with antidepressant medication and/or counselling.

What is a stroke unit?

This is a hospital ward where you will be cared for by a specialist stroke team, led by a physician specialising in stroke medicine (normally a geriatrician, neurologist or consultant in stroke or disability medicine, or a named consultant with expertise in stroke). The rest of the team should include a clinical specialist nurse with expertise in stroke, a speech and language therapist, a physiotherapist, an occupational therapist, a dietician, a clinical psychologist, a pharmacist, a social worker, a stroke care co-ordinator (this may be a specific post or a role that any team member could undertake) and if necessary a trained bi- or multilingual co-worker to reflect your language needs. There is good evidence that people who are admitted to a stroke unit are less likely to die, and more likely to be able to stay in their own home, following a stroke. At the moment, relatively few patients are treated in these units as they are not available in all hospitals. In this section, we tell you which hospitals have one.

What will be done for me while I am in hospital?

Rehabilitation is a key part of stroke treatment. Your treatment will vary according to your needs, but could include the speech and language therapy if you have communication or swallowing difficulties, physiotherapy to improve mobility and occupational therapy to assess and manage any problems you may have with activities of daily living or getting back to work. You may also be offered clinical psychology to help with any depression or problems with intellectual function. If you need it, you will also be given equipment to help support you in an independent lifestyle, nutritional advice for any dietary problems and specialist treatment for any bladder or bowel problems.

What will be done for me when I leave hospital?

The care and help you receive when you leave hospital should reflect the rehabilitative work already begun and provide the necessary support to help your recovery. For this to happen effectively, both you and your carers should be involved in planning your further care with your primary care team. This assessment should identify what you're likely to need immediately when you go home, and go on to consider what kind of issues will impact on your future independence. After this, you will be given an individual care plan that tells you what services you should receive, which professionals are responsible for providing those services and what the aims and potential outcomes of your rehabilitation are.

You should be assigned a stroke care co-ordinator who will be responsible for co-ordinating your individual care plan and ensuring that arrangements for your support are in place before you leave hospital. In addition to this, you and your family should be provided with information and advice on how to prevent further strokes. Your co-ordinator is also responsible for notifying your GP of your potential risk of having another stroke and the steps that have been, or will be taken, to reduce this.

What if I need long-term support?

You should be able to contact your stroke care co-ordinator for advice and to discuss your changing needs but your long-term care should include:

• Care in your own home provided by hospital outreach teams.

- Regular reviews of medication and nutritional well-being.
- Advice, treatment and support to reduce the risk of a further stroke.
- Social and emotional support to minimise the loss of independence following the stroke.
- Ensuring that your accommodation after discharge – whether ordinary housing, sheltered accommodation or a care home – meets your needs and that adaptations and community equipment services are provided where appropriate.

The support offered by the NHS can be complemented by a number of voluntary organisations and support groups such as the Stroke Association, Different Strokes. Your stroke team will probably already have links with these.

Can Complementary Therapy help with stroke?

Trials are currently being conducted in the UK to discover whether acupuncture can be effective in the treatment of stroke. Because acupuncture releases endorphins, the treatment may help alleviate post-stroke depression and encourage exercise. Other alternative treatments thought to help reduce stress and alleviate symptoms are massage and meditation. Some alternative medicines have dangerous side-effects when taken with conventional medicines, and you should always consult your consultant or GP before taking any form of alternative medicine.

Focus on Stroke

The following table shows what the facilities your hospital provides for stroke patients. Stroke patients often require two stages of treatment: immediate care followed by rehabilitation. Some hospitals offer care for the immediate trauma of a stroke but refer patients to another hospital for rehabilitative care, sometimes as an outpatient programme. Other hospitals provide both acute care and rehabilitation services. The following table tells what types of care your hospital can provide:

- **Acute Stroke Unit:** provides specialist care immediately following a stroke. This type of unit will usually admit patients directly from home to the unit and keep people for a short period while they provide immediate treatment. Patients will then be transfered to other services as soon as possible, usually within seven days.

- **Stroke Rehabilitation Unit:** accepts patients after a minimum delay (of seven days) and focuses on rehabilitation. Rehabilitation stroke units offer specialist therapy provided by a range of health professional. These are trained s to help the patient overcome or cope with the stroke damage and the difficulties this creates for daily living. Effective rehabilitation should actively involve the patient in planning their care.

- **Combined Stroke Unit:** These units manage the stroke patient throughout the course of their hospital stay, and will plan for a properly coordinated transfer of care between hospital and the community. Care will be provided by stroke specialist staff.

Early diagnosis of stroke and identification of the extent of stroke damage are important components of patient care. The availability of CT scans, an essential diagnostic procedure, is a key issue for stroke patients. The government recommendation for stroke cases is that all stroke patients receive a CT scan within 48 hours of being admitted. However, early diagnosis of the type of stroke can be important in determining and administering appropriate treatment. We have therefore included a column to show which hospitals are able to provide a CT scan within 24 hours.

We also give you the mortality rate for stroke patients admitted as an emergency (stroke mortality rate). These figures only apply to hospitals that have an A&E department or a stroke unit. We also identify the hospitals with rates significantly above or below average. However, some hospitals with a high or low number may not be significantly below or above average if they handle relatively few cases.

Stroke

If the hospital has not provided us with information, a dash appears instead of a Yes or No.

		stroke mortality rate	acute stroke unit	stroke rehab. unit	combined stroke unit	CT scan within 24 hours	CT scan within 48 hours
Eastern							
LOW	Bedford Hospital	83	Yes	Yes	Yes	No	Yes
	Basildon Hospital	84	No	Yes	Yes	No	Yes
AVERAGE	Watford General Hospital	95	No	No	No	No	No
	Hemel Hempstead General Hospital	95	No	No	No	No	No
	Princess Alexandra Hospital	102	Yes	No	No	No	Yes
	Luton & Dunstable Hospital	102	No	Yes	No	No	No
	Hinchingbrooke Hospital	102	No	No	No	No	Yes
	James Paget Hospital	103	No	No	Yes	No	No
	Norfolk & Norwich University Hospital	103	Yes	No	No	No	No
	Queen Elizabeth Hospital	105	No	No	Yes	No	No
	Southend Hospital	107	No	Yes	No	No	Yes
	Addenbrooke's Hospital	107	No	No	Yes	No	Yes
	West Suffolk Hospital	108	Yes	Yes	No	No	Yes
HIGH	Colchester General Hospital	109	No	No	No	Yes	Yes
	Peterborough District Hospital	112	Yes	No	No	Yes	Yes
	Ipswich Hospital	113	No	No	Yes	No	No
	Lister Hospital	114	No	Yes	No	No	No
	Queen Elizabeth II Hospital	114	No	Yes	No	No	No
	Broomfield Hospital	118	No	No	No	No	No
London							
LOW	Royal London Hospital	72	Yes	No	No	Yes	No
	Middlesex & University College Hospitals	77	No	No	Yes	Yes	Yes
	Chelsea and Westminster Hospital	79	No	No	Yes	No	Yes
	Northwick Park Hospital	81	No	Yes	No	Yes	Yes
	Central Middlesex Hospital	81	No	Yes	No	Yes	Yes

Stroke

	stroke mortality rate	acute stroke unit	stroke rehab. unit	combined stroke unit	CT scan within 24 hours	CT scan within 48 hours
LOW Queen Mary's Hospital (Hampstead)	86	Yes	Yes	No	Yes	Yes
Royal Free Hospital	86	Yes	Yes	No	Yes	Yes
St Thomas' Hospital	88	No	Yes	No	No	Yes
AVERAGE Homerton Hospital	90	No	Yes	No	No	No
St Mary's Hospital	91	No	No	Yes	No	Yes
St George's Hospital (London)	92	Yes	Yes	No	No	Yes
Hillingdon Hospital	92	No	No	Yes	No	No
Queen Mary's Hospital (Sidcup)	94	No	Yes	No	No	No
University Hospital Lewisham	96	No	Yes	No	No	Yes
Ealing Hospital	96	No	No	No	No	No
King's College Hospital	99	Yes	Yes	No	No	Yes
Epsom General Hospital	99	No	No	No	No	No
St Helier Hospital	99	No	No	No	No	No
Bromley Hospital	100	No	No	No	-	-
Orpington Hospital	100	No	Yes	No	No	Yes
Whipps Cross University Hospital	101	No	Yes	No	No	No
Charing Cross Hospital	101	No	No	Yes	No	Yes
King George Hospital	102	No	No	Yes	Yes	Yes
Barnet Hospital	103	-	-	-	-	-
Chase Farm Hospital	103	-	-	-	-	-
Kingston Hospital	104	No	No	No	Yes	Yes
Oldchurch Hospital	105	No	No	No	Yes	Yes
Whittington Hospital	107	No	No	No	No	Yes
Mayday Hospital	108	No	Yes	No	No	No
North Middlesex University Hospital	111	No	No	No	No	Yes
West Middlesex University Hospital	113	No	Yes	No	No	No
HIGH Queen Elizabeth Hospital	120	No	Yes	No	No	No
Newham General Hospital	124	No	Yes	No	No	No

North West

	stroke mortality rate	acute stroke unit	stroke rehab. unit	combined stroke unit	CT scan within 24 hours	CT scan within 48 hours
LOW Ormskirk and District General Hospital	89	No	Yes	No	Yes	Yes
Southport & Formby District General	89	No	No	No	Yes	Yes
University Hospital Aintree	91	Yes	Yes	No	No	No
AVERAGE Trafford General Hospital	94	No	No	Yes	No	No
Chorley & South Ribble District General	99	No	No	No	No	No

Stroke

	stroke mortality rate	acute stroke unit	stroke rehab. unit	combined stroke unit	CT scan within 24 hours	CT scan within 48 hours
AVERAGE						
Royal Lancaster Infirmary	101	No	No	No	No	Yes
Furness General Hospital	101	No	No	No	No	No
Wythenshawe Hospital	101	Yes	Yes	No	Yes	Yes
Royal Liverpool University Hospital	103	Yes	No	No	No	Yes
Hope Hospital	104	No	Yes	No	No	No
Tameside General Hospital	104	No	Yes	No	No	No
Royal Preston Hospital	105	No	No	Yes	No	No
Fairfield General Hospital	105	No	No	No	No	No
North Manchester General Hospital	105	No	Yes	Yes	No	Yes
Warrington Hospital	105	No	No	Yes	No	No
Burnley General Hospital	107	No	No	Yes	No	No
Royal Oldham Hospital	109	No	Yes	No	No	No
Rochdale Infirmary	112	No	No	No	No	Yes
Macclesfield District General Hospital	113	No	Yes	No	No	Yes
HIGH						
Wirral (Arrowe Park & Clatterbridge)	111	Yes	Yes	No	Yes	Yes
Queens Park Hospital	111	No	Yes	No	No	No
St Helens Hospital (Merseyside)	112	No	Yes	No	No	No
Whiston Hospital	112	Yes	No	No	No	Yes
Royal Albert Edward Infirmary	113	No	Yes	No	No	No
Stepping Hill Hospital	115	No	Yes	No	No	Yes
Leighton Hospital	117	No	No	Yes	No	Yes
Royal Bolton Hospital	120	No	Yes	No	No	No
Countess of Chester Hospital	121	No	No	No	No	Yes
Blackburn Royal Infirmary	125	No	No	Yes	Yes	Yes
Blackpool Victoria Hospital	125	Yes	No	No	No	No
Manchester Royal Infirmary	126	No	Yes	No	No	Yes
Northern and Yorks						
Friarage Hospital	79	No	No	Yes	No	No
Airedale General Hospital	80	No	No	No	No	No
LOW Huddersfield Royal Infirmary	85	-	-	-	-	-
St Luke's Hospital (Huddersfield)	85	-	-	-	-	-
Hexham General Hospital	85	No	No	Yes	No	No
North Tyneside General Hospital	85	Yes	Yes	No	No	No
Wansbeck General Hospital	85	Yes	Yes	No	No	No
Wharfdale General Hospital	88	-	-	-	-	-
Leeds General Infirmary	88	-	-	-	-	-
Seacroft Hospital	88	-	-	-	-	-

Stroke

	stroke mortality rate	acute stroke unit	stroke rehab. unit	combined stroke unit	CT scan within 24 hours	CT scan within 48 hours
AVERAGE						
St James's University Hospital	88	-	-	-	-	-
Calderdale Royal Hospital	88	No	Yes	No	No	No
Newcastle Hospitals*	90	Yes	No	No	No	Yes
Hull Royal Infirmary	91	Yes	Yes	No	No	No
HIGH						
Harrogate District Hospital	91	No	Yes	No	Yes	Yes
Queen Elizabeth Hospital	92	Yes	No	No	Yes	Yes
St Luke's Hospital (Bradford)	94	No	Yes	No	Yes	Yes
Bradford Royal Infirmary	94	No	No	No	Yes	Yes
University Hospital of North Durham	96	No	No	No	No	Yes
York District Hospital	98	No	Yes	No	No	Yes
South Tyneside District Hospital	99	No	Yes	No	No	Yes
West Cumberland Hospital	99	No	Yes	No	-	-
Cumberland Infirmary	99	No	Yes	No	-	-
Dewsbury and District Hospital	100	No	No	No	No	No
Bridlington & District Hospital	100	-	-	-	-	-
Scarborough General Hospital	100	-	-	-	-	-
Pontefract General Infirmary	101	No	No	No	No	No
Pinderfields General Hospital	101	No	No	No	No	No
James Cook University Hospital	102	No	Yes	No	No	No
Middlesbrough General Hospital	102	No	No	No	No	No
Sunderland Royal Hospital	108	No	No	Yes	No	No
University Hospital of North Tees	108	No	Yes	No	No	No
University Hospital of Hartlepool	108	No	Yes	No	Yes	No
Bishop Auckland General Hospital	110	No	No	Yes	Yes	Yes
Darlington Memorial Hospital	110	No	No	Yes	Yes	Yes
South East						
LOW						
Stoke Mandeville Hospital	86	No	Yes	No	Yes	Yes
St Richard's Hospital	89	No	Yes	No	No	Yes
AVERAGE						
Royal Surrey County Hospital	92	No	No	No	No	Yes
Frimley Park Hospital	93	Yes	No	No	No	Yes
Queen Alexandra Hospital	95	No	No	No	-	-
St Peter's Hospital	95	No	No	No	No	Yes
Ashford Hospital	95	No	No	Yes	-	-
North Hampshire Hospital	96	No	No	Yes	No	No
Northampton General Hospital	96	No	No	Yes	No	Yes

* Newcastle Hospitals comprises: Freeman Hospital, Royal Victoria Infirmary and Newcastle General Hospital.

Stroke

		stroke mortality rate	acute stroke unit	stroke rehab. unit	combined stroke unit	CT scan within 24 hours	CT scan within 48 hours
AVERAGE	Princess Royal Hospital	96	No	Yes	No	No	Yes
	Conquest Hospital	97	No	Yes	No	No	Yes
	Worthing Hospital	98	No	Yes	No	No	Yes
	Royal Hampshire County Hospital	100	No	No	Yes	No	Yes
	Maidstone Hospital	102	No	No	No	No	Yes
	Kent and Sussex Hospital	102	No	No	No	No	Yes
	Royal Berkshire & Battle Hospitals	102	Yes	No	No	No	Yes
	John Radcliffe Hospital	102	Yes	No	No	Yes	Yes
	Horton Hospital	102	Yes	-	-	-	-
	Radcliffe Infirmary	102	No	Yes	No	No	No
	Queen Elizabeth The Queen Mother Hos.	103	No	Yes	No	No	No
	Kent & Canterbury Hospital	103	No	Yes	No	No	No
	William Harvey Hospital	103	No	No	No	-	-
	Heatherwood Hospital	103	No	Yes	No	No	Yes
	Wexham Park Hospital	103	No	Yes	No	No	Yes
	Royal Sussex County Hospital	104	No	No	No	No	No
	St Mary's Hospital (Newport)	105	No	Yes	No	No	No
	East Surrey and Crawley Hospitals	105	No	No	Yes	Yes	Yes
	Crawley Hospital	105	No	Yes	No	No	Yes
	Kettering General Hospital	105	No	No	Yes	No	Yes
	Southampton General Hospital	106	-	-	-	-	-
	Wycombe Hospital	106	-	-	-	-	-
	Darent Valley Hospital	109	No	No	No	No	Yes
	Medway Maritime Hospital	111	No	No	No	No	No
HIGH	Eastbourne District General Hospital	111	No	Yes	No	No	No
	Milton Keynes General NHS Hospital	127	No	No	Yes	No	Yes
	South West						
LOW	Bristol Royal Infirmary	74	Yes	No	Yes	No	No
	Weston General Hospital	76	No	No	Yes	Yes	Yes
	Royal United Hospital	81	Yes	No	No	No	Yes
	Taunton & Somerset Hospital	89	Yes	No	No	-	-
	Poole Hospital	89	Yes	No	No	No	No
	Torbay District General Hospital	90	No	No	Yes	-	-
AVERAGE	West Cornwall Hospital	92	No	No	No	-	-
	Royal Cornwall Hospital	92	No	No	Yes	No	No
	Royal Bournemouth Hospital	92	Yes	Yes	No	No	No

Stroke

	stroke mortality rate	acute stroke unit	stroke rehab. unit	combined stroke unit	CT scan within 24 hours	CT scan within 48 hours
Cheltenham General Hospital	93	Yes	Yes	No	No	No
Cirencester Hospital	93	-	-	-	-	-
North Devon District Hospital	95	No	Yes	No	No	Yes
Dorset County Hospital	98	No	Yes	No	No	-
Royal Devon & Exeter Hospital	98	No	No	Yes	No	No
Frenchay Hospital	98	No	No	Yes	No	No
Southmead Hospital	98	No	No	No	No	No
Derriford Hospital	101	Yes	No	No	Yes	Yes
Salisbury District Hospital	106	No	No	Yes	No	Yes
Yeovil District Hospital	110	No	No	No	Yes	Yes
Princess Margaret Hospital	110	-	-	-	-	-
Gloucestershire Royal Hospital	110	No	No	Yes	No	Yes

AVERAGE applies to rows Cheltenham General Hospital through Princess Margaret Hospital. **HIGH** applies to Gloucestershire Royal Hospital.

Trent

	stroke mortality rate	acute stroke unit	stroke rehab. unit	combined stroke unit	CT scan within 24 hours	CT scan within 48 hours
Royal Hallamshire Hospital	73	No	Yes	No	No	Yes
Nottingham City Hospital	74	Yes	Yes	Yes	No	No
King's Mill Hospital	92	No	No	No	No	Yes
Skegness & District Hospital	95	-	-	-	-	-
Pilgrim Hospital	95	No	No	No	No	No
Louth County Hospital	95	No	No	No	-	-
Lincoln County Hospital	95	No	No	No	No	No
Grantham & District Hospital	95	No	No	No	No	No
Glenfield Hospital	99	No	No	Yes	No	Yes
Leicester Royal Infirmary	99	Yes	Yes	No	No	Yes
Leicester General Hospital	99	No	No	Yes	No	Yes
Northern General Hospital	101	No	No	Yes	No	Yes
Diana, Princess of Wales Hospital	104	No	Yes	No	No	No
Rotherham District General Hospital	109	-	-	-	-	-
Bassetlaw District General Hospital	111	No	No	No	No	Yes
Derbyshire Royal Infirmary	110	No	Yes	No	No	Yes
Doncaster Royal Infirmary & Montagu Hos.	112	No	No	No	No	No
Chesterfield & N. Derbyshire Royal Hos.	114	Yes	No	No	No	No
Queen's Medical Centre	117	No	No	Yes	No	No
Barnsley District General Hospital	119	Yes	Yes	Yes	No	Yes
Scunthorpe General Hospital	122	No	No	No	No	Yes

LOW applies to Royal Hallamshire Hospital and Nottingham City Hospital. **AVERAGE** applies to King's Mill Hospital through Bassetlaw District General Hospital. **HIGH** applies to Derbyshire Royal Infirmary through Scunthorpe General Hospital.

Stroke

	stroke mortality rate	acute stroke unit	stroke rehab. unit	combined stroke unit	CT scan within 24 hours	CT scan within 48 hours
West Midlands						
Royal Shrewsbury Hospital	88	No	No	Yes	No	Yes
Queen's Hospital (Burton)	89	No	No	No	No	No
Solihull Hospital	93	No	Yes	No	No	Yes
Birmingham Heartlands Hospital	93	No	No	Yes	No	No
County Hospital (Hereford)	90	No	No	No	No	No
General Hospital (Hereford)	90	-	-	-	-	-
Staffordshire General Hospital	92	No	Yes	No	No	Yes
Warwick Hospital	95	No	No	No	Yes	No
Selly Oak Hospital	105	Yes	No	No	No	No
Queen Elizabeth Hospital (Birmingham)	105	Yes	No	No	No	No
Princess Royal Hospital	107	No	Yes	Yes	No	No
New Cross Hospital	107	No	No	No	No	Yes
City Hospital	108	No	No	No	Yes	Yes
North Staffordshire Hospital	108	No	No	Yes	No	Yes
Dudley Group of Hospitals*	108	No	Yes	No	No	No
Coventry and Warwickshire Hospital	108	No	No	No	-	-
Hospital of St Cross	108	No	No	No	-	-
Walsgrave Hospital	108	Yes	No	No	No	No
Alexandra Hospital	111	No	No	No	No	No
Worcester Royal Infirmary	111	No	No	No	No	No
Good Hope District General Hospital	112	No	Yes	No	-	-
George Eliot Hospital	120	No	No	No	Yes	Yes
Sandwell General Hospital	121	No	Yes	No	No	No
Manor Hospital (Walsall)		No	Yes	No	-	-

LOW applies to rows: Royal Shrewsbury Hospital, Queen's Hospital (Burton), Solihull Hospital, Birmingham Heartlands Hospital

AVERAGE applies to rows: County Hospital (Hereford) through Dudley Group of Hospitals*

HIGH applies to rows: Coventry and Warwickshire Hospital through Sandwell General Hospital

* Dudley Group of Hospitals comprises: Russells Hall, Wordsley, Corbett and Guest Hospitals.

Scotland Stroke

	stroke mortality rate	CT scan within 48 hours
Aberdeen Royal Infirmary	84	-
Ayr Hospital	74	-
Borders General Hospital	75	Yes
Crosshouse Hospital	75	-
Dr Gray's Hospital	84	Yes
Dumfries and Galloway Royal Infirmary	76	Yes
Falkirk royal infirmary	76	-
Gartnavel General Hospital	80	-
Glasgow Royal Infirmary	73	-
Hairmyres Hospital	78	-
Inverclyde Royal Hospital	72	No
Lorn and Islands District General Hospital	72	Yes
Monklands Hospital	71	-
Ninewells Hospital	77	Yes
Perth Royal Infirmary	74	Yes
Queen Margaret Hospital	65	-
Raigmore Hospital	76	No
Royal Alexandra Hospital	74	No
Royal Infirmary of Edinburgh	67	-
Southern General Hospital	85	-
St John's Hospital at Howden	72	Yes
Stirling Royal Infirmary	79	Yes
Stobhill Hospital	76	-
Stracathro Hospital	84	Yes
Vale of Leven District General Hospital	-	No
Victoria Hospital	69	-
Victoria Infirmary	75	-
Western General Hospital	81	-
Western Infirmary	80	-
Woodend Hospital	84	-

Wishaw Hospital is not included in this table. This hospital opened in 2001 and consequently no data has been collated for it as yet.

N. Ireland and Wales Stroke

	acute stroke unit	stroke rehab. unit	combined stroke unit	CT scan within 48 hours
N. Ireland				
Altnagelvin Area Hospital	No	No	Yes	No
Antrim Hospital*	No	No	No	No
Belfast City Hospital	No	Yes	No	Yes
Causeway Hospital	-	-	-	-
Craigavon Area Hospital	No	Yes	No	-
Daisy Hill Hospital	Yes	Yes	Yes	Yes
Mater Hospital	No	No	No	Yes
Mid-Ulster Hospital	No	No	No	No
The Royal Hospitals	Yes	Yes	No	Yes
Ulster Hospital	No	No	Yes	No
Whiteabbey Hospital*	No	No	No	No
Wales				
Bronglais General Hospital	No	No	Yes	Yes
Caerphilly District Miners' Hospital	Yes	No	No	No
Glan Clwyd District General Hospital	Yes	Yes	No	Yes
Llandough Hospital	No	Yes	No	No
Llandudno General Hospital	No	No	No	No
Morriston Hospital	No	No	No	No
Nevill Hall Hospital	No	No	Yes	Yes
Prince Charles Hospital	No	No	No	No
Prince Philip Hospital	No	No	No	-
Princess of Wales Hospital	No	No	No	Yes
Royal Glamorgan Hospital	No	Yes	No	-
Royal Gwent Hospital	Yes	No	No	No
Singleton Hospital	No	No	Yes	Yes
University Hospital of Wales	No	No	No	-
West Wales General Hospital	No	No	No	-
Withybush General Hospital	No	Yes	No	Yes
Wrexham Maelor Hospital	-	-	-	-
Ysbyty Gwynedd	No	No	No	Yes

* These hospitals are currently establishing stroke units.

Cancer

Cancer

One person in three will develop cancer at some time in their lives. Many of these cancers will be curable. Even so, cancer is the second biggest killer, after heart disease, in the UK.

Cancer can affect any part of the body, but all cancers develop as a result of the same process. Like all living things, humans are made of billions of microscopic building blocks called cells. Normally each cell has a set lifespan, during which it grows, divides, shrinks and dies. When a cell is affected by cancer, this process goes wrong and the cell keeps on dividing at an immature stage of its development until it forms a ball of cells called a tumour. Not all tumours are cancerous. Some are benign, which means that they do not eat into the surrounding tissues and do not spread around the body. Cancerous tumours are malignant.

As well as using up the body's energy supplies to feed its own growth, a cancer can cause damage by eating into neighbouring organs and tissues, and by spreading through the bloodstream or lymphatic system or across body cavities to cause secondary cancers, or metastases. Some cancers also produce substances that interfere with the body's ability to regulate its internal environment.

Quick diagnosis of cancer is the key to survival and the Government has introduced targets whereby certain suspected cancer patients are referred to a consultant within 2 weeks of seeing their GP. If your GP suspects you have cancer, you will naturally want waiting times to be kept to a minimum. In this section we tell you which hospitals meet the 2-week referral target. If your hospital provides a one-stop clinic, you can receive results, for example, from mammograms on the same day.

If you are diagnosed with cancer, it is essential that your hospital provides you with the right kind of emotional support. Hospitals that provide integrated care are more likely to provide you with seamless care from diagnosis through every stage of your treatment.

Multi-disciplinary teams (teams of specialised health professionals working together) also ensure that you will receive all your care in the same place (see below).

Improving cancer services – and making them more consistent across the country – is a central priority of the NHS. There is an increasing realisation among health professionals that specialisation is important in the assessment and treatment of almost all cancers, in particular through the use of specialist multidisciplinary teams. The NHS Executive's Improving Outcomes series, together with the NHS Cancer Plan, present benchmark standards for improving care in this area. They suggest that:

- Cancer services are best provided by **multi-disciplinary teams** of clinicians – doctors, nurses, radiographers and other specialists – who work together effectively. Team working brings together staff with the necessary knowledge, skills and experience to ensure high quality diagnosis, treatment and care. It also improves the co-ordination and continuity of care for patients. For common cancers, such as breast cancer, patients treated by specialist teams are more likely to survive. (*NHS Cancer Plan*, 2000)

- Radiotherapy should be made more readily available to those who could benefit from it i.e. at weekends or on an inpatient or hotel basis. (*Improving Outcomes in Lung Cancer*, NHS Executive, 1998)

- Palliative care should be an integral part of patient management from the outset. It should be the responsibility of a multiprofessional team which has close links with the specialist cancer team, sharing at least one member in common. (*Improving Outcomes in Lung Cancer*, NHS Executive, 1998)

- The new patient workload of each oncology consultant should be less than 315 cases per year (recommendation made by the Royal College of Radiologists, 1999)

Case history

Lucy Edwards

When Lucy Edwards saw her consultant for the first time, she was still reeling from the shock and distress of discovering she had breast cancer. 'I was 30, and learned a few minutes before that what I'd thought was a cyst turned out to be cancer – at the one-stop-clinic in Norwich you can be examined and diagnosed the same day. The consultant was very cool and pragmatic, but I was crying. The hospital breast care nurse sat with me and supported me, while he was very cool and dispassionate.'

While the consultant explained Lucy's choices to her, he also wrote them down. Lucy was so numb with shock it was hard to take in what he was saying. When she left, the consultant shook her hand and said a few encouraging words but it took Lucy a long time to build up a relationship with him. She now trusts his medical judgement completely but feels 'his bedside manner could be better.'

Lucy very much wanted a family, so chose a form of chemotherapy which would not affect her fertility. However, her consultant hadn't suggested that she have some ovarian tissue frozen privately to enable her to have babies later and was angry at having to find this out for herself. 'He said he wasn't aware of the scheme. But when I told him I wanted to do this he was supportive and we scheduled my treatment around it.'

Throughout her treatment, Lucy could contact her breast cancer nurse at all times. Any questions she had were passed straight on to her consultant. At first, her tumour responded well, but when later the cancer returned she had to have a mastectomy. 'The surgeon who did this was a lot warmer – he could actually make jokes and make me smile. It really does help a lot when someone does that.'

After this operation, Lucy was ready to ask her consultant 'the hard questions'. She asked if he thought it would come back and he said yes. They decided to leave more chemotherapy in reserve. Lucy found this 'very strange – from having so much treatment I was now having none. It felt a bit like flying without a safety net.'

Two years later Lucy's progress has been good. Rather than seeing her consultant monthly, she now sees him every nine months. 'If I have another lump, he is confident I am body-aware and would spot it quickly. He also advised against regular blood tests, as they are not always accurate and can cause distress.' She has some criticisms of her consultant's approach, mainly to do with his tone and manner. 'When talking about life or death situations, the consultant sounded almost blithe about it; maybe he's just more honest about death than I was used to. He said I should not try for a baby for five years. When I asked, why five? He used the words "to ensure the survival of the mother", which I found a bit chilling.' she says. 'Consultants can forget you are not a medical professional and cannot understand their arguments quickly. They can also sound very cold but I can understand why. I feel it is not his job to become emotionally involved, though it can be very frustrating for the patient. The relationship between us is now warmer because it has been built up over time.'

What other words do health professionals use when they mean cancer?

Nowadays most health professionals aren't afraid to use the word 'cancer' when talking to patients. Other terms you might hear are 'neoplasm', 'growth', 'neoplastic growth', 'mitotic lesion', and 'malignancy'. Sometimes much more vague terms are used, such as 'ulcer', 'lump' or 'polyp'. If you aren't sure what the doctor or nurse is trying to tell you, ask whether they mean that you have cancer.

Will I be told if I have cancer?

Yes, unless you have made an explicit request that you should not be told. In the past, many doctors thought the best policy was to keep a diagnosis of cancer from the patient. It is now known that almost every patient wants to be told the truth about their diagnosis and outlook. This is a good thing, because you can only participate fully in decisions about your care if you know what is wrong with you.

What causes cancer?

Nobody knows exactly what happens to 'switch off' the protective mechanisms that stop immature cells from dividing, programme cell death and mop up cells that are not behaving normally – processes which are taking place in all of us all of the time. However, we do know that certain factors can put people at higher than average risk of developing cancer. These include:

Smoking This is by far the biggest single cause of cancer. Apart from being the direct cause of over 90 per cent of lung cancers (and lung cancer is the commonest cause of death from cancer in the UK), smoking substantially increases the risk of cancers of the mouth, throat, oesophagus, stomach, pancreas, kidney, bladder, cervix, and certain types of leukaemia in adults.

Exposure to asbestos and certain toxic chemicals on a regular basis, usually through work.

Sun exposure particularly in childhood and in fair-skinned races. The commonest cancer in the UK is non-melanoma skin cancer (rodent ulcers and squamous cell carcinoma). This occurs almost entirely on parts of the body that have been exposed to sunlight regularly. Fortunately, it can almost always be treated successfully. The other sun-related cancer is malignant melanoma, which can be extremely aggressive.

Obesity If you are more than a little overweight, your risk of bowel cancer and, in women, cancer of the breast and womb, increase considerably.

Diet Some cancers have been linked to a diet high in fat and low in fresh fruit and vegetables. A high fibre diet probably reduces the risk of bowel cancer, although recent research has cast some doubt on this. Eating a lot of smoked or heavily pickled foods can contribute to stomach cancer.

Alcohol especially when taken in excess and combined with smoking, can contribute to cancer of the mouth, throat, oesophagus and colon.

Some strains of **human papilloma virus (HPV)** have been implicated in cancer of the cervix. This virus is sexually transmitted, and the risk is increased in women who started having sex at a young age, have had many sexual partners, and have often had sex without a condom. The same viruses contribute to a high incidence of cancer of the anus in homosexual men. Other viruses such as **HIV, Hepatitis C** and, in developing countries, the glandular fever virus, can increase the risk of certain types of cancer.

Family history Some cancers run in families. Cancers of the breast, womb and ovary are genetically linked in some cases, and some families have an inherited tendency to develop bowel cancer at an early age. However, breast and bowel cancer are very common and most cases occur in people who have no family history.

Having certain other diseases For example, people with

ulcerative colitis are at high risk of developing bowel cancer, and people with pernicious anaemia are at increased risk of developing stomach cancer.

What can I do to reduce my risk of getting cancer?

Some risk factors cannot be avoided – getting older is in itself a risk factor for cancer, and you cannot change your family history. Even so, there are many things you can do to make sure your risk of developing cancer is as low as possible:

Don't smoke. If you don't smoke, don't start, and if you do smoke, try to stop. Even if you have been smoking for 40 or 50 years, your health will benefit – and your risk of cancer will fall.

Eat healthily. Eat at least 5 portions a day of fresh fruit and vegetables. If you eat a lot of red meat, reduce your consumption to less than 140g (5oz) a day and don't overcook it. Try to have fish, poultry or a vegetarian dish instead of red meat several times a week. Increase your intake of fibre and choose whole fresh foods in preference to processed foods. If you eat a healthy mixed diet, you should not need to take supplements.

Watch your weight. Try to keep your body mass index between 20 and 25. To calculate your body mass index, multiply your height in metres by itself and divide your weight in kilograms by the result. For example, if you are 1.6 metres tall and weigh 60kg, the square of your height in metres (1.6x1.6) is 2.56. To get your body mass index, divide 60 by 2.56, which gives 23.44.

Don't drink more that the recommended maximum amount of alcohol – 14 units a week for women and 28 units a week for men, spread over 4-5 days a week.

Practise safe sex. Be fussy about your choice of partners, and use condoms whenever possible. In future, a blood test for the harmful strains of human papilloma virus, and a vaccine, may become available for everyone.

Watch your sun exposure. In summer, wear sunscreen with a sun protection factor (SPF) of 15 or more and both UVA and UVB protection. Don't reduce the level of protection to try to get a tan – particularly avoid getting sun burnt. Keep babies out of the sun and keep children covered up – sunburn in childhood is a big risk factor for skin cancer. Stay out of the sun between 11am and 3pm.

Sunbeds, even when used as recommended, are just as harmful as natural sunlight.

Know your body. Become familiar with the feeling of your own abdomen and breasts or testes. Know what is a normal bowel habit for you, and what the moles on your skin look like. Report any changes to your GP.

Attend for screening tests. such as mammograms and smear tests, and any special screening tests you might be offered because of your family history or your occupation.

Relax. Don't let worry about cancer ruin your life.

What screening tests are offered for cancer?
At present, the only screening programmes available nationally are those for breast cancer, in which every woman aged between 50 and 64 is invited for a mammogram (an X-ray of the breast) every three years, and cancer of the cervix, in which every woman aged between 20 and 64 is invited for a smear test every 3 to 5 years.

Why are there no screening tests for other cancers?
To make screening worthwhile, the disease screened for has to be both common and serious, and the test has to fulfil certain criteria – it has to be accurate, acceptable to the population, and able to detect the disease at a stage where treatment will cure it. This means that a cure has to be available, and the cost of the treatment – both financial and in the inconvenience and side-effects people suffer as a result of the screening programme – has to be justifiable. However, some units will routinely offer all or some of the following screening tests:

- A blood test for prostate cancer for the over 50s.
- A blood test or colonoscopy for bowel cancer.
- A blood test for ovarian cancer. If you are in a high-risk category, you can have routine scanning for ovarian cancer at London teaching hospitals.

What should I do if I think I might have cancer?

If you find a lump, are inexplicably losing weight, suffering abnormal bleeding or a notice a change in bowel habits, tell your GP as soon as possible. Think in advance about any symptoms you may have. Do they differ from what is normal for you? When did you first suspect something was wrong? Have your symptoms changed since then? Have you had symptoms like these before? Is there any history of cancer in your family? Your GP will examine you and may organise blood tests or X-rays. If they think you could have cancer, they will refer you to see a consultant.

Will I have to wait long to see the consultant?

No – you shouldn't do. Priority is given to people with suspected cancer, both because cancer is more likely to be curable in the early stages and because the state of knowing that they might have cancer is difficult for most people to cope with. The Government has set targets for cancer waiting times, and all patients with suspected cancer who are referred urgently by their GP should be seen by the consultant within 2 weeks of the referral being received. To reduce delay, your GP should make the initial referral by telephone or fax.

Does this mean that everyone with cancer gets seen within two weeks?

No. Firstly it may be difficult for a GP to realise that cancer is the likely diagnosis – most cancers can present with a wide variety of symptoms which mimic commoner, less serious conditions. Also, not all hospitals are managing to meet the Government target of seeing all urgent cancer referrals within 2 weeks.

What sort of consultant will I see?

If you are referred urgently to hospital because cancer is suspected, and your cancer is operable, you will normally see a surgeon with a special interest in your type of cancer. Examples are:

- General surgeon with an interest in breast surgery
  Breast cancer.
- General surgeon with an interest in colorectal cancer
  Colon cancer, Rectal cancer.
- General surgeon, with an interest in the relevant area
  Stomach cancer, Oesophageal cancer, Pancreatic cancer, Thyroid cancer.
- Gynaecologist.
  Cancer of the cervix, ovary, womb or vulva.
- Urologist
  Cancer of the bladder, prostate, testis or kidney.
- Ear, nose and throat surgeon
  Cancer of the tonsil, throat, larynx (voice box) or the soft tissues of the neck.
- Orofacial surgeon
  Cancer of the mouth, tongue and salivary glands.
- Neurosurgeon
  Cancers of the brain, spinal cord and major nerves.
- Orthopaedic surgeon
  Bone cancer

Skin cancers are referred to a dermatologist and cancers of the blood (leukaemias) and lymphatic system (lymphomas), are referred to a blood consultant – a haematologist. Lung cancer, which is rarely suitable for surgery, is referred to a chest physician initially though a cardiothoracic surgeon would operate if required.

When you are referred, you should check that your specialist works as part of a **multi-disciplinary team**. This team will include clinicians with specialised knowledge of each aspect of diagnosis and treatment (eg a surgical specialist, oncologist, radiologist) and specialised nursing staff who will support, advise and assist you and provide information. This team should also work closely with other professionals involved in your care, specifically your GP. The advantage of a multi-disciplinary team is that it facilitates co-ordinated care. You are more likely to be offered a range of types of treatment at appropriate times and receive seamless care throughout all stages of your illness. On p141 we tell you which hospitals will provide you with multi-disciplinary care in the case of colo-rectal cancer.

What is an oncologist?
An oncologist is a specialist in the treatment of cancer and will co-ordinate all aspects of your treatment.

What is a radiotherapist?
A radiotherapist (clinical oncologist) is a doctor trained specifically in radiotherapy (see below).

How will my cancer be treated?
- **Surgery**
  To remove the tumour and control its spread.
- **Chemotherapy**
  Technically, the word 'chemotherapy' just means treating a disease with drugs, and is used by doctors to describe the treatment of non-cancerous conditions such as AIDS and tuberculosis. However, it is more commonly taken to refer to the treatment of cancer and here it means an attempt to destroy the

cancer cells using strong drugs. Doctors who specialise in chemotherapy are called medical oncologists, though haematologists use chemotherapy to treat cancers of the blood.

The decision about which of the many drugs to use, and at which strength, depends on the type of cancer and the individual patient.

Chemotherapy is usually given in hospital, in special oncology units which have day care facilities and a few inpatient beds and are staffed by specially trained nurses. Because the drugs used are so strong, staff who handle them need to have had appropriate training and to follow protocols. Most chemotherapy is given intravenously through a drip in the arm, but in some patients a central line going into a large vein in the chest is used, and some drugs have to be injected directly into body cavities or into the spine. A few chemotherapy drugs can be taken by mouth.

Like radiotherapy (see below), chemotherapy causes side-effects in most patients. These typically affect parts of the body where the cells divide frequently, such as the skin and the lining of the bowel. Common side-effects are nausea and vomiting, diarrhoea, skin rashes, pain on passing urine and hair loss but medication can be given to counteract some of these side-effects. All chemotherapy drugs stop the immune system from working properly and put the patient at risk of infections.

- **Radiotherapy**

Radiotherapy is a treatment given by a doctor called a clinical oncologist, usually after referral by another consultant. There are two different types of radiotherapy:

X-rays (much stronger than the ones used to take pictures of your bones) are directed towards the cancer. You will be fitted with a leaded shield to protect the other parts of your body, and the oncologist and radiotherapist calculate the strength of the X-rays, number of treatments and duration of each treatment

Case history

David Wright

The shock of learning that he had developed chronic lymphocytic leukaemia was heightened by a fearful irony in David Wright's case. As a successful tabloid editor he had spent years writing the only sort of headlines newspaper readers seem to be offered on 'taboo' subjects like cancer: 'Celebrity's Brave Battle For Life' . . . 'Leukaemia Child's Last-Chance Flight To US For Treatment'. Now it was David's turn to be gripped by the panic and helplessness so often associated with the merest mention of 'the Big C' and whose own headlines had unwittingly encouraged the public to see such situations as hopeless. 'All of those headlines I'd written over the years flashed through my head that day,' recalls David. 'Trouble was, apart from the odd "miracle recovery" story I couldn't remember any happy endings ... bad news sells better than good, I'm afraid.'

The good news in David's case was that his leukaemia – one of several forms of the disease – had been discovered during a routine medical arranged through his company's private health scheme. Within hours of the initial diagnosis he met with one of the country's leading haematologists at the renowned London Clinic. For the next 18 months his leukaemia's progress was simply monitored. Some instances of CLL never require actual treatment as the disease progresses so slowly; others can be controlled by drugs in tablet form, while the more aggressive cases require intravenous chemotherapy and stem cell transplants to control the growth of cancerous white cells or put the disease into remission.

'I went through the various stages of tablets and occasional one- or two-hour visits to a day clinic for intravenous chemo over a period of about three years,' says David, now 53. 'In between appointments I lived a more or less normal life.'

Eventually, David's team of three consultants – two of whom

also have practices at major NHS hospitals – decided that they would try an autograft: David's own stem cells were removed from his bone marrow then held in cold storage while he was given a huge dose of chemotherapy to kill off as many cancerous cells as possible before the stem cells were put back to begin the fight against the remaining cancer. 'That gave me about fifteen months' drug-free remission before we noticed that my lymph glands were swelling again,' says David. 'We'd achieved partial success in that my blood and bone marrow registered as normal, but the cancer cells were still developing in my lymph glands.' So, for the past eight months, David has been preparing for an allograft, or stem cell transplant from a donor, using cells from his brother, Richard, who proved to be a healthy 'match' (a one-in-four chance among siblings). Treatment has included mild intravenous chemotherapy and the introduction of antibodies to 'mop up' stubborn collections of cancerous cells before his brother's healthy stem cells are introduced to the battle to give David a healthy, normal immune system.

'There are risks I've not faced before,' says David, 'mainly through something called Graft Versus Host Disease because of the "invasion" of foreign tissue. But the possibility of long-term remission is too good to miss.' David is full of praise for the treatment he has received, both from the London Clinic's medical team and from the charity CancerBACUP, which counsels and advises cancer patients. 'But by far the most important team has been my wife, Gemma, and our two (now grown-up) kids, who have trawled the Internet, read the pamphlets and posed the questions I couldn't face asking. Between them all, they've taken the "fear factor" out of my condition.'

for every individual case. Each treatment is normally done as a day case.

Only a few types of cancer can be cured by radiotherapy alone (for example, Hodgkin's). More often, radiotherapy is used to reduce the bulk of the tumour before surgery, to kill off tiny groups of cancer cells that might have been left behind after surgery, or to relieve symptoms.

Radiotherapy does cause side-effects – unlike chemotherapy, these tend to occur largely around the part of the body that is treated and may include burning and soreness of the treated area.

Radioactive implants may be placed in or near the tumour mass to damage and kill the tumour cells. They are only used for a few types of cancer.

• **Hormonal Manipulation** Certain cancers depend on naturally occurring hormones to sustain their growth. By inhibiting these hormones, drugs such as Tamoxifen (used to treat breast cancer) blocks off the tumour's access to the hormone it requires to grow.

Do I get any say in the decisions about my treatment?

Yes. No form of treatment will be given without your consent, and if you choose not to have a particular form of treatment then that will be respected. On the other hand, you cannot insist on being given a treatment that is of no proven value in your type of cancer.

What can be done if I have incurable cancer?

There is a lot that can be done. Initially, you may be given palliative surgery, radiotherapy or chemotherapy to reduce the size of the tumour mass and relieve symptoms. After palliative treatment, many people remain well for months or even years. Your GP will also give you treatment for any pain or other symptoms caused by the cancer.

What can be done to look after people with terminal cancer at home?

When the cancer reaches the terminal phase, your GP and district nurses will try to help your family to care for you at home. Macmillan nurses are specialy trained to help patients with terminal cancer. Many treatments, including strong painkillers through a needle under the skin, can be given at home, and the local palliative care team may well have a home-care service. Other organisations, including Marie Curie nurses and social services, may also help. If you and your family are keen that you should die at home, every effort will be made to make sure that you remain at home.

How do I apply for a Macmillan nurse?

Most oncologists will routinely involve a Macmillan nurse as part of your care. However, if this is not the case, ask your GP, district nurse, consultant, or a senior hospital nurse such as a sister or ward manager, to make a referral.

What is a hospice?

Some palliative care teams are based at a hospice. A hospice is a residential and day-care facility for people with advanced cancer. Some hospices also take people with other terminal illnesses such as motor neurone disease. The palliative care team includes a doctor, often with a background in general practice. The hospice is staffed by nurses who are specially trained in palliative care, including Macmillan nurses. Lay workers, religious leaders and complementary therapists also visit. Hospices can offer day care, respite care, and can admit people who are in the terminal phase of their illness but cannot be managed at home. Hospices provide one of the best examples of holistic, patient-centred care in the NHS.

Can Complementary Therapy help with cancer?

Complementary therapies cannot cure cancer, but are used increasingly in NHS cancer units to ease anxiety, encourage relaxation and relieve pain. Breathing, relaxation and visualization techniques, hand or foot massage, reflexology and aromatherapy have been found to benefit patients suffering from nerves, needle phobia, nausea and morphine related constipation. What appears to be most effective is a combination of support groups, counseling, relaxation and self-hypnosis – all thought to enhance the immune system and help fight the disease. Diet is increasingly acknowledged as an important factor in the initial development of the disease. However, extreme dietary regimes or vitamin supplementation are not recommended as they may raise unrealistic hopes of recovery. Some alternative medicines have dangerous side-effects when taken with conventional medicines, and you should always consult your consultant or GP before taking any form of alternative medicine.

Focus on Cancer

As in all areas, hospitals can vary in their provision of cancer services; as an example the tables below tell you how your local hospital performs in its treatment of colorectal cancer. Colorectal cancer is one of the most common forms of cancer and as such the issues surrounding it are similar to the treatment of other cancers. If diagnosed early enough and effectively treated it can be cured, which enables us to test the whole range of facilities provided by the hospital.

Based on the issues our patient focus-groups regard as important, our table will tell you:

- Whether your hospital provides a service for this cancer
- Whether you will be given an appointment within 2 weeks of an urgent referral from your GP.

- If your hospital has a multi-disciplinary team for the treatment of this cancer. For England, Wales and Northern Ireland it is suggested that this team comprise a lower gastrointestinal surgeon, a radiologist with gastrointestinal expertise, a histopathologist, a physician gastroenterologist, a colonoscopist, an oncology nurse with a special interest in colorectal cancer, an oncologist and a palliative care specialist. Such teams for other cancers are expected to have similar members, with the relevant specialities. Scotland has wider criteria for multi-disciplinary care, but the minimum membership of a colorectal team is: surgeon, oncologist, pathologist and specialist nurse as a core for regular meetings with a radiologist and a colonoscopist who can be co-opted at any time.
- Whether your hospital can provide you with links to patient support groups.

Cancer

If the hospital has not provided information, a dash appears instead of yes or no.

	service	referal in 2 weeks	multi-disciplinary team	patient support
Eastern				
Addenbrooke's Hospital	Yes	98%	Yes	Yes
Basildon Hospital	Yes	100%	Yes	-
Bedford Hospital	Yes	100%	Yes	-
Broomfield Hospital	Yes	100%	Yes	Yes
Colchester General Hospital	Yes	94%	Yes	Yes
Hemel Hempstead General Hospital	Yes	88%	-	Yes
Hinchingbrooke Hospital	Yes	100%	Yes	Yes
Ipswich Hospital	Yes	32%	Yes	Yes
James Paget Hospital	Yes	99%	Yes	Yes
Lister Hospital	Yes	58%	Yes	Yes
Luton & Dunstable Hospital	Yes	100%	Yes	Yes
Mount Vernon Hospital	Yes	88%	-	Yes
Norfolk & Norwich University Hospital	Yes	98%	Yes	Yes
Orsett Hospital	-	100%	-	-
Peterborough District Hospital	Yes	100%	-	Yes

Cancer

	service	referal in 2 weeks	multi-disciplinary team	patient support
Princess Alexandra Hospital	Yes	72%	Yes	Yes
Queen Elizabeth Hospital	Yes	89%	Yes	Yes
Queen Elizabeth II Hospital	Yes	58%	Yes	Yes
Southend Hospital	Yes	96%	Yes	Yes
St Albans City Hospital	Yes	88%	-	Yes
St John's Hospital	-	100%	-	-
Stamford & Rutland Hospital	Yes	-	No	-
Watford General Hospital	Yes	88%	-	Yes
West Suffolk Hospital	Yes	72%	Yes	Yes

London

	service	referal in 2 weeks	multi-disciplinary team	patient support
Barking Hospital	-	91%	-	-
Barnet Hospital	-	98%	-	-
Bromley Hospital	-	100%	-	-
Central Middlesex Hospital	Yes	96%	Yes	Yes
Charing Cross Hospital	Yes	100%	Yes	Yes
Chase Farm Hospital	-	98%	-	-
Chelsea and Westminster Hospital	Yes	100%	Yes	Yes
Ealing Hospital	Yes	100%	Yes	Yes
Epsom General Hospital	Yes	97%	Yes	Yes
Farnborough Hospital	Yes	100%	Yes	Yes
Guy's Hospital	Yes	88%	Yes	Yes
Hammersmith Hospital	Yes	100%	Yes	Yes
Harold Wood Hospital	Yes	91%	Yes	Yes
Hillingdon Hospital	Yes	77%	-	No
Homerton Hospital	Yes	92%	Yes	Yes
King George Hospital	Yes	91%	Yes	Yes
King's College Hospital	Yes	100%	Yes	Yes
Kingston Hospital	Yes	100%	Yes	Yes
Mayday Hospital	Yes	98%	Yes	Yes
Middlesex & University College Hospitals	Yes	-	Yes	Yes
Newham General Hospital	Yes	95%	Yes	Yes
North Middlesex University Hospital	Yes	100%	Yes	Yes
Northwick Park Hospital	Yes	96%	Yes	Yes
Oldchurch Hospital	Yes	91%	Yes	Yes
Orpington Hospital	No	100%	-	No
Queen Elizabeth Hospital	Yes	-	Yes	Yes
Queen Mary's Hospital (Hampstead)	Yes	93%	Yes	Yes
Queen Mary's Hospital (Sidcup)	Yes	100%	Yes	Yes

Cancer

	service	referal in 2 weeks	multi-disciplinary team	patient support
Royal Free Hospital	Yes	93%	Yes	Yes
Royal London Hospital	Yes	100%	Yes	Yes
St Andrew's Hospital	-	95%	-	-
St Bartholomew's Hospital	Yes	100%	Yes	Yes
St George's Hospital (London)	Yes	100%	Yes	Yes
St Helier Hospital	Yes	97%	Yes	Yes
St Mary's Hospital	Yes	100%	Yes	Yes
St Thomas' Hospital	-	88%	-	-
University Hospital Lewisham	Yes	100%	Yes	Yes
West Middlesex University Hospital	Yes	100%	Yes	Yes
Whipps Cross University Hospital	Yes	100%	Yes	Yes
Whittington Hospital	Yes	92%	Yes	Yes

North West

	service	referal in 2 weeks	multi-disciplinary team	patient support
Blackburn Royal Infirmary	Yes	100%	Yes	No
Blackpool Victoria Hospital	Yes	100%	Yes	Yes
Broadgreen Hospital	-	89%	-	-
Burnley General Hospital	Yes	100%	Yes	No
Bury General Hospital	-	100%	-	-
Chorley & South Ribble District General Hospital	Yes	100%	Yes	Yes
Countess of Chester Hospital	Yes	87%	Yes	No
Fairfield General Hospital	Yes	100%	Yes	No
Furness General Hospital	Yes	96%	Yes	Yes
Halton General Hospital	Yes	90%	Yes	Yes
Hope Hospital	Yes	80%	Yes	Yes
Leigh Infirmary	-	83%	-	-
Leighton Hospital	Yes	69%	Yes	Yes
Macclesfield District General Hospital	Yes	88%	Yes	Yes
Manchester Royal Infirmary	Yes	81%	Yes	Yes
North Manchester General Hospital	Yes	82%	Yes	Yes
Ormskirk and District General Hospital	Yes	97%	Yes	Yes
Queens Park Hospital	Yes	100%	Yes	No
Rochdale Infirmary	Yes	100%	Yes	Yes
Rossendale General Hospital	Yes	100%	Yes	No
Royal Albert Edward Infirmary	Yes	83%	Yes	Yes
Royal Bolton Hospital	Yes	98%	Yes	Yes
Royal Lancaster Infirmary	Yes	96%	Yes	Yes
Royal Liverpool University Hospital	Yes	89%	Yes	Yes
Royal Oldham Hospital	Yes	97%	Yes	Yes

Cancer

	service	referal in 2 weeks	multi-disciplinary team	patient support
Royal Preston Hospital	Yes	100%	Yes	Yes
Southport & Formby District General Hospital	Yes	97%	Yes	Yes
St Helens Hospital (Merseyside)	Yes	75%	Yes	No
Stepping Hill Hospital	Yes	100%	Yes	Yes
Tameside General Hospital	Yes	100%	Yes	No
Trafford General Hospital	Yes	86%	Yes	Yes
University Hospital Aintree	Yes	99%	Yes	Yes
Warrington Hospital	Yes	90%	Yes	Yes
Westmorland General Hospital	Yes	96%	Yes	Yes
Whiston Hospital	Yes	75%	Yes	No
Wirral Hospital (Arrowe Park & Clatterbridge)	Yes	100%	Yes	Yes
Withington Hospital	No	89%	-	-
Wythenshawe Hospital	Yes	89%	Yes	Yes
Northern and Yorks				
Airedale General Hospital	Yes	100%	Yes	Yes
Bishop Auckland General Hospital	Yes	99%	Yes	Yes
Bradford Royal Infirmary	Yes	98%	Yes	Yes
Bridlington & District Hospital	-	-	-	-
Calderdale Royal Hospital	Yes	93%	Yes	Yes
Castle Hill Hospital	Yes	100%	Yes	Yes
Chapel Allerton Hospital	No	89%	-	-
Cumberland Infirmary	Yes	80%	Yes	Yes
Darlington Memorial Hospital	Yes	99%	Yes	Yes
Dewsbury and District Hospital	Yes	96%	Yes	Yes
Newcastle Hospitals*	Yes	100%	Yes	Yes
Friarage Hospital	Yes	100%	Yes	Yes
Harrogate District Hospital	Yes	97%	Yes	Yes
Hexham General Hospital	Yes	97%	No	Yes
Huddersfield Royal Infirmary	-	93%	-	-
Hull Royal Infirmary	Yes	100%	Yes	Yes
James Cook University Hospital	Yes	91%	Yes	Yes
Leeds General Infirmary	Yes	89%	Yes	-
Middlesbrough General Hospital	No	91%	-	No
North Tyneside General Hospital	Yes	97%	Yes	Yes
Pinderfields General Hospital	Yes	93%	Yes	Yes
Pontefract General Infirmary	Yes	93%	Yes	Yes
Princess Royal Hospital	Yes	100%	Yes	Yes

* Newcastle Hospitals comprises: Freeman Hospital, Royal Victoria Infirmary and Newcastle General Hospital.

Cancer

	service	referal in 2 weeks	multi-disciplinary team	patient support
Queen Elizabeth Hospital	Yes	72%	Yes	Yes
Royal Victoria Infirmary	-	100%	-	-
Ryhope Hospital	-	22%	-	-
Scarborough General Hospital	-	-	-	-
Seacroft Hospital	No	89%	-	-
South Tyneside District Hospital	Yes	96%	Yes	No
St James's University Hospital	-	89%	-	-
St Luke's Hospital (Huddersfield)	-	93%	-	-
St Luke's Hospital (Bradford)	Yes	98%	Yes	Yes
Sunderland Royal Hospital	Yes	22%	No	Yes
University Hospital of Hartlepool	Yes	91%	Yes	Yes
University Hospital of North Durham	Yes	100%	Yes	Yes
University Hospital of North Tees	Yes	91%	Yes	Yes
Wansbeck General Hospital	Yes	97%	Yes	Yes
West Cumberland Hospital	Yes	80%	Yes	Yes
Wharfdale General Hospital	No	89%	-	-
Whitby Hospital	-	-	-	-
York District Hospital	Yes	82%	Yes	Yes

South East

	service	referal in 2 weeks	multi-disciplinary team	patient support
Amersham Hospital	No	94%	-	-
Ashford Hospital	Yes	82%	Yes	No
Buckland Hospital	-	74%	-	-
Churchill Hospital	Yes	98%	Yes	Yes
Conquest Hospital	Yes	83%	Yes	Yes
Crawley Hospital	Yes	100%	Yes	No
Darent Valley Hospital	Yes	63%	Yes	Yes
East Surrey and Crawley Hospitals	Yes	100%	Yes	No
Eastbourne District General Hospital	Yes	100%	Yes	Yes
Frimley Park Hospital	Yes	100%	No	Yes
Heatherwood Hospital	Yes	98%	Yes	Yes
Horton Hospital	Yes	98%	Yes	Yes
John Radcliffe Hospital	Yes	98%	Yes	Yes
Kent & Canterbury Hospital	Yes	74%	Yes	Yes
Kent and Sussex Hospital	Yes	100%	Yes	Yes
Kettering General Hospital	Yes	100%	Yes	Yes
Maidstone Hospital	Yes	100%	Yes	Yes
Medway Maritime Hospital	Yes	100%	Yes	Yes
Milton Keynes General NHS Hospital	Yes	72%	Yes	Yes

Cancer

	service	referal in 2 weeks	multi-disciplinary team	patient support
North Hampshire Hospital	Yes	100%	Yes	No
Northampton General Hospital	Yes	61%	Yes	Yes
Pembury Hospital	-	100%	-	-
Princess Royal Hospital	Yes	50%	Yes	Yes
Queen Alexandra Hospital	Yes	82%	No	Yes
Queen Elizabeth The Queen Mother Hospital	Yes	74%	Yes	Yes
Queen Victoria Hospital	No	-	-	-
Radcliffe Infirmary	No	98%	-	No
Royal Berkshire & Battle Hospitals	Yes	75%	Yes	Yes
Royal Hampshire County Hospital	Yes	93%	Yes	No
Royal South Hants Hospital	-	97%	-	-
Royal Surrey County Hospital	Yes	100%	Yes	No
Royal Sussex County Hospital	Yes	91%	Yes	Yes
Southampton General Hospital	-	97%	-	-
Southlands Hospital	-	7%	-	-
St Mary's Hospital (Newport)	Yes	100%	Yes	Yes
St Mary's Hospital (Portsmouth)	Yes	82%	No	Yes
St Peter's Hospital	Yes	82%	Yes	No
St Richard's Hospital	Yes	100%	Yes	No
Stoke Mandeville Hospital	Yes	90%	Yes	Yes
Wexham Park Hospital	Yes	98%	Yes	Yes
William Harvey Hospital	Yes	74%	Yes	Yes
Worthing Hospital	Yes	7%	Yes	Yes
Wycombe Hospital	-	94%	-	-

South West

	service	referal in 2 weeks	multi-disciplinary team	patient support
Bristol General Hospital	-	61%	-	-
Bristol Royal Infirmary	Yes	61%	Yes	Yes
Cheltenham General Hospital	Yes	99%	Yes	-
Cirencester Hospital	-	99%	-	-
Derriford Hospital	Yes	100%	Yes	Yes
Dorset County Hospital	Yes	90%	No	Yes
Frenchay Hospital	Yes	92%	Yes	Yes
Gloucestershire Royal Hospital	Yes	100%	Yes	Yes
North Devon District Hospital	Yes	100%	Yes	Yes
Poole Hospital	Yes	97%	Yes	Yes
Princess Margaret Hospital	-	100%	-	-
Royal Bournemouth Hospital	Yes	86%	Yes	Yes
Royal Cornwall Hospital	Yes	76%	Yes	No

Cancer

	service	referal in 2 weeks	multi-disciplinary team	patient support
Royal Devon & Exeter Hospital	Yes	100%	Yes	No
Royal United Hospital	Yes	100%	Yes	Yes
Salisbury District Hospital	Yes	60%	Yes	Yes
Southmead Hospital	Yes	92%	Yes	Yes
St Michael's Hospital	-	61%	-	-
Standish Hospital	-	100%	-	-
Stroud General Hospital	-	-	-	-
Taunton & Somerset Hospital	Yes	95%	Yes	Yes
Torbay District General Hospital	Yes	100%	Yes	Yes
West Cornwall Hospital	Yes	76%	No	No
Weston General Hospital	Yes	100%	Yes	Yes
Yeovil District Hospital	Yes	91%	Yes	Yes

Trent

	service	referal in 2 weeks	multi-disciplinary team	patient support
Barnsley District General Hospital	Yes	100%	Yes	Yes
Bassetlaw District General Hospital	Yes	96%	Yes	Yes
Chesterfield & North Derbyshire Royal Hospital	Yes	98%	Yes	Yes
Derby City General Hospital	Yes	95%	Yes	Yes
Derbyshire Royal Infirmary	Yes	95%	Yes	Yes
Diana, Princess of Wales Hospital	Yes	98%	Yes	No
Doncaster Royal Infirmary & Montagu Hospital	Yes	96%	Yes	Yes
Glenfield Hospital	Yes	91%	Yes	No
Grantham & District Hospital	Yes	100%	No	Yes
King's Mill Hospital	Yes	100%	-	Yes
Leicester General Hospital	Yes	91%	Yes	No
Leicester Royal Infirmary	Yes	91%	Yes	No
Lincoln County Hospital	Yes	100%	Yes	Yes
Louth County Hospital	-	100%	-	-
Northern General Hospital	Yes	-	Yes	Yes
Nottingham City Hospital	No	93%	-	No
Pilgrim Hospital	Yes	100%	Yes	Yes
Queen's Medical Centre	Yes	28%	Yes	Yes
Rotherham District General Hospital	-	99%	-	-
Royal Hallamshire Hospital	Yes	-	Yes	Yes
Scunthorpe General Hospital	Yes	98%	Yes	No
Skegness & District Hospital	-	100%	-	-

Cancer

	service	referal in 2 weeks	multi-disciplinary team	patient support
West Midlands				
Alexandra Hospital	Yes	84%	Yes	Yes
Birmingham Heartlands Hospital	Yes	53%	Yes	Yes
City Hospital	Yes	100%	Yes	Yes
County Hospital (Hereford)	Yes	86%	Yes	Yes
Coventry and Warwickshire Hospital	Yes	55%	Yes	Yes
Dudley Group of Hospitals*	Yes	100%	Yes	Yes
General Hospital (Hereford)	-	86%	-	-
George Eliot Hospital	Yes	98%	Yes	Yes
Good Hope District General Hospital	Yes	90%	Yes	Yes
Hospital of St Cross	Yes	55%	Yes	Yes
Kidderminster Hospital	No	84%	-	No
Manor Hospital (Walsall)	Yes	96%	Yes	Yes
New Cross Hospital	Yes	100%	Yes	Yes
North Staffordshire Hospital	Yes	96%	Yes	Yes
North Staffordshire Royal Infirmary	-	96%	-	-
Princess Royal Hospital	Yes	97%	Yes	Yes
Queen Elizabeth Hospital (Birmingham)	Yes	85%	Yes	Yes
Queen's Hospital (Burton)	Yes	91%	Yes	Yes
Royal Shrewsbury Hospital	Yes	82%	Yes	Yes
Sandwell General Hospital	Yes	100%	Yes	Yes
Selly Oak Hospital	Yes	85%	Yes	Yes
Solihull Hospital	Yes	53%	Yes	Yes
Staffordshire General Hospital	Yes	91%	Yes	No
Walsgrave Hospital	Yes	55%	Yes	Yes
Warwick Hospital	Yes	46%	Yes	Yes
Worcester Royal Infirmary	Yes	84%	Yes	Yes

* Dudley Group of Hospitals comprises: Russells Hall, Wordsley, Corbett and Guest Hospitals.

Cancer

	service	multi-disciplinary team	patient support
N.Ireland			
Altnagelvin Area Hospital	Yes	No	No
Antrim Hospital	Yes	-	No
Belfast City Hospital	Yes	Yes	No
Causeway Hospital	Yes	Yes	-
Craigavon Area Hospital	Yes	-	-
Daisy Hill Hospital	Yes	Yes	es
Downe Hospital	-	-	-
Erne Hospital	-	-	-
Lagan Valley Hospital	-	-	-
Mater Hospital	Yes	Yes	No
Mid-Ulster Hospital	No	-	Yes
The Royal Hospitals	Yes	Yes	Yes
Tyrone County Hospital	-	-	-
Ulster Hospital	Yes	Yes	Yes
Whiteabbey Hospital	Yes	Yes	No
Scotland			
Aberdeen Royal Infirmary	-	-	-
Ayr Hospital	-	-	-
Balfour Hospital	Yes	No	No
Borders General Hospital	Yes	No	No
Crosshouse Hospital	-	-	-
Dr Gray's Hospital	Yes	Yes	Yes
Dumfries and Galloway Royal Infirmary	Yes	Yes	Yes
Falkirk Royal Infirmary	Yes	No	Yes
Gartnavel General Hospital	-	-	-
Gilbert Bain Hospital	-	-	-
Glasgow Royal Infirmary	-	-	-
Hairmyres Hospital	-	-	-
Inverclyde Royal Hospital	Yes	Yes	Yes
Lorn and Islands District General Hospital	Yes	No	No
Monklands Hospital	-	-	-
Ninewells Hospital	Yes	Yes	Yes
Perth Royal Infirmary	Yes	Yes	Yes
Queen Margaret Hospital	-	-	-
Raigmore Hospital	Yes	Yes	Yes
Royal Alexandra Hospital	Yes	Yes	-
Royal Infirmary of Edinburgh	-	-	-

Cancer

	service	multi-disciplinary team	patient support
Southern General Hospital	-	-	-
St John's Hospital at Howden	Yes	Yes	-
Stirling Royal Infirmary	Yes	No	Yes
Stobhill Hospital	-	-	-
Stracathro Hospital	No	-	Yes
Vale of Leven District General Hospital	Yes	No	Yes
Victoria Hospital	-	-	-
Victoria Infirmary	-	-	-
Western General Hospital	-	-	-
Western Infirmary	-	-	-
Western Isles Hospital	-	-	-
Woodend Hospital	-	-	-

Wishaw Hospital is not included in this table. This hospital opened in 2001 and consequently no data has been collated for it as yet.

Wales

	service	multi-disciplinary team	patient support
Bronglais General Hospital	Yes	Yes	Yes
Caerphilly District Miners' Hospital	No	-	No
Glan Clwyd District General Hospital	Yes	Yes	Yes
Llandough Hospital	Yes	Yes	Yes
Llandudno General Hospital	Yes	Yes	Yes
Morriston Hospital	Yes	Yes	-
Neath General Hospital	Yes	-	Yes
Nevill Hall Hospital	-	-	-
Prince Charles Hospital	Yes	Yes	Yes
Prince Philip Hospital	Yes	Yes	Yes
Princess of Wales Hospital	Yes	Yes	Yes
Royal Glamorgan Hospital	Yes	Yes	Yes
Royal Gwent Hospital	Yes	Yes	Yes
Singleton Hospital	Yes	Yes	Yes
University Hospital of Wales	Yes	Yes	Yes
West Wales General Hospital	Yes	Yes	Yes
Withybush General Hospital	Yes	Yes	Yes
Wrexham Maelor Hospital	-	-	-
Ysbyty Gwynedd	Yes	Yes	Yes

Specialist Cancer Hospitals

	service	referal in 2 weeks	multi-disciplinary team
London			
Royal Marsden Hospital	Yes	100%	Yes
North West			
Christie Hospital	Yes	100%	Yes
Northern and Yorks			
Northern Centre for Cancer Treatment	Yes	100%	Yes
South West			
Bristol Haemotology and Oncology Centre	Yes	100%	yes
Wales			
Velindre Hospital	Yes	-	Yes

Children

Children

One in four children has had an overnight hospital stay by the age of five and almost all children will end up in hospital at some time or another. Whenever a child is admitted to hospital it can be a difficult time for both the child and the parents. Being an adult and able to understand why you are being hospitalised and to ask questions about what is going on is one thing. Trying to explain the same thing to a child who does not have the same understanding or is unable to articulate the questions to which they want answers is another.

Children need their parents and feel more secure with you around and when they are admitted it is important to try to stay with them at all times. For this reason you may choose the hospital nearest to your home rather than one further away, but check with your GP what services your hospital provides and where your child will be best looked after. It is very important that the hospital let you stay with your child at all times. You should also take into account whether the hospital has a paediatrician available around the clock. It is also essential that your child be treated by the same individuals within the team, so you should ask your GP to refer you to a hospital where this will be the case. Will your child be allocated a 'named nurse' who will be the prime point of contact throughout your child's stay? As play is an important part of your child's recovery, you might want to check whether your hospital has a play room and staff that will be on hand to play with and supervise your child. If your child is a teenager, they may feel uncomfortable on either a children's or adult ward: does your hospital have a separate adolescent ward?

What are my child's rights within the NHS?
The entitlements of children under the Patient's Charter are set out in a Government document issued in 1996. The document is called Services for Children and Young People, and states they have a

right to be registered with a doctor and given information about their health care. If they are not, they too have a right to complain. They can also expect to see a health visitor and school nurse, who know their names, be consulted about their treatment and have their views respected. Their questions should be answered in a way that they can understand. In hospital they can expect:

- To be safe.
- To be in hospital only when necessary.
- To be on a ward for children and young people. Teenagers should be allowed to choose whether they want to be in a children's ward or an adult ward.
- To visit the ward before a planned admission to hospital.
- Staff to be polite and friendly.
- To know the names of staff – staff should wear name badges.
- To have a named nurse.
- To wear their own clothes and have some of their own belongings with them.
- To have their parents with them 24 hours a day if they wish.
- Where possible, to be accompanied to the anaesthetic room by a parent, and for the parent to remain with them until they fall asleep.
- To have a choice of healthy food.
- To have their privacy and dignity respected, and to be able to go somewhere quiet and private.
- To be able to continue their school work.
- To play and make friends with other children.
- Not to be in pain where this can be avoided.

If my child needs hospital treatment, who might they be referred to?

This depends on the nature of the problem. The following consultants may become involved with the care of children:

Case history

Alison Lewis

In June 2001 Alison Lewis, 41-year-old mother of four, was in a park in Exmouth when her 18-month-old son Hugh ran full face into a moving swing. She was horrified when there was so much blood coming from the bottom of his face that she couldn't actually see where it was coming from. 'I grabbed the nearest available thing to stop the bleeding which was an unused nappy. Within moments it was totally saturated,' she says. Alison got a passing stranger to call 999 and within 10 minutes an ambulance and a paramedic car arrived. Alison and Hugh travelled to Exmouth hospital by ambulance and her three other children followed in the paramedic car.

At the hospital, Hugh was examined by a nurse who then called out a doctor to see him. When the doctor arrived at A&E she examined Hugh and said that the wound needed specialist attention. As this could not be provided there, she referred them immediately to the A&E department of the Royal Devon and Exeter Hospital. Alison drove Hugh, together with her three other small children, to the hospital herself.

When she got there, there was a queue of 20 patients waiting to be assessed by the triage nurse. As Alison already had a letter from the doctor at Exmouth Hospital to give directly to the consultant, she assumed that she should simply bypass the queue and go to the A&E reception to register her son. However, at reception she was told that she should join the end of the triage queue.

Alison pointed out that he didn't need to see a nurse as he had been referred by a doctor at another hospital. Alison made the point that it was now almost 3 hours since the accident and that Hugh, traumatised, was still bleeding and shaking with shock.

However, A&E staff were adamant that hospital policy had to be observed and that Alison and Hugh should rejoin the queue. 'I was furious – it seemed ludicrous to have to go through the process twice, and it was very clear to me that Hugh needed urgent attention.'

Together with Hugh and her three children, Alison refused to move from the reception desk. Eventually she was approached by the A&E Sister who told her that due to pressure of numbers she would make an exception in this case. 'She was obviously too busy to argue and called the consultant,' says Alison. Three minutes later, Hugh was examined by a registrar who decided that Hugh needed surgery. He was quickly admitted to the children's ward and given a range of tests to get him ready for theatre. Three hours later Hugh was given eight stitches inside his mouth under general anaesthetic. He was discharged the following day.

Alison's advice to anyone in a similar situation is to be insistent that you or the person you are with needs urgent attention. 'I've heard several stories of people being turned away from A&E who were very ill. They obviously didn't feel able to stand up for their right to be seen and taken seriously,' she says.

A paediatrician, a doctor specialising in child health who will diagnose your child's problem and then involve other consultants in their care. For instance, if your child has appendicitis, they will be placed under the care of a general surgeon, if they have glue ear they will be looked after by an ear, nose and throat specialist, and if they have a broken limb, they will be under the care of an orthopaedic consultant. As with other specialties, the most senior paediatrician is a consultant, and their team will include junior doctors who are training to become paediatricians, child psychiatrists or GPs. Paediatricians look after children who are inpatients and see children as outpatients, sometimes in centres outside the hospital. Some paediatricians specialise in one aspect of child health, such as diabetes or bowel disease.

A surgeon, either a consultant paediatric surgeon or a general surgeon who also operates on children.

An A&E doctor, if you take your child directly to A&E.

A community paediatrician, who works on an outpatient basis in community clinics and child development centres. They work closely with other agencies such as health visitors and social services, and may have particular expertise in child protection matters.

A child psychiatrist, who manages mental health problems in children.

If my child needs an operation, who will do it?

Some operations on children are carried out by surgeons who also operate on adults, although these surgeons will have additional expertise in operating on children. Other procedures, such as heart surgery and transplant surgery, are done in specialist centres by surgeons with expertise in treating children. Your GP will know which surgeons in your area operate on children. Your child will be anaesthetised for the operation by an anaesthetist who has a special interest in children's anaesthesia.

Can I choose which surgeon my child is referred to?

If there is more than one surgeon in your area doing the type of operation your child needs, your preference should be taken into consideration.

What will happen if my GP refers my child to hospital as an emergency?

You child will be seen initially by a nurse, who will ask for some information and check their pulse and temperature, then by one of the junior members of the paediatric team on call – usually the senior house officer (SHO). In some units, all children are taken straight to the children's ward for assessment, while in others they will be seen initially in A&E.

An SHO will take a detailed history of your child's problem and ask you about their past medical history. It is always a good idea therefore to have any important information to hand, such as medication they are taking or any family history that may be relevant. The SHO will then examine your child and may take swabs and blood tests or arrange X-rays. They will also put up a drip if one is needed. Your child will then be given a bed and settled in by the nursing staff.

The commonest problems requiring admission in children are infectious diseases such as bronchiolitis and gastroenteritis, and in most cases the nurses and the SHO have the expertise to provide the necessary care. In less straightforward cases, a more senior paediatrician will be called to see your child urgently, no matter what time of day or night it is.

What will happen if I take my child to A&E?

Your child will be seen soon after arrival by the triage nurse, who will assess how urgently they need to see a doctor. Some A&E departments have special waiting areas, cheerfully decorated and full of toys, for children. In this section, we tell you which hospitals have separate children's waiting areas. They will then be seen by one of the A&E doctors, who will do one of the following:

- Treat the problem. The senior house officers in A&E can deal with most minor injuries and illnesses in children.
- Refer your child to a senior A&E doctor – for example, if they have a badly broken bone or a large wound that needs suturing.
- Refer your child to a paediatrician, a surgeon, or an appropriate specialist.
- Offer you advice on how to manage the problem, and advise you to take your child to the GP if you need further help.

Do children get priority in the A&E department?

Not necessarily. Priority is allocated according to medical need, not age. As with adults, it is recommended that the longest you should wait in A&E is 4 hours before being admitted to a ward or discharged.

Do all hospitals have a paediatrician on site? Why is this important?

A&E departments need to be ready to receive children who need urgent medical attention, and any hospital that has children as patients has to be prepared to deal with paediatric emergencies. Having a paediatrician on site is extremely helpful in these circumstances, as the management of medical emergencies in children is a specialised area. The Royal College of Surgeons advises that all hospitals that operate on children as inpatients or that treat children in A&E should have a paediatrician present in the hospital 24 hours a day. However, not all hospitals have this, and in this section, we tell you which ones that do.

Do all hospitals have intensive care facilities for children?

No. Specialised children's intensive care units are only found in some of the larger hospitals. In hospitals without these facilities, the child will either be managed in the adult intensive care unit or transferred by ambulance or by air to another hospital with appropriate facilities. Children's intensive care units are staffed by highly trained nurses, paediatricians and anaesthetists. Children there can be continually monitored, given treatment that needs to be carefully controlled, and have their breathing assisted by artificial ventilation. At the back of this Guide, we tell you whether your local hospital has intensive care facilities for children.

How should I tell my child about going into hospital?
If your child is going to be admitted to hospital, ask the outpatient staff for an information leaflet to help you tell your child what to expect. Alternatively, there are several good storybooks that can be used to prepare children for a visit to hospital – your library may have copies of these. These explain, in a simple factual way, what will happen. Children can be very scared but are often very brave and very resilient. Seeing your child in pain or distress is very hard but being there to reassure them is crucial. They will often take their lead from you so try not to become upset or worried yourself. You can also help them by discovering as much as possible about what is going to happen to them. You can try to explain it to them in simple terms if they are old enough to talk and when things are under way continue to explain and inform them as their treatment proceeds. However, it is important not to tell them that 'it won't hurt' if it will. Be honest – tell them that they will have a sore throat after having their tonsils out, but also tell them that they will be given medicine to make the pain better. If you are going to have to leave them at any time during their stay in hospital, tell them in advance, let them know the reason, and assure them that one of the nurses will be personally responsible for looking after them in your absence.

Can I stay in hospital with my child?

A hospital stay can be very distressing for a child and ward staff will encourage you to stay with your child and help to look after them while they are there. You are unlikely to find the accommodation luxurious, though. In most acute children's wards, parents are given a mattress or a sofa-bed at the child's bedside.

Focus on children – surgery

Not all hospitals operate on children, and of those that do, not all of them operate on children under general anaesthetic. Trusts that perform a high level of operations are likely to be more experienced at certain procedures and therefore you may prefer to make sure that your child is treated there. For this reason your child might be referred to one of the bigger regional hospitals such as Southampton or Bristol, rather than a smaller local hospital.

The Royal College of Surgeons recommends that hospitals performing such operations have a paediatrician on site round the clock, should complications occur. Equally it is good practice that there be two registered children's nurses per ward round the clock. The Royal College of Surgeons also recommends that major or complex surgery on children should be performed in hospitals that have paediatric intensive care departments. The hospital entries at the back of this Guide tell you which have these facilities.

Children's Surgery

If the hospital has not provided us with information, a dash appears instead of a Yes or No.

	pediatrician on site 24hrs	2 children's nurses per ward 24hrs
Eastern		
Addenbrooke's Hospital	Yes	Yes
Basildon Hospital	Yes	Yes
Bedford Hospital	Yes	Yes
Broomfield Hospital	No	Yes
Colchester General Hospital	Yes	Yes
Hemel Hempstead General Hospital	No	-
Hinchingbrooke Hospital	Yes	Yes
Ipswich Hospital	Yes	Yes
James Paget Hospital	Yes	Yes
Lister Hospital	Yes	Yes
Luton & Dunstable Hospital	Yes	Yes
Norfolk & Norwich University Hospital	Yes	Yes
Peterborough District Hospital	Yes	Yes
Princess Alexandra Hospital	Yes	Yes
Queen Elizabeth Hospital	Yes	Yes
Queen Elizabeth II Hospital	Yes	Yes
Southend Hospital	Yes	Yes
St John's Hospital	Yes	Yes
Watford General Hospital	Yes	-
West Suffolk Hospital	Yes	Yes
London		
Barnet Hospital	Yes	-
Bromley Hospital	No	Yes
Central Middlesex Hospital	Yes	Yes
Chase Farm Hospital	Yes	-
Chelsea and Westminster Hospital	Yes	Yes
Ealing Hospital	Yes	Yes
Epsom General Hospital	Yes	Yes
Farnborough Hospital	Yes	Yes
Guy's Hospital	Yes	Yes
Harold Wood Hospital	Yes	Yes
Hillingdon Hospital	Yes	Yes
Homerton Hospital	Yes	Yes
King George Hospital	Yes	Yes
King's College Hospital	Yes	Yes
Kingston Hospital	Yes	Yes

Children's Surgery

	pediatrician on site 24hrs	2 children's nurses per ward 24hrs
Mayday Hospital	Yes	Yes
Middlesex & University College Hospitals	Yes	Yes
Newham General Hospital	Yes	Yes
North Middlesex University Hospital	Yes	Yes
Northwick Park Hospital	Yes	Yes
Oldchurch Hospital	Yes	Yes
Queen Elizabeth Hospital	Yes	Yes
Queen Mary's Hospital (Sidcup)	No	Yes
Royal Free Hospital	Yes	Yes
Royal London Hospital	Yes	Yes
St Bartholomew's Hospital	Yes	Yes
St George's Hospital (London)	Yes	Yes
St Helier Hospital	Yes	Yes
St Mary's Hospital	Yes	Yes
St Thomas' Hospital	Yes	Yes
University Hospital Lewisham	Yes	Yes
West Middlesex University Hospital	Yes	Yes
Whipps Cross University Hospital	Yes	Yes
Whittington Hospital	Yes	Yes

South East

Ashford Hospital	No	-
Buckland Hospital	No	-
Conquest Hospital	Yes	Yes
Crawley Hospital	Yes	Yes
Darent Valley Hospital	Yes	Yes
East Surrey and Crawley Hospitals	No	Yes
Eastbourne District General Hospital	Yes	Yes
Frimley Park Hospital	Yes	Yes
Heatherwood Hospital	No	Yes
Horton Hospital	Yes	Yes
John Radcliffe Hospital	Yes	Yes
Kent & Canterbury Hospital	Yes	Yes
Kent and Sussex Hospital	Yes	Yes
Kettering General Hospital	Yes	Yes
Maidstone Hospital	Yes	Yes
Medway Maritime Hospital	Yes	Yes
Milton Keynes General NHS Hospital	Yes	Yes
North Hampshire Hospital	Yes	Yes

Children's Surgery

	pediatrician on site 24hrs	2 children's nurses per ward 24hrs
Northampton General Hospital	Yes	Yes
Princess Royal Hospital	No	No
Queen Alexandra Hospital	No	Yes
Queen Elizabeth The Queen Mother Hospital	No	Yes
Queen Victoria Hospital	Yes	Yes
Royal Berkshire & Battle Hospitals	Yes	Yes
Royal Hampshire County Hospital	Yes	Yes
Royal Surrey County Hospital	Yes	Yes
Southampton General Hospital	Yes	-
St Mary's Hospital (Portsmouth)	Yes	Yes
St Mary's Hospital (Newport)	Yes	Yes
St Peter's Hospital	Yes	Yes
St Richard's Hospital	No	Yes
Stoke Mandeville Hospital	Yes	Yes
Wexham Park Hospital	Yes	Yes
William Harvey Hospital	Yes	Yes
Worthing Hospital	Yes	Yes
Wycombe Hospital	Yes	-

South West

Cheltenham General Hospital	Yes	Yes
Derriford Hospital	Yes	Yes
Dorset County Hospital	Yes	No
Frenchay Hospital	Yes	Yes
Gloucestershire Royal Hospital	Yes	
North Devon District Hospital	No	Yes
Poole Hospital	Yes	Yes
Princess Margaret Hospital	No	-
Royal Bournemouth Hospital	No	-
Royal Cornwall Hospital	Yes	Yes
Royal Devon & Exeter Hospital	Yes	Yes
Royal United Hospital	Yes	Yes
Salisbury District Hospital	Yes	Yes
Southmead Hospital	Yes	Yes
Taunton & Somerset Hospital	Yes	Yes
Torbay District General Hospital	Yes	Yes
West Cornwall Hospital	No	-
Weston General Hospital	No	No
Yeovil District Hospital	Yes	Yes

Children's Surgery

	pediatrician on site 24hrs	2 children's nurses per ward 24hrs
North West		
Blackburn Royal Infirmary	No	Yes
Blackpool Victoria Hospital	Yes	Yes
Burnley General Hospital	Yes	Yes
Chorley & South Ribble District General Hospital	Yes	No
Countess of Chester Hospital	Yes	Yes
Fairfield General Hospital	Yes	Yes
Furness General Hospital	Yes	Yes
Halton General Hospital	No	-
Leighton Hospital	Yes	Yes
Macclesfield District General Hospital	No	Yes
Ormskirk and District General Hospital	Yes	Yes
Rochdale Infirmary	Yes	Yes
Royal Albert Edward Infirmary	Yes	-
Royal Bolton Hospital	Yes	Yes
Royal Lancaster Infirmary	Yes	Yes
Royal Oldham Hospital	Yes	-
Royal Preston Hospital	Yes	Yes
Southport & Formby District General Hospital	Yes	Yes
Stepping Hill Hospital	Yes	Yes
Tameside General Hospital	Yes	No
Trafford General Hospital	Yes	Yes
University Hospital Aintree	No	-
Warrington Hospital	Yes	Yes
Whiston Hospital	Yes	Yes
Wirral Hospital (Arrowe Park & Clatterbridge)	Yes	Yes
Wythenshawe Hospital	Yes	Yes
Northern and Yorks		
Airedale General Hospital	Yes	Yes
Bishop Auckland General Hospital	No	Yes
Bradford Royal Infirmary	Yes	Yes
Calderdale Royal Hospital	Yes	Yes
Cumberland Infirmary	No	Yes
Darlington Memorial Hospital	No	Yes
Dewsbury and District Hospital	Yes	Yes
Newcastle Hospitals*	Yes	Yes

* Newcastle Hospitals comprises: Freeman Hospital, Royal Victoria Infirmary and Newcastle General Hospital.

Children's Surgery

	pediatrician on site 24hrs	2 children's nurses per ward 24hrs
Friarage Hospital	Yes	Yes
Harrogate District Hospital	No	No
Hexham General Hospital	No	-
Huddersfield Royal Infirmary	Yes	-
Hull Royal Infirmary	Yes	Yes
James Cook University Hospital	Yes	Yes
Leeds General Infirmary	Yes	-
Middlesbrough General Hospital	No	No
North Tyneside General Hospital	No	Yes
Pinderfields General Hospital	Yes	Yes
Pontefract General Infirmary	Yes	Yes
Queen Elizabeth Hospital	Yes	Yes
Royal Victoria Infirmary	No	-
Scarborough General Hospital	No	-
South Tyneside District Hospital	Yes	Yes
St James's University Hospital	Yes	Yes
Sunderland Royal Hospital	Yes	Yes
University Hospital of Hartlepool	Yes	Yes
University Hospital of North Durham	Yes	Yes
University Hospital of North Tees	Yes	Yes
Wansbeck General Hospital	No	-
York District Hospital	Yes	Yes

Trent

Barnsley District General Hospital	Yes	Yes
Bassetlaw District General Hospital	Yes	Yes
Chesterfield & North Derbyshire Royal Hospital	Yes	Yes
Derby City General Hospital (Children's)	Yes	Yes
Diana, Princess of Wales Hospital	No	Yes
Doncaster Royal Infirmary & Montagu Hospital	Yes	Yes
Grantham & District Hospital	No	-
King's Mill Hospital	Yes	Yes
Leicester Royal Infirmary	Yes	Yes
Lincoln County Hospital	Yes	Yes
Northern General Hospital	No	-
Nottingham City Hospital	Yes	Yes
Pilgrim Hospital	No	Yes
Queen's Medical Centre	Yes	Yes
Rotherham District General Hospital	Yes	-

Children's Surgery

	pediatrician on site 24hrs	2 children's nurses per ward 24hrs
Royal Hallamshire Hospital	No	-
Scunthorpe General Hospital	Yes	Yes

West Midlands

Alexandra Hospital	Yes	Yes
Birmingham Heartlands Hospital	Yes	Yes
City Hospital	Yes	Yes
County Hospital (Hereford)	No	Yes
Coventry and Warwickshire Hospital	No	Yes
Dudley Group of Hospitals*	Yes	Yes
George Eliot Hospital	-	Yes
Good Hope District General Hospital	No	Yes
Hospital of St Cross	No	-
Manor Hospital (Walsall)	No	Yes
New Cross Hospital	Yes	Yes
North Staffordshire Hospital	Yes	Yes
Princess Royal Hospital	Yes	Yes
Queen's Hospital (Burton)	Yes	Yes
Royal Shrewsbury Hospital	Yes	No
Sandwell General Hospital	Yes	Yes
Staffordshire General Hospital	Yes	Yes
Walsgrave Hospital	Yes	Yes
Warwick Hospital	Yes	Yes
Worcester Royal Infirmary	Yes	Yes

Wales

Glan Clwyd District General Hospital	Yes	Yes
Llandough Hospital	Yes	Yes
Morriston Hospital	No	Yes
Neath General Hospital	Yes	Yes
Nevill Hall Hospital	Yes	Yes
Prince Charles Hospital	Yes	Yes
Princess of Wales Hospital	Yes	Yes
Royal Glamorgan Hospital	Yes	Yes
Royal Gwent Hospital	Yes	Yes
Singleton Hospital	Yes	Yes
University Hospital of Wales	Yes	Yes

* Dudley Group of Hospitals comprises: Russells Hall, Wordsley, Corbett and Guest Hospitals.

Children's Surgery

	pediatrician on site 24hrs	2 children's nurses per ward 24hrs
West Wales General Hospital	Yes	Yes
Withybush General Hospital	No	Yes
Wrexham Maelor Hospital	Yes	-
Ysbyty Gwynedd	Yes	Yes

N. Ireland

Altnagelvin Area Hospital	Yes	Yes
Antrim Hospital	Yes	Yes
Belfast City Hospital	Yes	No
Causeway Hospital	No	Yes
Craigavon Area Hospital	Yes	Yes
Daisy Hill Hospital	Yes	Yes
Erne Hospital	Yes	-
Mater Hospital	No	-
Mid-Ulster Hospital	No	-
Ulster Hospital	Yes	Yes

Scotland

Ayr Hospital	Yes	No
Balfour Hospital	Yes	No
Borders General Hospital	Yes	Yes
Crosshouse Hospital	Yes	No
Dr Gray's Hospital	Yes	No
Dumfries and Galloway Royal Infirmary	Yes	Yes
Falkirk Royal Infirmary	Yes	Yes
Inverclyde Royal Hospital	Yes	Yes
Lorn and Islands District General Hospital	Yes	No
Monklands Hospital	Yes	No
Ninewells Hospital	Yes	Yes
Perth Royal Infirmary	Yes	Yes
Queen Margaret Hospital	Yes	No
Raigmore Hospital	Yes	Yes
Royal Alexandra Hospital	Yes	No
St John's Hospital at Howden	Yes	Yes
Stirling Royal Infirmary	Yes	Yes
Stracathro Hospital	Yes	No
Vale of Leven District General Hospital	Yes	Yes
Victoria Hospital	Yes	Yes

Children's Surgery

	pediatrician on site 24hrs	2 children's nurses per ward 24hrs
SPECIALIST CHILDREN'S HOSPITALS		
London		
Great Ormond Street Hospital for Children	Yes	Yes
North West		
Alder Hey Children's Hospital	Yes	Yes
St Mary's Hospital for Women and Children (Manchester)	Yes	Yes
Booth Hall Children's Hospital	Yes	Yes
Royal Manchester Children's Hospital	Yes	Yes
South East		
Royal Alexandra Hospital for Sick Children	Yes	Yes
South West		
Bristol Royal Hospital for Sick Children	Yes	Yes
Trent		
Sheffield Childrens Hospital	Yes	Yes
Derbyshire Children's Hospital	Yes	Yes
West Midlands		
Diana, Princess of Wales Children's Hospital	Yes	Yes
N.Ireland		
Royal Belfast Hospital for Sick Children	Yes	Yes
Scotland		
Royal Aberdeen Children's Hospital	Yes	Yes
Royal Hospital for Sick Children (Edingburgh)	Yes	Yes
Royal Hospital for Sick Children (Glasgow)	Yes	Yes

Older People

Older People

Older People

As well as children, one of the biggest users of the NHS are older people. At any time, around 65 per cent of hospital beds are occupied by people aged over 65. Patient group research carried out for Dr Foster showed a high level of dissatisfaction among older people about the way they are treated. One of those interviewed said: 'When age comes into it, they look at you and think, you've gone past your sell-by date.' As a result, older people believe this means the specific requirements of their illnesses are not met and there is a significant lack of information offered to them about their condition and treatment.

The research carried out among this group provided some disturbing and wide-ranging fears. On the whole, older people feel they are given less consideration than they deserve. One patient said: 'I've paid into the NHS all my life so I'm entitled to something out of it.' At present, pensioners believe that their GP will choose the hospital they go to and do not believe they have access to the information that would enable them to make that choice. Our research also showed older people worry they are 'ghettoised' in age-defined wards, that falls may not be investigated further, that their intake of medication may not be monitored and reviewed and that, because of their age, they may not be resuscitated. However, there is good evidence that treating high blood pressure and stopping smoking confer health benefits in the over 80s. As the proportion of older people in the population grows, the health needs of this group will become increasingly important.

Most people over the age of 65 have at least one chronic health problem – typically heart disease, diabetes, osteoarthritis or smoker's lung. They may have suffered a stroke. Alzheimer's disease and other forms of dementia are also becoming increasingly common. These conditions, more than any others, have an enormous impact on the lives of everyone close to the sufferer.

Being admitted to hospital puts frail older people at risk of disruption to their social networks, disorientation and hospital acquired infections, perhaps leaving them less able to care for themselves than before. It is increasingly important therefore that where possible, older people are treated and cared for in the community rather than as inpatients on a hospital ward. The Government has issued National Service Frameworks specifically aimed to improve intermediate care services which emphasise the promotion of faster recovery from illness, the prevention of unnecessary acute hospital admissions, support of timely discharge and the maximization of independent living.

The aims of the National Service Frameworks for older people include:

- To root out age discrimination and provide NHS services regardless of age.
- The provision of person-centered care and to ensure that NHS and social care services treat older people as individuals.
- The provision of a new range of intermediate care services at home or in designated care settings to promote older people's independence and avoid unnecessary hospital admission.
- The promotion of an active healthy life in old age through a co-ordinated programme of action led by the NHS with support from councils.
- Older people in hospital should be given appropriate specialist care by hospital staff who have the right set of skills to meet their needs.
- Older people thought to have had a stroke should have access to diagnostic services, be treated appropriately by a specialist stroke service, and subsequently, with their carers, participate in a multidisciplinary programme of secondary prevention and rehabilitation.
- Older people who have had a fall should receive effective

Case history

Peter Reid

When Martin Reid's father, Peter, started showing symptoms of Alzheimer's disease, it was very hard to diagnose. Mr Reid first started to realise he might be ill when he found it increasingly hard to concentrate. Reading books or remembering directions became difficult or impossible. Even simple tasks like telling the time or dealing with money required an enormous effort.

His GP sent him to see a neurologist at the local hospital who at first was unsure whether it was a psychological or physical problem. Mr Reid was still in his fifties, which is very young to be suffering from a disease such as Alzheimer's. He was referred on to a psychiatrist who took the view that it might be nothing more than depression. However, as his condition deteriorated over the next two years, it became clear that he was suffering from a degenerative brain disease.

Mr Reid was referred for tests to the National Hospital for Neurology and Neurosurgery in London. 'Because of his age, the doctors were very uncertain of the diagnosis and in the end it was never clear whether he had Alzheimer's or a related condition,' says Martin. But it was clear that he was going to continue to get worse and that there were probably no effective treatments. By now he was unable to recognise people or places easily. He would enjoy watching TV but could no longer understand the storyline of a film.

He took part in a drug trial at St Mary's Hospital in Paddington. 'With drug trials, you are never told whether you are receiving the drug or the placebo, but whatever he was taking, it appeared to make no difference,' says Martin. 'My mother wanted to keep my father at home for as long as possible and continued to look after him long after his doctors and nurses recommended that he go into long-term care.

Alzheimer's patients can sometimes become depressed, angry or even violent from their frustration at becoming increasingly helpless. Fortunately, my father remained relatively cheerful through most of his illness as gradually he lost the power to talk or dress himself. But eventually there came a point where my mother was no longer able to look after him.'

At this point, the health system can be extremely unpredictable. Currently, patients who are no longer regarded as requiring medical care are not entitled to free care from the NHS. Recent changes mean that the cost of nursing such people is paid for by the health service, but that they must pay for their accommodation themselves if they have sufficient resources. Mr Reid could easily have been regarded as such a case. However, he was lucky, as because he was relatively young he continued to be treated as a medical patient and therefore remained under the care of the NHS. He was looked after in a small hospital that housed about 15 people suffering from similar conditions. Martin says, 'he was expected to die within 18 months of being moved into the hospital. In fact he lived on for a further four years, during which time he was cared for extremely well by a wonderful team of nurses.'

treatment and rehabilitation and, with their carers, receive
advice on prevention through a specialised falls service.

- Older people with mental health problems should have access to
integrated mental health services, provided by the NHS and
councils to ensure effective diagnosis, treatment and support, for
them and for their carers.

In this section, we focus on two acute conditions, broken hip and
stroke. In both cases, the kind of care received on admission is crucial
to survival, recovery and getting back home as soon as possible.

Can I get any special check-ups because of my age?

If you are over 75, your GP or practice nurse should offer you a check-
up once a year if you are living at home. Visiting you at home for this
routine check gives the nurse a useful opportunity to assess whether
you might benefit from referral to other services, such as district
nurses, social services, physiotherapy, occupational therapy and
hearing services. You should also be offered immunisation against flu
every year. If you do not receive a letter from your GP offering you an
appointment, you should ring up to arrange one.

Can I be refused hospital treatment because of my age?

Your age has to be taken into consideration when making decisions
about whether it is advisable for you to have an operation or some
types of drug treatment (some procedures and treatment may carry
risks that outweigh the benefits), but you should never be refused
treatment solely because of your age.

Who decides whether I should be resuscitated if I have a cardiac arrest while I'm in hospital?

You do. Any decision as important as this should only be made after
a doctor and a senior nurse have discussed the issue with you. If you
are unconscious all appropriate efforts should be made to resuscitate
you, in consultation with your nearest relative. However, you will

not be resuscitated if you are unresuscitatable after a cardiac arrest and that a futile resuscitation attempt would be disrespectful to the dead. Nor will you be resuscitated if your condition is terminal, and resuscitation is likely to cause distress or damage without any real prolongation of life. In these circumstances, you will be allowed to die – though nothing should be done to hasten your death.

When I leave hospital, I won't be able to look after myself at home for a few weeks. How will help be arranged, and will I have to pay?

If you are being admitted for a planned operation and know when you will be coming home, tell your GP or community nurse in advance – they will be able to refer you to the local social services department, and a social worker will visit or contact you to discuss what help you are likely to need and arrange for it to begin when they are notified that you are home. If you do not have an opportunity to do this – for example, if you are admitted as an emergency – ask the ward manager to arrange for you to see the hospital social worker. They can liaise with the community service to organise your care. This will depend on your needs and you may be offered a period of residential care or visits from a home carer in your own home. Whether, and how much, you have to pay depends on your financial situation. The social worker will be able to give you specific information.

Can I, or my carer, organise social services input without going through my GP?

You can do this independently, but most social services departments are quite fragmented and it is unlikely to be as simple as making one telephone call to a central office. It can be frustrating to be passed from one extension to another, and be told that the only person who can deal with your query is unavailable, when you are in the middle of a crisis.

Case history

Betty Morgan

After Betty Morgan, 76, had an operation for skin cancer, it was up to her daughter, Jennifer Brown, to get her home support. With hindsight, Jennifer, 55, says that she should have done things differently, specifically, that she should have asked more questions.

Mrs Morgan spent a week in a London hospital in October 2001 to have a squamous cell skin cancer removed from her shin. The operation left her feeling weak, in some pain and unsteady on her legs, one of which was bandaged. She was given a walking stick, but found it difficult to use because of a previous stroke which had left one hand semi-paralysed.

'Once I got my mother home, I suddenly realised how incapacitated she was. She couldn't make herself a cup of tea. She couldn't climb the stairs and she has no downstairs toilet in her house. She couldn't even get out of her chair – no one had told me she'd need a special chair,' says Jennifer. She felt her mother hadn't been assessed properly or the extent of her difficulties realised. 'I had assumed that there would be social services support when she came home. I was wrong. We had no problems with the medical side of things – a district nurse visited each day to change my mother's dressing – but it was the care support that let us down.'

Social services said that they could arrange nothing without notification from the hospital that Mrs Morgan had been discharged and needed help. When Mrs Morgan's GP called social services, she was told that if Mrs Morgan was that bad she should be readmitted to hospital. 'That was the last thing she wanted,' says Jennifer, 'the thought of going back into hospital was horrific and it would have set her back enormously. She wanted to be in her own home and she didn't need medical help – she needed a carer for a couple of weeks.'

Jennifer drove for almost an hour each day before going to work to get her mother out of bed, help her downstairs and make breakfast. She organised a rota of friends and people from the local church to visit her mother each evening and help her upstairs. 'This was getting tiring, so I organised for a carer from a private firm to visit my mother for half an hour each morning,' says Jennifer. As this cost £8 a day and Mrs Morgan was on income support, this wouldn't have been possible without Jennifer's help.

Two weeks after Mrs Morgan had been discharged from hospital, social services finally offered help. Jennifer says, 'they were very helpful, but by this point the worst was over. I only wished I'd been more assertive and contacted them before my mother was discharged. But I'd never been in this situation before and didn't know what to do.'

Jennifer's advice to others is to make sure that arrangements for care at home are in place before a patient leaves hospital and to contact social services directly. She also found charities like Age Concern helpful in giving advice and that the Red Cross will loan out equipment like a commode for a fee.

I've heard that if the social services know that my relative has me to look after them, they won't offer as much help. Is this true?

This does happen. Social services have limited human and financial resources, and may cut corners where they see that a client is being looked after by caring friends or relatives. Even if you are keen to do as much as possible for your relative you must be realistic about the amount of additional help you will need. If there are tasks that you are not fit to do, or if there are times when other commitments mean that you will not be able to attend to them, tell the social worker this when your relative is being assessed. Caring for a relative at home is possibly the most stressful job of all, and you will be able to do it better, and for longer, if you have plenty of professional help from the start.

How do I make a living will, and is it legally binding?

A living will is a statement of your wishes should you become incapable of making decisions on your own behalf, such as after a severe stroke. You do not need a solicitor to make one, although your solicitor will be happy to help you draw up and store a living will. A written statement of your wishes, signed by yourself and independently witnessed, is sufficient. A properly drawn up living will (also known as an advance directive) is legally binding, although your medical attendants may seek further legal advice before, for example, withdrawing treatment that is keeping you alive. Keep a copy with your personal documents, and ensure that your nearest relative knows of its existence.

What is an Enduring Power of Attorney?

Enduring Power of Attorney is a way of making sure in advance that, if you become mentally incapacitated, your financial affairs will be in the hands of the person or people of your choice. It is not just for older people – every adult should make one. Enduring Power of

Attorney is made by filling in a form available from solicitors and legal stationers. It should then be signed by the donor, the attorney and at least one independent witness, and kept securely until it is needed, for instance if the donor shows signs of becoming mentally incapacitated. The attorney should register the Enduring Power of Attorney with the Public Trust Office using forms EP1 and EP2, available from legal stationers. After a 35-day delay to allow the donor and relatives to register any objections, the attorney is granted the powers listed in the Enduring Power of Attorney form.

If I need long-term nursing care who will pay for it?

If you have more than £18,000 in financial assets, including your home, you will have to contribute towards the cost of nursing care. This means that if you have no money in the bank, but own a house worth more than £18,000, you will have to sell your house to pay for your care. However, new rules mean that the first three months of residential or nursing care is provided without you having to sell your house. They also state that you will have your level of 'nursing' need assessed and a sum will be paid by the Government direct to the nursing home coresponding to your need and the nursing home will reduce your overall bill by the same amount. In England you will still be responsible for funding your own 'personal' care needs as well as general living costs. The situation in Scotland is different. The Scottish parliament has stated its intention of providing free long-term care (including nursing and personal care costs) for all older people who need it, irrespective of how much money they have. Older people who do not have assets of £18,000 will have the costs of their care needs met by either local Social Services or Primary Care Trusts.

Is there any way around this?

Yes. You could take out an insurance policy that will pay the cost of your nursing care. Policies of this type are expensive and are

Case history

Mary Watts

When Mary Watts was told she needed a hip operation because of osteo-arthritis, she was shocked. 'I was lying on a bed in a tiny cubicle and the consultant, who I had never met, just came in and leaned on the table. His attitude was very cool and matter of fact. He told me, in a very cool manner, that there would be a wait of a year for my hip replacement. I felt very vulnerable – I would prefer to have had the discussion across a desk.'

Mary had a full-time job in North London and was in frequent pain. 'The consultant did not say anything positive or compassionate. I saw him for no longer than 15 minutes. I dressed and came out of the cubicle and he said something like "see you in a year, then". It was a very lonely experience.'

Mary had no confidence in the consultant or in the hospital, which she describes as 'miserable, unfriendly and unwelcoming'. Instead she opted to go private, paying £7000 for a hip operation which was done a few weeks later. Mary did not have health insurance, so had to pay for the operation herself, but the hospital gave her a discount from a special bursary they had for Londoners.

Whereas she felt that the attitude of the NHS consultant was far too matter of fact, the private consultant treated her as an individual and gave her lots of positive advice. Now fully recovered and back to work, Mary does not regret the expense of her operation. 'I had total confidence in the private hospital: I was frightened and I needed compassion and individual attention, as well as having the op done swiftly.'

unlikely to benefit you personally. If you are in long-term nursing care, you will not need your house or other financial assets. Your heirs may want to take out long-term care insurance on your behalf if they are unhappy with the idea of the assets that they would otherwise inherit being stripped by the state.

How do I arrange a place in residential care?

Your local authority is responsible for making an assessment of the sort of care you need and suggesting a suitable home. They will also work out the funding arrangements. It is possible to go into a private residential or nursing home and pay the fees yourself. This can be useful for short periods, but if you expect to stay in the home indefinitely you should seek a local authority assessment so that you can be sure that your fees will be paid even if your savings run out.

What happens to my benefits when I go into hospital?

You should notify your social security office when you go into hospital, and when you return home. Your benefits will not normally be affected by a short stay in hospital unless you are admitted to hospital from a local authority residential care home, in which case there is an immediate reduction. If you are receiving Attendance Allowance or Disability Living Allowance, payments will stop four weeks after you are admitted to hospital. If you are receiving the Disabled Person's Tax Credit, payments continue to be made until the end of the 26-week period of the award. If you are in hospital when your claim is due for renewal, this may affect the amount you receive. If you are receiving Incapacity Benefit, Severe Disablement Allowance, the State Retirement Pension or Widows' Pension, your payment will be reduced after you have been in hospital for 6 weeks, and reduced again after 52 weeks. If you are receiving Income Support, your payment will be reduced after 4 weeks and again at intervals thereafter. If someone for whom you receive Invalid Care Allowance goes into hospital, the allowance normally stops immediately. Further details are available on the DSS website, www.dss.gov.uk.

Focus on older people – hospital care

One factor that concerns older people is how they are treated when they are in hospital. For example, if you are an 80-year-old woman with a minor illness, you may find it unsettling to be in a geriatric ward with patients suffering more serious illnesses and may prefer to be surrounded by a range of people of different ages and with different health problems. Alternatively, you may feel more comfortable surrounded by people of the same age. A range of care is available for older people, and the following tables tell you which type your hospital provides:

Needs based care
Older patients are allocated on admission either to specialist wards for older people or to general wards. Bed allocation is based on their clinical need rather than chronological age.

Age-defined care
Patients are admitted to specialist geriatric or general medical wards depending on an agreed age criteria. This age criteria may vary between hospitals. There can be benefits to this kind of placement, for example, being cared for by a team that specialise in the various effects of ageing.

Integrated care
Patients of all ages are cared for on acute wards and all physicians receive patients irrespective of age.

Hospital care

If the hospital has not provided information, a dash appears instead of yes or no.

	age-defined care	integrated care	needs-based care
Eastern			
Addenbrooke's Hospital	-	-	Yes
Basildon Hospital	Yes	-	-
Bedford Hospital	-	-	Yes
Broomfield Hospital	No	No	Yes
Colchester General Hospital	No	No	Yes
Hemel Hempstead General Hospital	Yes	-	Yes
Hinchingbrooke Hospital	-	Yes	-
Ipswich Hospital	-	Yes	-
James Paget Hospital	No	Yes	No
Lister Hospital	Yes	Yes	No
Luton & Dunstable Hospital	Yes	No	No
Mount Vernon Hospital	Yes	-	Yes
Norfolk & Norwich University Hospital	No	No	Yes
Orsett Hospital	-	-	-
Peterborough District Hospital	-	-	-
Princess Alexandra Hospital	Yes	No	No
Queen Elizabeth Hospital	-	Yes	-
Queen Elizabeth II Hospital	Yes	No	No
Southend Hospital	No	Yes	-
St Albans City Hospital	Yes	-	Yes
St John's Hospital	-	-	-
Stamford & Rutland Hospital	Yes	Yes	Yes
Watford General Hospital	Yes	-	Yes
West Suffolk Hospital	No	Yes	-
London			
Barking Hospital	Yes	No	No
Barnet Hospital	-	-	-
Bromley Hospital	-	Yes	-
Central Middlesex Hospital	No	Yes	Yes
Charing Cross Hospital	-	-	Yes
Chase Farm Hospital	-	-	-
Chelsea and Westminster Hospital	No	Yes	No
Ealing Hospital	-	Yes	-
Epsom General Hospital	No	Yes	No
Farnborough Hospital	-	-	-
Guy's Hospital	-	-	-

Hospital care

	age-defined care	integrated care	needs-based care
Hammersmith Hospital	No	No	Yes
Harold Wood Hospital	-	Yes	-
Hillingdon Hospital	Yes	-	-
Homerton Hospital	No	Yes	No
King George Hospital	-	Yes	Yes
King's College Hospital	No	Yes	Yes
Kingston Hospital	Yes	-	Yes
Mayday Hospital	Yes	No	No
Middlesex & University College Hospitals	-	Yes	Yes
Newham General Hospital	Yes	No	Yes
North Middlesex University Hospital	Yes	Yes	-
Northwick Park Hospital	No	Yes	Yes
Oldchurch Hospital	-	Yes	Yes
Orpington Hospital	No	Yes	No
Queen Elizabeth Hospital	-	-	Yes
Queen Mary's Hospital (Sidcup)	Yes	Yes	Yes
Queen Mary's Hospital (Hampstead)	Yes	-	-
Royal Free Hospital	Yes	-	-
Royal London Hospital	No	No	Yes
St Andrew's Hospital	-	-	-
St Bartholomew's Hospital	No	No	Yes
St George's Hospital (London)	No	No	Yes
St Helier Hospital	Yes	Yes	Yes
St Mary's Hospital	Yes	-	-
St Thomas' Hospital	-	-	Yes
University Hospital Lewisham	-	-	Yes
West Middlesex University Hospital	No	Yes	No
Whipps Cross University Hospital	Yes	No	No
Whittington Hospital	-	-	Yes

North West

	age-defined care	integrated care	needs-based care
Blackburn Royal Infirmary	No	No	Yes
Blackpool Victoria Hospital	No	Yes	Yes
Broadgreen Hospital	-	Yes	-
Burnley General Hospital	No	Yes	No
Bury General Hospital	-	-	-
Chorley & South Ribble District General Hospital	No	Yes	No
Countess of Chester Hospital	No	No	Yes
Fairfield General Hospital	No	Yes	Yes

Hospital care

	age-defined care	integrated care	needs-based care
Furness General Hospital	-	-	Yes
Halton General Hospital	No	No	Yes
Hope Hospital	Yes	No	Yes
Leigh Infirmary	-	Yes	No
Leighton Hospital	No	Yes	No
Macclesfield District General Hospital	No	Yes	Yes
Manchester Royal Infirmary	No	Yes	No
North Manchester General Hospital	No	Yes	Yes
Ormskirk and District General Hospital	No	Yes	No
Queens Park Hospital	No	No	Yes
Rochdale Infirmary	-	Yes	-
Rossendale General Hospital	No	Yes	No
Royal Albert Edward Infirmary	Yes	No	No
Royal Bolton Hospital	-	-	-
Royal Lancaster Infirmary	-	-	Yes
Royal Liverpool University Hospital	Yes	-	Yes
Royal Oldham Hospital	No	Yes	No
Royal Preston Hospital	-	Yes	-
Southport & Formby District General Hospital	No	Yes	No
St Helens Hospital (Merseyside)	No	Yes	No
Stepping Hill Hospital	Yes	Yes	No
Tameside General Hospital	-	Yes	-
Trafford General Hospital	-	Yes	-
University Hospital Aintree	-	-	Yes
Warrington Hospital	-	-	Yes
Westmorland General Hospital	-	Yes	Yes
Whiston Hospital	No	Yes	No
Wirral Hospital (Arrowe Park & Clatterbridge)	Yes	No	Yes
Withington Hospital	-	-	-
Wythenshawe Hospital	-	-	-
Northern and Yorks			
Airedale General Hospital	Yes	-	Yes
Bishop Auckland General Hospital	-	Yes	Yes
Bradford Royal Infirmary	Yes	No	No
Bridlington & District Hospital	-	-	-
Calderdale Royal Hospital	Yes	-	Yes
Castle Hill Hospital	Yes	-	-
Chapel Allerton Hospital	-	-	-

Hospital care

	age-defined care	integrated care	needs-based care
Cumberland Infirmary	No	No	Yes
Darlington Memorial Hospital	-	-	Yes
Dewsbury and District Hospital	Yes	-	-
Newcastle Hospitals*	No	Yes	No
Friarage Hospital	-	Yes	Yes
Harrogate District Hospital	No	No	Yes
Hexham General Hospital	No	No	Yes
Huddersfield Royal Infirmary	-	-	-
Hull Royal Infirmary	Yes	-	-
James Cook University Hospital	No	No	Yes
Leeds General Infirmary	-	-	-
Middlesbrough General Hospital	No	No	Yes
North Tyneside General Hospital	No	No	Yes
Pinderfields General Hospital	Yes	-	-
Pontefract General Infirmary	No	Yes	No
Princess Royal Hospital	Yes	-	-
Queen Elizabeth Hospital	-	-	Yes
Royal Victoria Infirmary	-	-	-
Ryhope Hospital	-	-	-
Scarborough General Hospital	-	-	-
Seacroft Hospital	-	-	-
South Tyneside District Hospital	No	No	Yes
St James's University Hospital	-	-	-
St Luke's Hospital (Huddersfield)	-	-	-
St Luke's Hospital (Bradford)	Yes	-	-
Sunderland Royal Hospital	Yes	No	Yes
University Hospital of Hartlepool	-	-	Yes
University Hospital of North Durham	No	No	Yes
University Hospital of North Tees	-	-	Yes
Wansbeck General Hospital	-	-	Yes
West Cumberland Hospital	No	Yes	No
Wharfdale General Hospital	-	-	-
Whitby Hospital	-	-	-
York District Hospital	Yes	-	Yes

* Newcastle Hospitals comprises: Freeman Hospital, Royal Victoria Infirmary and Newcastle General Hospital.

Hospital care

	age-defined care	integrated care	needs-based care
South East			
Amersham Hospital	Yes	-	-
Ashford Hospital	-	Yes	-
Buckland Hospital	-	-	Yes
Churchill Hospital	-	-	Yes
Conquest Hospital	Yes	No	-
Crawley Hospital	No	Yes	Yes
Darent Valley Hospital	Yes	Yes	Yes
East Surrey and Crawley Hospitals	Yes	No	No
Eastbourne District General Hospital	No	No	Yes
Frimley Park Hospital	-	Yes	-
Heatherwood Hospital	-	-	Yes
Horton Hospital	-	-	-
John Radcliffe Hospital	-	-	-
Kent & Canterbury Hospital	Yes	-	Yes
Kent and Sussex Hospital	No	Yes	No
Kettering General Hospital	No	Yes	-
Maidstone Hospital	No	Yes	No
Medway Maritime Hospital	-	-	-
Milton Keynes General NHS Hospital	No	Yes	Yes
North Hampshire Hospital	No	Yes	Yes
Northampton General Hospital	No	Yes	Yes
Pembury Hospital	-	-	-
Princess Royal Hospital	No	Yes	-
Queen Alexandra Hospital	Yes	-	Yes
Queen Elizabeth The Queen Mother Hospital	Yes	-	Yes
Queen Victoria Hospital	-	Yes	-
Radcliffe Infirmary	No	Yes	No
Royal Berkshire & Battle Hospitals	No	No	Yes
Royal Hampshire County Hospital	-	Yes	-
Royal South Hants Hospital	-	-	-
Royal Surrey County Hospital	Yes	-	Yes
Royal Sussex County Hospital	No	Yes	No
Southampton General Hospital	-	-	-
Southlands Hospital	-	-	-
St Mary's Hospital (Newport)	Yes	-	Yes
St Mary's Hospital (Portsmouth)	No	Yes	Yes
St Peter's Hospital	-	Yes	Yes
St Richard's Hospital	-	Yes	-

Hospital care

	age-defined care	integrated care	needs-based care
Stoke Mandeville Hospital	No	Yes	Yes
Wexham Park Hospital	-	-	Yes
William Harvey Hospital	Yes	-	Yes
Worthing Hospital	-	-	Yes
Wycombe Hospital	-	-	-
South West			
Bristol General Hospital	-	-	-
Bristol Royal Infirmary	No	No	Yes
Cheltenham General Hospital	-	Yes	-
Cirencester Hospital	-	-	-
Derriford Hospital	No	No	Yes
Dorset County Hospital	-	-	Yes
Frenchay Hospital	-	-	Yes
Gloucestershire Royal Hospital	No	Yes	Yes
North Devon District Hospital	Yes	Yes	Yes
Poole Hospital	Yes	-	Yes
Princess Margaret Hospital	-	-	-
Royal Bournemouth Hospital	No	Yes	No
Royal Cornwall Hospital	No	Yes	Yes
Royal Devon & Exeter Hospital	No	No	Yes
Royal United Hospital	-	-	Yes
Salisbury District Hospital	No	No	Yes
Southmead Hospital	-	-	Yes
St Michael's Hospital	-	-	-
Standish Hospital	-	-	-
Stroud General Hospital	-	-	-
Taunton & Somerset Hospital	No	No	Yes
Torbay District General Hospital	No	No	Yes
West Cornwall Hospital	No	Yes	Yes
Weston General Hospital	No	Yes	-
Yeovil District Hospital	No	Yes	No
Trent			
Barnsley District General Hospital	No	Yes	No
Bassetlaw District General Hospital	Yes	Yes	-
Chesterfield & North Derbyshire Royal Hospital	No	Yes	No
Derby City General Hospital	-	Yes	-
Derbyshire Royal Infirmary	-	Yes	-

Hospital care

	age-defined care	integrated care	needs-based care
Diana, Princess of Wales Hospital	Yes	No	No
Doncaster Royal Infirmary & Montagu Hospital	Yes	Yes	No
Glenfield Hospital	No	Yes	No
Grantham & District Hospital	No	Yes	-
King's Mill Hospital	-	Yes	-
Leicester General Hospital	No	Yes	No
Leicester Royal Infirmary	No	Yes	No
Lincoln County Hospital	Yes	-	-
Louth County Hospital	-	-	-
Northern General Hospital	No	Yes	Yes
Nottingham City Hospital	-	Yes	Yes
Pilgrim Hospital	No	Yes	-
Queen's Medical Centre	No	No	Yes
Rotherham District General Hospital	-	-	-
Royal Hallamshire Hospital	No	Yes	Yes
Scunthorpe General Hospital	No	No	Yes
Skegness & District Hospital	-	-	-

West Midlands

	age-defined care	integrated care	needs-based care
Alexandra Hospital	Yes	No	No
Birmingham Heartlands Hospital	-	-	Yes
City Hospital	-	Yes	-
County Hospital (Hereford)	No	No	Yes
Coventry and Warwickshire Hospital	No	No	Yes
Dudley Group of Hospitals*	No	Yes	No
General Hospital (Hereford)	-	-	-
George Eliot Hospital	-	Yes	-
Good Hope District General Hospital	-	-	Yes
Hospital of St Cross	No	No	Yes
Kidderminster Hospital	No	-	-
Manor Hospital (Walsall)	No	No	Yes
New Cross Hospital	-	-	Yes
North Staffordshire Hospital	No	Yes	Yes
North Staffordshire Royal Infirmary			
Princess Royal Hospital	No	No	Yes
Queen Elizabeth Hospital (Birmingham)	No	Yes	Yes
Queen's Hospital (Burton)	Yes	No	No
Royal Shrewsbury Hospital	-	Yes	-

* Dudley Group of Hospitals comprises: Russells Hall, Wordsley, Corbett and Guest Hospitals.

Hospital care

	age-defined care	integrated care	needs-based care
Sandwell General Hospital	No	Yes	No
Selly Oak Hospital	No	Yes	Yes
Solihull Hospital	-	-	Yes
Staffordshire General Hospital	No	Yes	Yes
Walsgrave Hospital	No	No	Yes
Warwick Hospital	No	Yes	Yes
Worcester Royal Infirmary	No	-	-

N. Ireland

Altnagelvin Area Hospital	-	-	Yes
Antrim Hospital	No	Yes	-
Belfast City Hospital	-	-	Yes
Causeway Hospital	-	Yes	-
Craigavon Area Hospital	No	No	Yes
Daisy Hill Hospital	No	Yes	No
Downe Hospital	-	-	-
Erne Hospital	-	-	-
Lagan Valley Hospital	-	-	-
Mater Hospital	-	Yes	-
Mid-Ulster Hospital	No	Yes	-
The Royal Hospitals	-	-	Yes
Tyrone County Hospital	-	-	-
Ulster Hospital	Yes	No	No
Whiteabbey Hospital	-	Yes	-

Wales

Bronglais General Hospital	No	No	Yes
Caerphilly District Miners' Hospital	No	Yes	-
Glan Clwyd District General Hospital	Yes	-	-
Llandough Hospital	No	Yes	Yes
Llandudno General Hospital	Yes	-	-
Morriston Hospital	No	No	Yes
Neath General Hospital	No	Yes	No
Nevill Hall Hospital	-	-	Yes
Prince Charles Hospital	No	Yes	No
Prince Philip Hospital	-	Yes	-
Princess of Wales Hospital	No	Yes	No
Royal Glamorgan Hospital	No	Yes	No
Royal Gwent Hospital	No	Yes	-

Hospital care

	age-defined care	integrated care	needs-based care
Singleton Hospital	No	No	Yes
University Hospital of Wales	No	Yes	No
West Wales General Hospital	-	Yes	-
Withybush General Hospital	No	Yes	No
Wrexham Maelor Hospital	-	-	-
Ysbyty Gwynedd	No	Yes	Yes

Focus on older people – broken hip

Approximately 70,000 people fracture a hip each year, 85 per cent of whom are women. Some fracture their hip simply by walking, others by falling. On average 10 per cent of these patients die within a month of the injury and 20 to 25 percent die within a year.

The hospital you go to and the type of care you receive while there are crucial to your survival and recovery.

The most common causes of death after admission for a broken hip are pneumonia, blood clots and infections due to reduced mobility. The following procedures have been identified as helping to reduce the risk of death due to broken hip and hospitals that follow them are therefore likely to have a lower mortality rate:

- You are moved out of casualty within one hour
- You receive antibiotics to ward off infections
- You are operated on within 24 hours
- You are encouraged to become mobile as soon as possible after surgery
- Your orthopaedic surgeon works closely with your geriatrician and other doctors to plan future care.

The figures in the table are based on the mortality rate for patients coming into hospital with broken hips. A Trust with an average performance has an index of 100. Figures smaller than 100 indicate a lower mortality rate than expected for the types of patients treated and vice-versa. As an example, a Trust with a mortality index of 90 would have only had 90 deaths for every 100 deaths that you would expect in view of the type of patients they treat – a good performance (10 per cent better than average). The table has been split into three groups for every region, clearly showing whether the hospital has a significantly lower than average, average or asignificantly higher than average mortality rate. Hospitals with a very high or low number may not necessarily be significantly above or below average if, for example, they treat relatively few patients.

Hip mortality rate

If the hospital has not provided us with information, a dash appears instead of a figure.

	hip mortality rate
Eastern	
Peterborough District Hospital	49
Edith Cavell Hospital	49
Bedford Hospital	69
Colchester General Hospital	85
Norfolk & Norwich University Hospital	85
Orsett Hospital	104
Basildon Hospital	104
Queen Elizabeth Hospital	104
Princess Alexandra Hospital	106
St John's Hospital	107
Broomfield Hospital	107
Luton & Dunstable Hospital	110
West Suffolk Hospital	111
Hemel Hempstead General Hospital	113
Mount Vernon Hospital	113
St Albans City Hospital	113
Watford General Hospital	113
James Paget Hospital	118
Hinchingbrooke Hospital	131
Lister Hospital	121
Queen Elizabeth II Hospital	121
Southend Hospital	133
Addenbrooke's Hospital	140
Ipswich Hospital	142

LOW — Peterborough District Hospital, Edith Cavell Hospital
AVERAGE — from Norfolk & Norwich University Hospital to Hinchingbrooke Hospital
HIGH — Lister Hospital to Ipswich Hospital

London	
Hillingdon Hospital	25
King's College Hospital	35
Middlesex & University College Hospitals	43
St Bartholomew's Hospital	61
Royal London Hospital	61
Chelsea and Westminster Hospital	71

LOW — London group

	hip mortality rate
Guy's Hospital	71
St Thomas' Hospital	71
Homerton Hospital	83
North Middlesex University Hospital	88
Queen Mary's Hospital (Hampstead)	91
Royal Free Hospital	91
Whittington Hospital	95
Queen Mary's Hospital (Sidcup)	98
St Mary's Hospital	100
Kingston Hospital	105
Central Middlesex Hospital	107
Northwick Park Hospital	107
Chase Farm Hospital	116
Barnet Hospital	116
University Hospital Lewisham	119
Queen Elizabeth Hospital	121
Ealing Hospital	123
West Middlesex University Hospital	125
Orpington Hospital	125
Bromley Hospital	125
Farnborough Hospital	125
King George Hospital	126
Barking Hospital	126
Epsom General Hospital	128
St Helier Hospital	128
St Andrew's Hospital	134
Newham General Hospital	134
Whipps Cross University Hospital	137
Mayday Hospital	138
Harold Wood Hospital	140
Oldchurch Hospital	140
Hammersmith Hospital	140
Charing Cross Hospital	140
St George's Hospital (London)	143

LOW — Guy's Hospital, St Thomas' Hospital
AVERAGE — Homerton Hospital to West Middlesex University Hospital
HIGH — Orpington Hospital to St George's Hospital (London)

Hip mortality rate

		hip mortality rate
North West		
LOW	Warrington Hospital	75
	Leighton Hospital	78

		hip mortality rate
	Rochdale Infirmary	78
	Wirral Hospital (Arrowe Park & Clatterbridge)	84
	Withington Hospital	85
	Wythenshawe Hospital	85
	Blackburn Royal Infirmary	85
	Queens Park Hospital	85
	Chorley & South Ribble District General Hospital	86
	Royal Oldham Hospital	89
	University Hospital Aintree	91
	Hope Hospital	103
	Manchester Royal Infirmary	103
	Macclesfield District General Hospital	105
AVERAGE	Broadgreen Hospital	107
	Royal Liverpool University Hospital	107
	Countess of Chester Hospital	108
	Royal Preston Hospital	108
	Furness General Hospital	108
	Westmorland General Hospital	108
	Royal Lancaster Infirmary	108
	North Manchester General Hospital	112
	Ormskirk and District General Hospital	114
	Southport & Formby District General Hospital	114
	Royal Bolton Hospital	117
	Fairfield General Hospital	126
	Bury General Hospital	126
	Trafford General Hospital	147

		hip mortality rate
	Tameside General Hospital	129
	Stepping Hill Hospital	131
HIGH	Blackpool Victoria Hospital	134
	St Helens Hospital (Merseyside)	139
	Whiston Hospital	139

		hip mortality rate
HIGH	Burnley General Hospital	141
	Rossendale General Hospital	141
	Leigh Infirmary	166
	Royal Albert Edward Infirmary	166

		hip mortality rate
Northern and Yorks		
	University Hospital of North Tees	57
	University Hospital of Hartlepool	57
	Airedale General Hospital	67
	North Tyneside General Hospital	69
	Hexham General Hospital	69
	Wansbeck General Hospital	69
	Friarage Hospital	70
LOW	Newcastle Hospitals*	72
	Royal Victoria Infirmary	72
	Dewsbury and District Hospital	78
	Huddersfield Royal Infirmary	78
	St Luke's Hospital (Huddersfield)	78
	Castle Hill Hospital	78
	Princess Royal Hospital	78
	Hull Royal Infirmary	78

		hip mortality rate
	Darlington Memorial Hospital	82
	Bishop Auckland General Hospital	82
	York District Hospital	83
	Ryhope Hospital	84
	Sunderland Royal Hospital	84
	South Tyneside District Hospital	90
	Middlesbrough General Hospital	91
AVERAGE	James Cook University Hospital	91
	Cumberland Infirmary	97
	Harrogate District Hospital	98
	Seacroft Hospital	98
	Wharfdale General Hospital	98
	Chapel Allerton Hospital	98
	Leeds General Infirmary	98
	St James's University Hospital	98
	Pontefract General Infirmary	101

* Newcastle Hospitals comprises: Freeman Hospital, Royal Victoria Infirmary and Newcastle General Hospital.

Hip mortality rate

	hip mortality rate
AVERAGE	
Pinderfields General Hospital	101
St Luke's Hospital (Bradford)	106
Bradford Royal Infirmary	106
Calderdale Royal Hospital	110
University Hospital of North Durham	111
HIGH	
Scarborough General Hospital	139
Whitby Hospital	139
Bridlington & District Hospital	139
West Cumberland Hospital	143
Bensham Hospital	152
Queen Elizabeth Hospital	152

South East

	hip mortality rate
LOW	
Royal Sussex County Hospital	62
St Richard's Hospital	65
St Mary's Hospital (Portsmouth)	66
Queen Alexandra Hospital	66
Royal Hampshire County Hospital	67
Eastbourne District General Hospital	69
St Mary's Hospital (Newport)	75
Conquest Hospital	76
AVERAGE	
Princess Royal Hospital	76
Royal Surrey County Hospital	84
Heatherwood Hospital	91
Wexham Park Hospital	91
Southlands Hospital	94
Worthing Hospital	94
Darent Valley Hospital	96
Frimley Park Hospital	97
Royal Berkshire & Battle Hospitals	98
Battle Hospital	98
St Peter's Hospital	100
Ashford Hospital	100
Kettering General Hospital	108
Milton Keynes General NHS Hospital	109
Buckland Hospital	110
William Harvey Hospital	110

	hip mortality rate
AVERAGE	
Kent & Canterbury Hospital	110
Queen Elizabeth The Queen Mother Hospital	110
Pembury Hospital	110
Kent and Sussex Hospital	110
Maidstone Hospital	110
Amersham Hospital	111
Wycombe Hospital	111
Northampton General Hospital	112
North Hampshire Hospital	115
Stoke Mandeville Hospital	124
HIGH	
East Surrey and Crawley Hospitals	126
Crawley Hospital	126
John Radcliffe Hospital	133
Horton Hospital	133
Radcliffe Infirmary	133
Churchill Hospital	133
Medway Maritime Hospital	134
Royal South Hants Hospital	159
Southampton General Hospital	159

South West

	hip mortality rate
LOW	
Weston General Hospital	58
Royal Devon & Exeter Hospital	62
Salisbury District Hospital	77
AVERAGE	
Cheltenham General Hospital	81
Cirencester Hospital	81
Dorset County Hospital	83
West Cornwall Hospital	84
Royal Cornwall Hospital	84
North Devon District Hospital	85
St Michael's Hospital	90
Bristol General Hospital	90
Bristol Royal Infirmary	90
Standish Hospital	98
Gloucestershire Royal Hospital	98
Frenchay Hospital	98
Southmead Hospital	98

Hip mortality rate

		hip mortality rate
AVERAGE	Royal United Hospital	99
	Poole Hospital	111
	Taunton & Somerset Hospital	111
	Princess Margaret Hospital	112
	Derriford Hospital	117
HIGH	Torbay District General Hospital	144

Trent

		hip mortality rate
LOW	Scunthorpe General Hospital	62
	Derbyshire Royal Infirmary	67
	Derby City General Hospital	67
	Diana, Princess of Wales Hospital	74
	King's Mill Hospital	74
	Barnsley District General Hospital	77
	Skegness & District Hospital	85
	Pilgrim Hospital	85
	Grantham & District Hospital	85
	Louth County Hospital	85
	Lincoln County Hospital	85
AVERAGE	Rotherham District General Hospital	78
	Doncaster Royal Infirmary & Montagu Hospital	82
	Northern General Hospital	101
	Queen's Medical Centre	107
	Bassetlaw District General Hospital	115
HIGH	Leicester Royal Infirmary	119
	Glenfield Hospital	119
	Leicester General Hospital	119
	Chesterfield & North Derbyshire Royal Hospital	155

West Midlands

		hip mortality rate
LOW	General Hospital (Hereford)	74
	County Hospital (Hereford)	74
	Walsgrave Hospital	75
	Hospital of St Cross	75
	Coventry and Warwickshire Hospital	75
	New Cross Hospital	77
AVERAGE	Queen's Hospital (Burton)	86
	Alexandra Hospital	95
	Worcester Royal Infirmary	95
	Kidderminster Hospital	95
	Dudley Group of Hospitals*	96
	Princess Royal Hospital	97
	North Staffordshire Royal Infirmary	99
	North Staffordshire Hospital	99
	Staffordshire General Hospital	101
	Royal Shrewsbury Hospital	105
	Warwick Hospital	114
	Manor Hospital (Walsall)	114
HIGH	Queen Elizabeth Hospital (Birmingham)	114
	Selly Oak Hospital	114
	Sandwell General Hospital	123
	Good Hope District General Hospital	129
	City Hospital	129
	Birmingham Heartlands Hospital	143
	Solihull Hospital	143
	George Eliot Hospital	150

* Dudley Group of Hospitals comprises: Russells Hall, Wordsley, Corbett and Guest Hospitals.

Hip mortality rate

	hip mortality rate
Scotland	
Aberdeen Royal Infirmary	90
Ayr Hospital	93
Balfour Hospital	-
Borders General Hospital	89
Crosshouse Hospital	91
Dr Gray's Hospital	95
Dumfries and Galloway Royal Infirmary	89
Dunoon & District General Hospital	-
Falkirk Royal Infirmary	93
Gartnavel General Hospital	91
Gilbert Bain Hospital	-
Glasgow Royal Infirmary	95
Hairmyres Hospital	92
Inverclyde Royal Hospital	92
Lorn and Islands District General Hospital	-
Monklands Hospital	92
Ninewells Hospital	91
Perth Royal Infirmary	93
Queen Margaret Hospital	91
Raigmore Hospital	93
Royal Alexandra Hospital	92
Royal Infirmary of Edinburgh	90
Southern General Hospital	91
St John's Hospital at Howden	90
Stirling Royal Infirmary	90
Stobhill Hospital	-
Stracathro Hospital	92
Vale of Leven District General Hospital	-
Victoria Hospital	-
Victoria Infirmary	92
Western General Hospital	-
Western Infirmary	91
Woodend Hospital	-

Private Medicine

Private medicine

More and more patients are choosing to use private medicine. Once only available to a privileged minority, it is increasingly joining the mainstream. Under Government plans to reduce waiting times, more NHS patients will be treated in the private sector.

The cost of treatment in NHS hospitals is met from public funds, whereas in a private hospital you, or an insurance company on your behalf, pay for your own treatment. Most people who choose to go into a private hospital do so either to avoid long NHS waiting lists or because the facilities are better – for example, private hospitals can offer almost every patient a single room with a bathroom, telephone and television, and are more flexible about meals and visiting times. People also like the ability to choose their consultant and to know that they will be seen and operated on by him or her. Treatments not available on the NHS, such as fertility treatment or complementary therapies like acupuncture and osteopathy, are another draw towards the private sector.

However, for many conditions, private treatment may not be the answer, especially if you are seriously ill. Although private hospitals are regulated in terms of the quality of their infrastructure, staffing and record keeping, clinical care standards are not monitored. Many private hospitals may have intensive care and high dependency facilities but these are smaller than NHS hospitals and have fewer facilities. Any conditions that need special treatment facilities, such as kidney dialysis, are not usually catered for in private hospitals, nor do all private hospitals have intensive care beds and this could be a problem should you need life-saving equipment and care. Similarly, private hospitals may not be sufficiently equipped to carry out complex procedures and you should make sure that the hospital you choose has sufficient expertise in your condition. In the data section of this Guide, we tell you what procedures each private hospital specialises in.

Can I get better treatment in a private hospital?

You may get quicker treatment but the standard of medical care you receive will not necessarily be better than in an NHS hospital. Most are staffed by NHS consultants but you will have the reassurance of knowing that a named consultant will be personally responsible for you throughout and will not delegate your care to junior colleagues. A private hospital that draws most of its staff from a major teaching Trust is liable to be a good one. Because facilities for treating seriously ill patients are limited in private hospitals, you should consider using the private facilities in a local NHS hospital for complex surgery, or be aware of the proximity of the nearest NHS intensive care unit should you need to be transferred there in an emergency.

How do I arrange to go to a private hospital? Can I refer myself?

As with NHS hospitals, you need to be referred by your GP. The referral procedure varies between hospitals and consultants. All private hospitals produce directories of the consultants who work there, complete with details of how to make a referral. Your GP should have access to this information, and it is available to the public too – telephone the customer services department of the hospital with your queries. If you have private medical insurance, then your insurer will also be able to advise you on which consultants you can see – depending on the type of insurance you have there may be rules about which hospitals you can be treated in.

Can I choose which hospital I go to and which consultant I see?

If your private medical insurers are paying for your treatment, they will have 'networks' of hospitals with which they have contracts and you are limited to those hospitals. Many have an option whereby you can pay a higher premium which removes all restrictions on which hospitals you can be treated in.

Case history

John and Eileen Lambie

When 64-year-old Eileen Lambie needed to go into hospital for cancer, she opted for a private hospital because she would have her own room, and it would be easier for friends and family to visit her. Although he was retired, John's health insurance was covered by his company. When Eileen started to develop problems in her abdomen, an X-ray revealed a large growth in her bladder which proved to be malignant.

Eileen's problems began after an operation to remove her bladder. Three weeks after the operation, her consultant went on leave, and John says that the locum in charge of her care 'neglected her abominably', seeing her only a few times over a period of weeks. Eileen became very ill – she was unable keep down food or drink, and was sustained by drip. Her family's request for a second opinion was refused as unnecessary, and her symptoms were dismissed as psychosomatic. Despite her ill health, she was sent home, where she deteriorated further.

Her GP was horrified at her condition, and she was admitted to another private hospital (John refused to let her go back to the hospital she was first treated in). There, doctors discovered that her illness was being caused by an excess of calcium in the blood – something John says should have been routinely checked for. She was given treatment to deal with this, but she died a couple of months later. John believes that her life wouldn't have been saved by better treatment, but she would have been spared 'weeks and weeks of misery'.

John tried to find out why his wife had been treated so badly. 'I began to enquire about private hospitals, and was shattered to discover the lack of responsibility and accountability in private acute hospitals. The hospital took the attitude that the management had no responsibility for clinical care, and although the RMO (resident medical officer) lives in the hospital, they don't routinely examine patients – they only carry out the instructions of consultants.'

John formed a lobby group, the Action for the Proper Regulation of Private Hospitals (APRoP). It has had input into the development of the Care Standards Act, and the new National Care Standards Commission, which are meant to improve standards in private hospitals. But John still believes there are gaps in the way private hospitals are regulated, and particularly in the back-up and support they can offer. 'A fatal weakness of the private sector is that there is no team. In the specialist unit of an NHS hospital, there is a team of doctors and nurses all specialising in a particular field, who can all provide the necessary back-up.'

John's advice to people who need to go to hospital for a major procedure is to go to the private wing of an NHS hospital, where, in theory, you should be able to draw on the back-up of the public hospital in an emergency. He also recommends that if you are having a general anaesthetic that you ensure you have a friend or relative to stay with you immediately after the operation, so that they can alert staff if there are any problems.

My GP won't refer me privately to the consultant/hospital of my choice. What can I do about it?

You do not have a right to be referred privately to a consultant on demand – your GP has to agree that the referral is medically necessary and that the consultant is appropriate. The hospital or consultant of your choice may not be equipped to give you the best treatment for your problem. A few hospitals and consultants will only accept patients who have private medical insurance. If your GP suggests a different consultant or hospital, ask why. If you are not satisfied with the answer and your GP still won't refer you, then you can see another doctor within your practice, or change to another practice in your area.

Are the consultants who work privately as up-to-date as the NHS consultants?

Very few consultants do nothing but private work, and most have an active NHS commitment too. They are therefore obliged to spend a certain amount of time each year updating their skills and knowledge. GPs normally advise patients seeking a private referral to see a consultant who also has a reputation as a good NHS doctor. You should be cautious about seeing consultants who only perform private work.

Does the NHS sometimes use private hospitals?

Sometimes it will take advantage of the spare operating theatre capacity in private hospitals, usually for minor surgical procedures that do not require an overnight stay. It may also use their diagnostic equipment (eg MRI scanner) and make use of the availability of beds.

Can I be a private patient in an NHS hospital?

Yes. Most NHS hospitals accept private patients. Some will have a private suite or wing which will often be as comfortable as a private hospital. Others use amenity beds, which are better-equipped single rooms on the main wards. This can be a less expensive option to going into a private hospital. A large NHS hospital may also be better equipped to treat high-risk patients as they routinely accept critically ill patients through A&E. Many NHS hospitals also offer tests such as X-rays and scans on a private basis.

What is private medical insurance?

This is an arrangement where you, or your employer on your behalf, pay a yearly fee to an insurance company and, in return, the insurance company will pay for private medical treatment if you become ill or need an operation. These schemes allow you to avoid NHS waiting lists and you can be sure that you will be seen by a named consultant. Some of the best known private medical insurers are PPP (part of the AXA insurance group) and BUPA. Some major insurance companies like Norwich Union and Standard Life also offer private medical insurance. Levels of cover range from the most basic, such as only paying for inpatient treatment in a private bed in an NHS hospital, through to comprehensive policies which include things like normal pregnancy care, complementary medicine and a yearly routine health check. As you might expect, you pay more to have access to a wider range of facilities. You also pay a higher premium if you are older. Private medical insurance does not generally cover treatment for problems that were already diagnosed before you took out the policy, or for long-term hospital treatment for chronic diseases (such as kidney dialysis). Nor does it automatically allow you to see any consultant or go to any hospital unless you pay a high premium.

I'm not insured for private treatment. Can I pay for my own treatment as I need it? Are there any situations where it might be worth going private at my own expense?

You do not need private medical insurance to have private treatment. Most hospitals will allow you to pay for your own treatment. Many charge a fixed price to have an operation and any care you might need afterwards. Some have finance arrangements to let you borrow the cost of your treatment at a low rate of interest. The main reason to have private treatment at your own expense would be if you needed an operation for which there can be a long wait on the NHS – joint replacement surgery or cataract extraction are typical examples – or if you wanted a procedure that neither the NHS nor private medical insurance would fund, such as fertility treatment or liposuction.

What are private insurance networks?

Some insurers have contracts with particular hospitals or consultants. This allows the insurance company to be confident that the consultant is reputable, and to get a good deal on charges for consultations, tests and operations so that they can offer you competitive premiums. These contracts work both ways, and some hospitals and consultants will only accept private patients whose treatment costs will be met by insurance. However, there are many perfectly reputable consultants who do not have contracts with private health insurers.

Can I switch between private and NHS for the same condition?

You can have a private consultation with a consultant then go on an NHS waiting list for surgery. You can also see a consultant on the NHS for the initial consultation and have your operation done privately by the same consultant. If you need a test for which there is a long wait on the NHS, such as an MRI scan, you may be able to speed things up by having the test done privately.

How can I compare private hospitals?

Private hospitals are listed separately in the data section of this Guide with an explanation of what to look out for when choosing one.

What sort of problems are dealt with particularly well in private hospitals?

It depends on the hospital. Routine operations of all types and treatment of skin and eye problems are areas where private hospitals can offer advantages over NHS hospitals. Many private hospitals will not accept high-risk patients as they are not equipped to deal with the possible complications of surgery in these patients. If you do have an operation in a private hospital and experience major complications, you will usually need to be transferred to an NHS hospital for intensive care.

How much emergency cover does a private hospital need?

All of the private hospitals surveyed in this Guide had at least one doctor available on site 24 hours a day – generally known as a resident medical officer (RMO). This is important, but it is also vital that both the doctors and the nurses have appropriate training for dealing with emergencies. The number of trained staff a hospital needs on site depends on how large the hospital is and what type of patients it is treating. A large hospital performing a lot of heart bypass surgery will obviously need more than a small hospital specialising in minor surgery. Most private hospitals, by and large, have less doctors on site 24 hours a day than the large NHS hospitals. However, they treat far less critically ill and unstable patients than NHS hospitals and do not generally admit patients as emergencies. The on-site staff are also able to call the consultants responsible for your care to come in from home if necessary. The type of doctors and nurses available on site should also be suitable for the types of patients treated. As an example, a hospital performing a lot of throat surgery involving tracheostomy tubes (breathing tubes in the neck) would benefit from having nurses on site who are experienced in managing these devices. Also, if a hospital is undertaking major surgery, having an anaesthetist on site may be an advantage as these doctors generally have the highest level of training for emergencies and particularly for putting patients on ventilators. It is important that you are satisfied that the cover provided is suitable for you personally.

What makes a good private intensive care, high-dependency or coronary care unit?

There are currently no official definitions for each of these types of unit, though this is changing. In general, as well as having suitable monitoring and emergency facilities, these units should have plenty of space between beds and the staff should always be able to see the patients. Most importantly, however, the staff should have appropriate experience – they should be familiar with the equipment they are using and they should have experience of this type of care as well as appropriate training. This is particularly true in intensive care units and coronary care units. Ideally, the resident doctor would have at least 6 months' experience of working on an intensive care unit (which is a specialised field) or of treating heart patients, and the nurses would be similarly experienced. It is also an advantage if an intensive care unit is under the overall control of a consultant who specialises in this area. There is a big difference between a room where appropriate equipment is wheeled in and switched on once a year and a full-time working intensive care unit.

If I have an operation in a private hospital, what will happen if there are complications?

If you need to be in a high dependency unit or intensive care unit, smaller hospitals may not have the facilities or the skilled staff to cope and you may need to be transferred to an NHS hospital. Hospitals should not admit patients who are likely to have complications they are not equipped to manage.

What questions should I ask about the on-site doctors?

It is important that resident medical officers are chosen with some care and made familiar with the workings of the hospital. Questions you might ask could include: How many RMOs are there on-site 24 hours a day? How much previous experience are they required to have? Is that experience relevant to my condition if it is in a specialised area? Are they required to have recent Advanced Life Support training? Do they have a formal induction day on arrival at the hospital? How long is their minimum contract period?

What questions should I ask about the on-site nurses?

It is important that there is adequate nursing cover overnight and that the nurses have suitable experience. Questions you might ask could include: How many nurses are present on each ward overnight? How experienced are those nurses? Is that experience relevant to my condition? How many are required to have Advanced Life Support training? How often do they check the patients' rooms?

What sort of equipment should the hospital have?

Hospitals should have suitable emergency equipment available and it should be accessible within minutes from all parts of the hospital where patients are treated – the equipment is usually kept on a resuscitation trolley. The equipment should be appropriate for the types of patients treated, for example, if children are treated then the equipment should come in children's sizes. It is also important that it is checked daily and that staff are familiar with it. The hospital should also have a system for alerting staff to emergencies and this should also be tested daily. Patient rooms should have buttons allowing patients and staff to call for help.

What types of critical care beds does a private hospital need?

High dependency units are used most commonly in private hospitals for looking after patients following major surgery.

Similarly, coronary care units are used mainly for patients who have had heart bypass surgery and sometimes for looking after patients who have had coronary angioplasty. Intensive care units are only needed for the very sickest patients. The type of care a patient is likely to need after surgery is greatly influenced by how well they are prior to the surgery as well as by how major or complex the surgery is. Therefore, as with staffing levels in private hospitals, the most important thing is that the facilities available are appropriate to the types of patients being treated and particularly that you feel that they are appropriate for your own case. If a hospital does not have a particular type of critical care bed available, the most important thing is that they have agreed transfer arrangements in place with another local hospital so that if an emergency arises requiring a critical care bed then the patient can be efficiently transported to that hospital.

How much does private treatment cost?
This depends on which hospital or consultant you go to, what treatment you have and how long you need to stay in hospital. Typically, a consultation with a physiotherapist or an osteopath will cost £25–£35, a consultation with a doctor will cost £70–£150, a minor operation such as a day-case hernia repair will cost around £1,500 and a coronary artery bypass graft (heart bypass operation) will cost at least £12,000.

Section Three:
Comparing Hospitals

How to Compare NHS Hospitals

In the following pages there are descriptions of most NHS hospitals in the UK with key facts and figures about each. In order to supplement the information we have already given you in the Guide, we tell you whether your hospital meets certain standards in terms of facilities, mortality and waiting times. NHS Hospitals are run by NHS Trusts, which may run more than one hospital. The statistics published here relate to NHS Trusts, not individual hosptials, and will therefore reflect the service provided by all the hospitals in that Trust. Services may be organised across more than one hospital by a Trust. Throughout the tables, where the hospital has not supplied us with figures, we have put a dash in the field where the figure should be.

 A&E This tells you whether the hospital has an A&E unit.

 Children's A&E This tells you whether the hospital has an A&E for children with separate waiting and treatment area.

 ITU This tells you whether the hospital has an intensive care unit which provides very high levels of care for the most seriously ill patients. Higher standards of equipment and staffing are provided and patients can be kept on ventilators.

 Children's ITU This tells you whether the hospital has an intensive care unit exclusively for children.

 24hr X-ray This tells you whether the hospital has X-ray facilities available around the clock. This is particularly important for emergency diagnoses.

 CT scanner This tells you if the hospital has a CT (computed tomography) scanner on site. These produce sophisticated X-rays for bone and soft tissue. One specific function is to image the brain, and so are an essential tool for identifying bleeding in the brain or diagnosing stroke. If

your hospital does not have a CT scanner, you would need
to be referred to a different hospital for this type of
diagnostic test. For routine diagnoses, a hospital without a
CT scanner may be reluctant to refer you for a test at all.

 CT Scanner 24 hours This tells you whether your hospital
has a CT scanner available around the clock. This is
particularly important in emergency diagnoses (for instance,
in the case of suspected stroke) after A&E admittance.

MRI Scanner This tells you whether the hospital has an
MRI (magnetic resonance imaging) scanner. These scanners
are considerably better than normal X-rays for imaging soft
tissues and are very good at showing the spine and joints.
For routine diagnoses, a hospital without an MRI scanner
may be reluctant to refer you for a test at all.

Overall Mortality Index (Death Rate)

This figure (for England only) compares the relative rates of
mortality in hospital trusts after allowing for factors such as
differences in types of patients treated. It is one indicator of the
quality of clinical care in the hospital. A trust with an average
performance has an index of 100. Figures greater than 100 indicate
a higher mortality rate than expected for the types of patients
treated and vice versa. We give you the regional average so that
you can see how your hospital is performing within your area.

Vacancy Rate

This tells you the percentage of consultant posts that have been
vacant for over three months (for England only). A high vacancy
rate may suggest that certain specialists at that hospital will have
longer waiting lists than at others. The national average is 3 per
cent. We give you the regional average so that you can see how
your hospital is performing within your area.

Doctors per 100 beds

This tells you the number of full-time doctors employed per 100 beds in the trust, across all levels of seniority. This has been shown to have a strong relationship to the mortality rate: trusts with high numbers of doctors generally have low mortality rates. The figures are strongly affected by the type of work done at the Trust. Trusts with community services will have lower numbers of doctors per bed than purely acute Trusts. Teaching hospitals will have high numbers. We give averages for Northern Ireland, Wales and Scotland. In England, averages are given for each region and type of hospital with different averages for teaching hospitals, large acute hospitals and small acute hospitals.

These numbers are calculated differently for different countries and are not comparable across borders.

Nurses per 100 beds

This tells you the number of full-time nurses employed per 100 beds in the trust. This does not have a strong relationship to mortality rate, but may influence the amount of attention you receive from nursing staff and so affect your satisfaction with your hospital stay. Averages are calculated as for doctors per 100 beds. We give you the regional average so that you can see how your hospital is performing within your area.We also give you national averages for Scotland, Wales and Northern Ireland.

These numbers are calculated differently for different countries and are not comparable across borders.

Cancelled Operations

This tells you the number of operations that were cancelled on the day for reasons other than the patient was unfit for surgery (for England only). The national average is 3 per cent. We give you the regional average so that you can see how your hospital is performing within your area.

Complaints

This tells you the number of written complaints received by a trust for every 1000 patients admitted. A low figure may suggest that patients tend to be satisfied with the care they receive at this hospital. The national average for England is 3 per cent. We give you the regional average so that you can see how your hospital is performing within your area. We also give you national averages for Scotland, Wales and Northern Ireland.

Complaints Clear-up

This tells you the percentage of complaints for which the trust provided a full response within 20 working days. A low may be interpreted as some measure of the seriousness with which the trust considers complaints. The national average for England is 47 per cent. We give you the regional average so that you can see how your hospital is performing within your area. We also give you national averages for Scotland, Wales and Northern Ireland.

WAITING TIME PERFORMANCE
Inpatients

This tells you the average waiting time for all specialties from the decision to admit the patient to hospital admission (excluding emergencies). For England, Scotland and Northern Ireland, it is the percentage of patients admitted within six months; for Wales, within 12 months. The national average for England is 74 per cent. We give you the regional average so that you can see how your hospital is performing within your area. We also give you national averages for Scotland, Wales and Northern Ireland.

Outpatients

This tells you average waiting time for all specialties from the day a patient gets an appointment to see a specialist until seeing that specialist. For England it is the percentage of patients seen within 12 weeks, for Scotland, it is the percentage of patients seen within

13 weeks; in Northern Ireland, two months; in Wales, within six months. The national average for England is 78 per cent. We give you the regional average so that you can see how your hospital is performing within your area. We also give you national averages for Scotland, Wales and Northern Ireland.

How to compare private hospitals

In the first two sections of this Guide, we have explained the main differences between the public and private health care sectors. In the following tables we tell give you a range of information to help you compare private hospitals. In the tables, if the hospital has not provided us with information, we have put a dash in the field where this should be.

When choosing which private hospital you go to, you should take the following into consideration:

Does your hospital offer a wide range of diagnostic services?
These range from relatively simple tests such as blood tests – which are often sent to be analysed at another location – through to X-rays and more complex scanning. The availability of the most complex and specialised tests will depend on the particular areas of expertise for each hospital. Complex heart testing for instance is only carried out in a few centres. Where a hospital does not have a particular diagnostic technique available, the consultant you see there will still be able to refer you to another hospital which does provide the service, if they feel that is necessary. CT (computed tomography) and MRI (magnetic resonance imaging) scanners are considerably better than normal X-rays for imaging soft tissues. They are particularly important for imaging the brain and, in the case of MRI, for imaging the spine and joints.

Most private hospitals are able to offer CT or MRI scanning though relatively few have these scanners on site. They often use a mobile scanning unit which visits the hospital periodically – this may mean that you are only able to have a scan on certain days.

 MRI Scanner This tells you whether the hospital has an MRI scanner.

 mob MRI Scanner This tells you whether the hospital has access to a mobile MRI scanner.

 CT Scanner This tells you whether the hospital has a CT scanner.

Does the hospital have intensive care facilities should you need to be put on a ventilator after surgery?

If you become seriously ill during surgery and need to be ventilated you will need intensive care facilities. We tell you which hospitals have these. High dependency units allow increased levels of care, though patients generally cannot be put on a ventilator as they can in an intensive care unit.

 ITU This icon tells you whether your hospital has an intensive care unit.

 HDU This icon tells you whether your hospital has a high dependency unit.

INSURERS

Which insurance companies accredit your hospital?

Listed are which of the six major private health insurers accredit this hospital for treatment – BUPA, PPP Healthcare, Standard Life, Norwich Union Healthcare, Royal Sun Alliance and WPA. This shows you whether you are insured for treatment at that hospital. If the insurers are asterisked, then they recognise that particular hospital as a network member and the hospital may offer you reduced rates for treatment.

Prices

We give you prices for hip replacement and cataract removal. This enables you to compare treatment costs between private hospitals in your area.

Beds

This figure tells you how large the hospital is. A large hospital would have 60 or more beds and a small hospital as few as 10.

Do the nurses have Advanced Life Support training?

Advanced Life Support (ALS) training is the gold standard for training doctors and nurses to manage the early stages of an emergency. We tell you how many staff with this training the hospital requires to be present on site 24 hours a day. It is important to note that this number should be taken in the context of the size of the hospital and the type of patients it treats.

Does the hospital specialise in heart disease?

Most private hospitals have doctors specialising in heart disease available for you to see in the outpatients clinic. However, fewer of them are able to provide the more complex investigations and treatments for heart disease such as heart bypass surgery. The hospitals that do provide these services usually have a special interest in the area and are equipped to provide complex investigations and surgery with the back up of a coronary care unit.

 This tells you whether your hospital performs coronary angioplasty.

 This tells you whether your hospital performs coronary artery bypass graft (CABG).

 This tells you whether your hospital has a cardiac rehabilitation unit.

If you are being privately treated for cancer, does the hospital offer radiotherapy or chemotherapy?

We tell you whether your hospital offers the core cancer services (chemotherapy, radiography and palliative care). Private hospitals usually offer surgical treatment of a wide variety of cancers. However, less of them offer radiotherapy and chemotherapy. Because these treatments are expensive, some patients prefer to receive these them under the NHS. However, others will want to be able to receive all their treatment at one hospital. We tell you which private hospitals can provide these treatments.

 This tells you whether your hospital offers radiotherapy.

 This tells you whether your hospital offers chemotherapy.

 This tells you whether your hospital offers paliative care.

BUPA uses a system of accreditation for breast cancer and bowel cancer units. To achieve BUPA approval a unit must have consultants available who are specialists in this field and who regularly submit the results of their work to be audited. It must also be able to provide a seamless transition between all the stages of treatment so that, for instance, patients needing radiotherapy after surgery are referred straight on for this service. If the hospital does not have all the necessary facilities, then it must have arrangements in place with other local hospitals that are able to provide them.

 This tells you whether your hospital has a BUPA approved breast cancer unit.

 This tells you whether your hospital has a BUPA approved bowel cancer unit.

The East

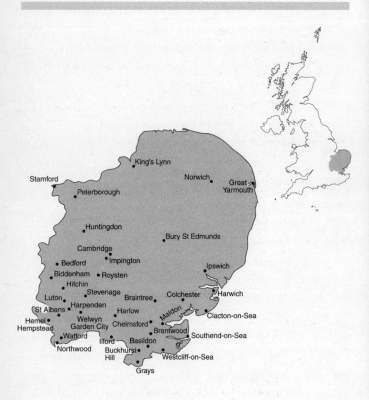

King's Lynn
Stamford
Norwich
Great
Yarmouth
Peterborough
Huntingdon
Bury St Edmunds
Cambridge
Impington
Bedford
Biddenham
Roysten
Hitchin
Ipswich
Stevenage
Luton
Braintree
Colchester
Harpenden
Harwich
St Albans
Harlow
Clacton-on-Sea
Hemel
Welwyn
Maldon
Hempstead
Garden City
Chelmsford
Watford
Brentwood
Southend-on-Sea
Northwood
Ilford
Basildon
Buckhurst
Westcliff-on-Sea
Hill
Grays

NHS

Basildon	Basildon Hospital
Bedford	Bedford Hospital
Bury St Edmonds	West Suffolk Hospital
Cambridge	Addenbrooke's Hospital
Chelmsford	Broomfield Hospital
Chelmsford	St John's Hospital
Colchester	Colchester General Hospital
Grays	Orsett Hospital
Great Yarmouth	James Paget Hospital
Harlow	Princess Alexandra Hospital, The
Hemel Hempstead	Hemel Hempstead General Hospital
Huntingdon	Hinchingbrooke Hospital
Ipswich	Ipswich Hospital
King's Lynn	Queen Elizabeth Hospital
Luton	Luton & Dunstable Hospital
Northwood	Mount Vernon Hospital
Norwich	Norfolk & Norwich Hospital
Peterborough	Peterborough General Hospital
Peterborough	Edith Cavell Hospital
St Albans	St Albans City Hospital
Stamford	Stamford & Rutland Hospital
Stevenage	Lister Hospital
Watford	Watford General Hospital
Welwyn Garden City	Queen Elizabeth II Hospital
Westcliff-on-Sea	Southend Hospital

Private

Biddenham	BMI Manor Hospital
Bury St Edmunds	Bury St Edmunds Nuffield
Cambridge	BUPA Cambridge Lea Hospital
Chelmsford	Springfield Hospital
Colchester	Oaks Hospital
Harpenden	BUPA Hospital Harpenden
Hitchin	Pinehill Hospital
Ipswich	Suffolk Nuffield at Christchurch Park Hospital
Ipswich	Suffolk Nuffield at Foxhall
King's Lynn	Sandringham Private Hospital
Northwood	BMI Bishops Wood Hospital
Norwich	BUPA Hospital Norwich
Peterborough	Fitzwilliam
Sawbridgeworth	Rivers Hospital
Southend-on-Sea	BUPA Wellesley Hospital
Watford	BUPA Hospital Bushey

Basildon · **Basildon Hospital**

Nethermayne, Basildon
Essex, SS16 5NL
Phone: 01268 533 911

Trust: Basildon and Thurrock General
Hospitals NHS Trust

Basildon Hospital opened in 1973 and is the main district hospital for the area. It is currently undergoing a £30 million development programme. So far a major extension to the children's ward has been completed and a new self-contained Breast Cancer Unit opened last year. The hospital has a stroke unit and all suspected stroke patients receive a CT scan within 48 hours of admission as recommended. The death rate for emergency stroke admissions is low. There is a separate waiting area for children in A&E although no separate treatment area.

Number of beds		650
✚ ⚕ ✖ ☎ ◉		
		regional
Overall mortality	108	104
Vacancy rates	5	3
Doctors per 100 beds	31	31
Nurses per 100 beds	95	98
Cancelled operations	0.8	2
Complaints	2	3
Complaints clear up	38	63
waiting times		
Inpatient	77	71
Outpatient	90	75

Bedford · **Bedford Hospital**

Kempston Road, Bedford
MK42 9DJ
Phone: 01234 355122

Trust: Bedford Hospital NHS Trust

Bedford Hospital is a large hospital. In A&E 99 per cent of patients are dealt with within 4 hours and the death rates for emergency admissions for hip fractures and strokes are low. The hospital's overall death rate is also low. A cancer care unit is being built as a centre of excellence for Bedfordshire. Bedford was this year acclaimed as a Beacon Site for cleanliness in the NHS.

Number of beds		475
✚ ⊕ ⚕ ✖ ☎ ◉		
		regional
Overall mortality	87	104
Vacancy rates	0	3
Doctors per 100 beds	39	36
Nurses per 100 beds	137	111
Cancelled operations	6	2
Complaints	3	3
Complaints clear up	65	63
waiting times		
Inpatient	58	71
Outpatient	69	75

Bury St Edmunds · **West Suffolk Hospital**

Hardwick Lane, Bury St Edmunds
Suffolk, IP33 2QZ
Phone: 01284 713000

Trust: West Suffolk Hospitals NHS Trust

West Suffolk Hospital recently upgraded its A&E department and now plans to build a 6-bed high dependency unit. Nine out of ten patients requiring emergency treatment in A&E are seen within the recommended time of 4 hours. The hospital has multidisciplinary teams for breast, colorectal, lung and stomach cancer treatment. CT scans for stroke patients are given within the recommended time of 48 hours.

Number of beds		680
⊕ ⊕ ⊛ ⊗ ⊕ ⊙		
		regional
Overall mortality	109	104
Vacancy rates	4	3
Doctors per 100 beds	26	31
Nurses per 100 beds	79	98
Cancelled operations	0.5	2
Complaints	4	3
Complaints clear up	81	63
waiting times		
Inpatient	62	71
Outpatient	75	75

Cambridge · **Addenbrooke's Hospital**

Hills Road, Cambridge
Cambridgeshire, CB2 2QQ
Phone: 01223 245151

Trust: Addenbrooke's NHS Trust

Addenbrooke's is a large regional teaching hospital linked to Cambridge University. The overall hospital death rate is average although the death rate for emergency hip fracture admissions is above average. The hospital's A&E has separate children's treatment and waiting areas. The hospital has a new stroke unit and administers a CT scan to patients within the recommended 48 hours of admission. The death rate for emergency stroke patients is average.

Number of beds		1300
⊕ ⊕ ⊛ ⊕ ⊗ ⊕ ⊙		
		regional
Overall mortality	98	104
Vacancy rates	5	3
Doctors per 100 beds	42	42
Nurses per 100 beds	129	129
Cancelled operations	1	2
Complaints	4	3
Complaints clear up	62	63
waiting times		
Inpatient	69	71
Outpatient	73	75

Chelmsford · **Broomfield Hospital**

Court Road, Chelmsford
Essex, CM1 7ET
Phone: 01245 440 761

Trust: Mid-Essex Hospital Services NHS Trust

Broomfield Hospital is the main district general hospital for the populations of Chelmsford, Witham, Maldon and Braintree. It is also home to the St Andrew's Centre and a large modern specialist plastic surgery and burns unit. It has become one of the biggest and most modern units of its kind, providing a range of services to an area encompassing Essex, north London and beyond.

Number of beds			596

⊕ ⊕ ⊛ ⊗ ⊕ ⊚

			regional
Overall mortality		118	104
Vacancy rates		2	3
Doctors per 100 beds		31	38
Nurses per 100 beds		92	114
Cancelled operations		0.9	2
Complaints		4	3
Complaints clear up		47	63
waiting times			
Inpatient		68	71
Outpatient		72	75

Chelmsford · **St John's Hospital**

Wood Street, Chelmsford
Essex, CM2 9BG
Phone: 01245 491 149

Trust: Mid-Essex Hospital Services NHS Trust

The services of St John's Hospital are due to be transferred to nearby Broomfield Hospital, but it currently provides paediatric, gynaecology and ENT facilities. There is no A&E at the hospital. The death rate for the Trust that runs the hospital is high.

Number of beds			183

⊗

			regional
Overall mortality		118	104
Vacancy rates		2	3
Doctors per 100 beds		31	38
Nurses per 100 beds		92	114
Cancelled operations		0.0	2
Complaints		4	3
Complaints clear up		47	63
waiting times			
Inpatient		68	71
Outpatient		72	75

Colchester · **Colchester General Hospital**

Turner Road, Colchester
Essex, CO4 5JL
Phone: 01206 747 474

Trust: Essex Rivers Healthcare NHS
   Trust

Colchester General Hospital is a large acute hospital serving north Essex. It has an A&E department with separate facilities for children. A £79 million redevelopment was announced this year that will see all Essex County Hospital services transferred to Colchester General. The Essex Rivers Healthcare Trust has a low death rate for emergency hip fracture admissions, but deaths following emergency stroke admissions are high and the overall death rate is high. The hospital does not have a separate stroke unit.

Number of beds		543
✛ ⊕ ♦ ✖ ☎		
		regional
Overall mortality	110	104
Vacancy rates	4	3
Doctors per 100 beds	30	38
Nurses per 100 beds	97	114
Cancelled operations	0.1	2
Complaints	4	3
Complaints clear up	71	63
waiting times		
Inpatient	72	71
Outpatient	73	75

Grays · **Orsett Hospital**

Rowley Road, Grays
Essex, RM16 3EU
Phone: 01268 533 911

Trust: Basildon and Thurrock General
   Hospitals NHS Trust

Orsett Hospital, in Grays, Essex, will have its inpatient wards transferred to Basildon Hospital in 2002. Its day surgery unit, outpatient clinics and diagnostic services and a minor injuries unit will continue to serve the people of Thurrock. The hospital does not have an A&E department.

Number of beds		200
		regional
Overall mortality	108	104
Vacancy rates	5	3
Doctors per 100 beds	31	31
Nurses per 100 beds	95	98
Cancelled operations	-	2
Complaints	2	3
Complaints clear up	38	63
waiting times		
Inpatient	77	71
Outpatient	90	75

Great Yarmouth · **James Paget Hospital**

Lowestoft Road, Great Yarmouth
Norfolk, NR31 6LA
Phone: 01493 452452

Trust: James Paget Healthcare NHS
Trust

The James Paget Hospital serves the inhabitants of Great Yarmouth, Lowestoft and the Waveney valley. Its A&E department has undergone an £800,000 refurbishment. Several major cancer types are treated at the hospital, and specialist multidisciplinary teams care for most patients. The A&E department has separate children's areas for waiting and treatment, but suspected heart attack patients do not currently receive thrombolytic drugs within the target 30 minutes of arrival.

Number of beds		502
⊕ ⊕ ⊛ ⊗ ⊚ ⊚		
		regional
Overall mortality	100	104
Vacancy rates	9	3
Doctors per 100 beds	32	31
Nurses per 100 beds	108	98
Cancelled operations	4	2
Complaints	4	3
Complaints clear up	86	63
waiting times		
Inpatient	75	71
Outpatient	76	75

Harlow · **Princess Alexandra Hospital**

Hamstel Road, Harlow
Essex, CM20 1QX
Phone: 01279 444 455

Trust: The Princess Alexandra Hospital
NHS Trust

The Princess Alexandra hospital has an A&E department, a coronary care unit and provides care for cancer patients with a well-known Breast Cancer Unit. The hospital has a low death rate for people needing emergency treatment for a broken hip. There are dedicated stroke facilities and suspected stroke patients receive a CT scan within the recommended 48 hours.

Number of beds		447
⊕ ⊛ ⊗ ⊚ ⊚		
		regional
Overall mortality	108	104
Vacancy rates	1	3
Doctors per 100 beds	36	36
Nurses per 100 beds	97	111
Cancelled operations	-	2
Complaints	5	3
Complaints clear up	61	63
waiting times		
Inpatient	64	71
Outpatient	79	75

Hemel Hempstead · **Hemel Hempstead General**

Hillfield Road, Hemel Hempstead
Hertfordshire, HP2 4AD
Phone: 01442 213 141

Trust: West Hertfordshire Hospitals
NHS Trust

Hemel Hempstead General Hospital provides general acute services. Just 60 per cent of patients using the A&E department are dealt with within 4 hours, and suspected heart attack patients do not currently receive thrombolytic drugs within an average of 30 minutes of arrival. The hospital performs surgery on children but does not have a paediatrician on site 24 hours a day.

Number of beds		297
		regional
Overall mortality	103	104
Vacancy rates	1	3
Doctors per 100 beds	47	38
Nurses per 100 beds	126	114
Cancelled operations	2	2
Complaints	2	3
Complaints clear up	69	63
waiting times		
Inpatient	64	71
Outpatient	75	75

Huntingdon · **Hinchingbrooke Hospital**

Hinchingbrooke Park, Huntingdon
Cambridgeshire, PE29 6NT
Phone: 01480 416416

Trust: Hinchingbrooke Healthcare NHS
Trust

This modern hospital caters for around 165,000 people spread across a 325 square mile area. Mortality rates and waiting times figures are average. Hinchingbrooke has multidisciplinary teams for most cancer treatment, and is one of only a few hospitals to provide CT scans for all suspected stroke patients within 24 hours of admission. However, not all suspected heart attack patients receive thrombolytic drugs within 30 minutes of arrival. The hospital has a paediatric ITU and a paediatrician available 24 hours a day.

Number of beds		460
		regional
Overall mortality	103	104
Vacancy rates	0	3
Doctors per 100 beds	34	36
Nurses per 100 beds	101	111
Cancelled operations	3	2
Complaints	2	3
Complaints clear up	60	63
waiting times		
Inpatient	75	71
Outpatient	72	75

Ipswich · **Ipswich Hospital**

Heath Road, Ipswich
Suffolk, IP4 5PD
Phone: 01473 712233

Trust: Ipswich Hospital NHS Trust

The Ipswich Hospital is one of the largest district general hospitals in the Eastern region, providing a full range of services such as oncology and radiotherapy. It has high death rates in both hip surgery and stroke. There are multidisciplinary teams for lung, breast, colorectal and stomach cancers and thrombolytic drugs are administered to heart attack patients within 30 minutes of arrival.

Number of beds		728
➕ ⊕ ✇ ✖ ☏ ☺		
		regional
Overall mortality	105	104
Vacancy rates	3	3
Doctors per 100 beds	32	38
Nurses per 100 beds	111	114
Cancelled operations	2	2
Complaints	4	3
Complaints clear up	65	63
waiting times		
Inpatient	71	71
Outpatient	73	75

King's Lynn · **Queen Elizabeth Hospital**

Gayton Road, King's Lynn
Norfolk, PE30 4ET
Phone: 01553 613613

Trust: King's Lynn and Wisbech

The Queen Elizabeth Hospital, King's Lynn, has recently spent £4 million creating a new critical care unit and opened a £1 million cancer and palliative care centre. It has MRI and CT scanning facilities but cannot guarantee stroke patients a CT scan within 48 hours. The hospital has single-sex wards throughout the hospital, except for ITU and CCU. It does not yet deliver thrombolysis within 30 minutes of the patient entering the hospital premises.

Number of beds		707
➕ ⊕ ✇ ✖ ☏ ☺		
		regional
Overall mortality	103	104
Vacancy rates	0	3
Doctors per 100 beds	30	31
Nurses per 100 beds	94	98
Cancelled operations	5	2
Complaints	3	3
Complaints clear up	55	63
waiting times		
Inpatient	68	71
Outpatient	75	75

Luton · **Luton & Dunstable Hospital**

Lewsey Road, Luton
Bedfordshire, LU4 0DZ
Phone: 01582 491122

Trust: Luton and Dunstable NHS Trust

The Luton & Dunstable Hospital is undergoing a £30 million re-development including the construction of a 3-storey medical wing, which will provide 4 wards and specialist facilities for older patients. Breast, lung, stomach and colorectal cancers are treated at the hospital and multidisciplinary teams are in place for all of these as recommended. However, suspected stroke patients are not guaranteed a CT scan within 48 hours of admission. Death rates for the hospital are in line with the national average.

Number of beds		524
⊕ ⊕ ⊕ ⊗ ⊕ ⊛		
		regional
Overall mortality	103	104
Vacancy rates	3	3
Doctors per 100 beds	39	31
Nurses per 100 beds	119	98
Cancelled operations	1	2
Complaints	3	3
Complaints clear up	84	63
waiting times		
Inpatient	87	71
Outpatient	73	75

Northwood · **Mount Vernon Hospital**

Rickmansworth Road, Northwood
Middlesex, HA6 2RB
Phone: 01923 826 111

Trust: West Hertfordshire Hospitals
NHS Trust

Mount Vernon Hospital covers four sites, but has no A&E department. Its dedicated cancer centre, which was given a Government beacon award, offers alternative therapies. Staff have also received a Nye Bevan award for their work. Although all the major cancers are treated, multidisciplinary teams are not used.

Number of beds		145
⊕ ⊛		
		regional
Overall mortality	103	104
Vacancy rates	1	3
Doctors per 100 beds	47	38
Nurses per 100 beds	126	114
Cancelled operations	-	2
Complaints	2	3
Complaints clear up	69	63
waiting times		
Inpatient	64	71
Outpatient	75	75

Norwich · **Norfolk & Norwich Hospital**

Brunswick Road, Norwich
Norfolk, NR1 3SR
Phone: 01603 286286

Trust: Norfolk and Norwich University
Hospital NHS Trust

The Norfolk and Norwich Hospital will close in 2002 and its services will be transferred to the new Norfolk and Norwich University Hospital. At present the hospital has single-sex wards and offers coronary angiography, meeting a key Government standard for this procedure. However, heart attack patients do not currently receive thrombolytic drugs within the target average of 30 minutes from arrival. Death rates are average and waiting times slightly better than average.

Number of beds		973
➊ ⊕ ✿ ⊗ 🚑 ◐		
		regional
Overall mortality	94	104
Vacancy rates	2	3
Doctors per 100 beds	43	38
Nurses per 100 beds	143	114
Cancelled operations	0.7	2
Complaints	3	3
Complaints clear up	82	63
waiting times		
Inpatient	77	71
Outpatient	78	75

Peterborough · **Peterborough District Hospital**

Thorpe Road, Peterborough
Cambridgeshire, PE3 6DA
Phone: 01733 874000

Trust: Peterborough Hospitals NHS
Trust

Peterborough District Hospital has recently used a £615,000 Government cash injection to modernise its A&E. It is now child friendly with designated waiting and treatment areas for children. Among emergency admissions, patients with a broken hip have a low death rate, but deaths following strokes are high even though the hospital has an acute stroke unit and performs CT scans on all suspected stroke patients within 24 hours of admission.

Number of beds		363
➊ ⊕ ✿ ⊗ 🚑 ◐		
		regional
Overall mortality	102	104
Vacancy rates	2	3
Doctors per 100 beds	30	31
Nurses per 100 beds	100	98
Cancelled operations	-	2
Complaints	3	3
Complaints clear up	67	63
waiting times		
Inpatient	82	71
Outpatient	75	75

Peterborough · **Edith Cavell Hospital**

Bresson Gate, Peterborough
Cambridgeshire, PE3 9GZ
Phone: 01733 874000

Trust: Peterborough Hospitals NHS
Trust

Edith Cavell Hospital is the second site of Peterborough District Hospitals NHS Trust. Most acute services are provided by Peterborough District Hospital although patients for several specialties including ENT, rheumatology and care for the elderly are referred to the Edith Cavell. Across the Trust staffing levels and waiting times are close to the national average. The overall death rate is also average.

Number of beds		-
✕ ◉		
		regional
Overall mortality	102	104
Vacancy rates	2	3
Doctors per 100 beds	30	31
Nurses per 100 beds	100	98
Cancelled operations	-	2
Complaints	3	3
Complaints clear up	67	63
waiting times		
Inpatient	82	71
Outpatient	75	75

St Albans · **St Albans City Hospital**

Waverley Road, St Albans
Hertfordshire, AL3 5TL
Phone: 01727 866 122

Trust: West Hertfordshire Hospitals
NHS Trust

St Albans City Hospital does not have an A&E department but has a minor injuries unit. The hospital has a one-stop breast cancer clinic where patients urgently referred by their GP will receive the necessary tests and diagnosis, with a decision on treatment and counselling support all on the same day. It is run by West Hertfordshire Hospitals NHS Trust, which has average death rates.

Number of beds		94
◑		
		regional
Overall mortality	103	104
Vacancy rates	1	3
Doctors per 100 beds	47	38
Nurses per 100 beds	126	114
Cancelled operations	-	2
Complaints	2	3
Complaints clear up	69	63
waiting times		
Inpatient	64	71
Outpatient	75	75

Stamford · **Stamford & Rutland Hospital**

Ryhall Road, Stamford
Lincolnshire, PE9 1UA
Phone: 01780 764151

Trust: North West Anglia Healthcare
NHS Trust

Stamford and Rutland hospital is a small acute hospital managed by the North West Anglia Healthcare NHS Trust. The hospital has a minor injuries department and X-ray services are available 24 hours a day. Only elective surgery is undertaken at the hospital. Clinics for cancer patients are run here but treatment is provided by neighbouring hospitals in particular the Peterborough Hospitals NHS Trust. Waiting times at the hospital are shorter than average particularly for inpatient admission.

Number of beds		90
➕ ✖		
		regional
Overall mortality	-	104
Vacancy rates	-	3
Doctors per 100 beds	-	38
Nurses per 100 beds	-	114
Cancelled operations	-	2
Complaints	-	3
Complaints clear up	26	63
waiting times		
Inpatient	87	71
Outpatient	71	75

Stevenage · **Lister Hospital**

Coreys Mill Lane, Stevenage
Hertfordshire, SG1 4AB
Phone: 01438 314333

Trust: East and North Hertfordshire
NHS Trust

Lister Hospital completed a £1.5 million overhaul and refurbishment of its A&E department in February 2001. The hospital meets a government recommended standard for coronary angiographies, by peforming at least 500 catheterisations per year. But heart attack patients aren't currently given thrombolysis within an average of 30 minutes of arrival at A&E. The hospital has high death rates for those admitted as emergencies with broken hips or strokes.

Number of beds		430
➕ 🔧 ✖ 🔵 🔵		
		regional
Overall mortality	107	104
Vacancy rates	2	3
Doctors per 100 beds	32	38
Nurses per 100 beds	108	114
Cancelled operations	1	2
Complaints	4	3
Complaints clear up	86	63
waiting times		
Inpatient	74	71
Outpatient	71	75

Watford · **Watford General Hospital**

60 Vicarage Road, Watford
Hertfordshire, WD1 8OHB
Phone: 01923 244 366

Trust: West Hertfordshire Hospitals
**   NHS Trust**

Watford General is a medium-sized district general hospital serving West Hertfordshire. The Trust that runs the hospital has average death rates. A&E waiting times are slow compared to other hospitals and inpatient waiting times are longer than average. A paediatrician is on site 24 hours a day as recommended by the Royal College of Surgeons and single-sex wards are available throughout the hospital.

Number of beds		352
✚ ⊕ 〽 ✖ ☏		
		regional
Overall mortality	103	104
Vacancy rates	1	3
Doctors per 100 beds	47	38
Nurses per 100 beds	126	114
Cancelled operations	2	2
Complaints	2	3
Complaints clear up	69	63
waiting times		
Inpatient	64	71
Outpatient	75	75

Welwyn Garden City · **Queen Elizabeth II Hospital**

Howlands, Welwyn Garden City
Hertfordshire, AL7 4HQ
Phone: 01707 328 111

Trust: East and North Hertfordshire
**   NHS Trust**

The A&E department of the Queen Elizabeth II hospital has undergone a £750,000 extension, in order to improve the department's ability to cater for major accident and trauma victims. The hospital has a stroke rehabilitation department, but suspected stroke patients do not always receive CT scans within 48 hours of arrival. The Trust has a high death rate among patients admitted as emergencies with a stroke or a broken hip.

Number of beds		367
✚ 〽 ✖ ☏ ◉		
		regional
Overall mortality	107	104
Vacancy rates	2	3
Doctors per 100 beds	32	38
Nurses per 100 beds	108	114
Cancelled operations	1	2
Complaints	4	3
Complaints clear up	86	63
waiting times		
Inpatient	74	71
Outpatient	71	75

Westcliff-on-Sea · **Southend Hospital**

Prittlewell Chase, Westcliff-on-Sea
Essex, SS0 0RT
Phone: 01702 435 555

Trust: Southend Hospital NHS Trust

Southend Hospital has recently refurbished a range of facilities including its pathology laboratories and the A&E department. Death rates for emergency broken hip admissions are high but the overall death rate is average. The hospital provides coronary angiography and meets a key Government target for this procedure by performing at least 500 catheterisations a year. There are dedicated stroke and renal units, and the hospital provides CT scans for all suspected stroke patients within the recommended 48 hours of admission.

Number of beds		804
✚ ⊕ ♨ ✖ ☎ ◉		
		regional
Overall mortality	95	104
Vacancy rates	4	3
Doctors per 100 beds	29	38
Nurses per 100 beds	113	114
Cancelled operations	4	2
Complaints	3	3
Complaints clear up	21	63
waiting times		
Inpatient	68	71
Outpatient	80	75

Biddenham · **BMI Manor Hospital**

Church End, Biddenham
Bedford, MK40 4AW
Phone: 01234 364 252

The BMI Manor Hospital, which has 25 beds, offers a broad range of services to its patients including diagnostic procedures, cosmetic surgery and cancer services.

General Healthcare Group Ltd

Insurers: BUPA*, PPP*, Norwich, Standard Life, Royal Sun Alliance, WPA,

price guide	£
Hip replacement	8055
Cataract removal	1990-2500

Number of beds	25
Doctors per beds	1
heart services	-
Cancer services	

Bury St Edmunds · **Bury St Edmunds Nuffield**

St Mary's Square, Bury St Edmunds
West Suffolk, IP33 2AA
Phone: 01284 701371

Over the past two years clinical facilities have been upgraded providing "state of the art" theatres and diagnostic imaging. There is also a physiotherapy department. The hospital has a Fixed Price scheme for patients who do not have private medical insurance.

Nuffield Hospitals

Insurers: BUPA*, PPP*, Norwich*, Standard Life*, Royal Sun Alliance*, WPA

price guide	£
Hip replacement	6800-7000
Cataract removal	2100-2400

Number of beds	40
ALS staff	2
heart services	-
Cancer services	

Cambridge · **BUPA Cambridge Lea Hospital**

30 New Road, Impington
Cambridge, CB4 9EL
Phone: 01223 266900

BUPA Cambridge Lea Hospital has strong links with Addenbrooke's NHS Trust, including an MRI scanner partnership and two joint specialist nursing posts.

BUPA Hospitals

Insurers: BUPA, PPP, Norwich, Standard Life, Royal Sun Alliance, WPA

price guide	£
Hip replacement	7861-7861
Cataract removal	2450-2450

Number of beds	60
Doctors per beds	3
heart services	
Cancer services	

Chelmsford · **Springfield Hospital**

Lawn Lane, Springfield
Chelmsford, Essex, CM1 7GU
Phone: 01245 234000

Springfield Hospital is situated in a
semi-rural location on the outskirts of
Chelmsford. It is modern and well
equipped, managing a range of
surgical and medical conditions with
contemporary technology.

Capio Healthcare UK

Insurers: BUPA*, PPP*, Norwich*,
Standard Life*, Royal Sun Alliance*, WPA*

price guide	£
Hip replacement	8040-8844
Cataract removal	2733-3010

Number of beds	
ALS staff	1
heart services	–
Cancer services	

Colchester · **Oaks Hospital**

Oaks Place, Mile End Rd
Colchester, CO4 5XR
Phone: 01206 752121

The Oaks Hospital provides a range of
medical facilities including a private GP
clinic. Services include osteoporosis
treatment, prostate assessment, a pain
clinic and an occupational therapy
service for the disabled.

Capio Healthcare UK

Insurers: BUPA*, PPP*, Norwich*,
Standard Life*, Royal Sun Alliance*, WPA*

price guide	£
Hip replacement	7400
Cataract removal	2500

Number of beds	
ALS staff	1
heart services	–
Cancer services	

Harpenden · **BUPA Hospital Harpenden**

Ambrose Lane, Harpenden
Herts, AL5 4BP
Phone: 01582 763191

BUPA Hospital Harpenden offers a
range of facilities and is best known for
its Back and Neck Clinic, which uses
special exercise machines to
strengthen problem muscles.

BUPA Hospitals

Insurers: BUPA, PPP, Norwich, Standard Life,
Royal Sun Alliance, WPA

price guide	£
Hip replacement	7421-7421
Cataract removal	1900-2500

Number of beds	61
ALS staff	2
heart services	–
Cancer services	

Hitchin · **Pinehill Hospital**

Benslow Lane, Hitchin
Hertfordshire, SG4 9QZ
Phone: 01462 422 822

Pinehill Hospital, located on the outskirts of Hitchin, offers a range of surgical and medical services. Consultants are drawn mainly from the hospitals of the East and North Hertfordshire NHS Trust.

Capio Healthcare UK

Insurers: BUPA*, PPP, Norwich Standard Life*, Royal Sun Alliance, WPA

price guide	£
Hip replacement	7953-7992
Cataract removal	1500-1900

Number of beds	34
ALS staff	1
heart services	-
Cancer services	✪ ① ✔

Ipswich · **Suffolk Nuffield at Christchurch Park**

57-61 Fonnereau Rd, Ipswich
Suffolk, IP1 3JN
Phone: 01473 256071

The Suffolk Nuffield at Christchurch Park offers an allergy clinic, respite care and general health and breast screening. There is a sister hospital at Foxhall.

Nuffield Nursing Homes Trust

Insurers: BUPA*, PPP*, Norwich, Standard Life, Royal Sun Alliance, WPA

price guide	£
Hip replacement	7400-7550
Cataract removal	2200-2300

Number of beds	43
ALS staff	1
heart services	-
Cancer services	✪

Ipswich · **Suffolk Nuffield at Foxhall**

Foxhall Rd, Ipswich
Suffolk, IP4 5SW
Phone: 01473 279100

The Suffolk Nuffield at Foxhall has 71 admitting consultants drawn from nearby hospitals including the NHS Ipswich hospital. It has a sister hospital at Christchurch Park.

Nuffield Nursing Homes Trust

Insurers: BUPA*, PPP*, Norwich, Standard Life, Royal Sun Alliance, WPA

price guide	£
Hip replacement	7400-7550
Cataract removal	2200-2300

Number of beds	46
Doctors per beds	1
heart services	-
Cancer services	✪

King's Lynn · **Sandringham Private Hospital**

Gayton Rd, King's Lynn
Norfolk, PE30 4HJ
Phone: 01553 769770

Opened in 1990 in response to local needs, this purpose-built unit works in partnership with King's Lynn & Wisbech Hospitals NHS Trust to provide private healthcare to the community of East Anglia.

General Healthcare Group LTD

Insurers: BUPA*, PPP*, Norwich, Royal Sun Alliance, WPA

price guide	£
Hip replacement	5880-6409
Cataract removal	1782-2131

Number of beds	35
ALS staff	1

heart services	-
Cancer services	

Northwood · **BMI Bishops Wood Hospital**

Rickmanworth Rd, Northwood
Middlesex, HA6 2JW
Phone: 01923 835 814

Bishops Wood Hospital works in partnership with NHS Mount Vernon Hospital, making use of the hospital's specialist facilities. Bishops Wood also offers a range of complementary therapies including acupuncture, relaxation techniques and massage.

General Healthcare Group

Insurers: BUPA*, PPP*, Norwich*, Royal Sun Alliance*, WPA

price guide	£
Hip replacement	7410-9510
Cataract removal	2366-2496

Number of beds	47
ALS staff	4

heart services	-
Cancer services	

Norwich · **BUPA Hospital Norwich**

Old Watton Road, Colney
Norwich, NR4 7TD
Phone: 01603 456181

Located near the Norfolk & Norwich NHS hospital, this modern purpose-built hospital has nine dedicated day case beds and two special parent/child rooms.

BUPA Hospitals

Insurers: BUPA, PPP, Norwich, Standard Life, Royal Sun Alliance, WPA

price guide	£
Hip replacement	1941-2240
Cataract removal	7854-7854

Number of beds	67
ALS staff	1

heart services	-
Cancer services	

Peterborough · **Fitzwilliam**

Milton Way, South Bretton
Peterborough, Cambridgeshire, PE3 9AQ
Phone: 01733 21717

The Fitzwilliam Hospital offers a range
of surgical and medical procedures,
and extensive diagnostic and
treatment facilities, including X-ray,
physiotherapy, ultrasound, MRI, sports
injury clinic, IVF, health screening,
complementary therapies and
cosmetic surgery.

Community Hospitals Group

Insurers: BUPA, PPP, Norwich Union,
Standard Life, Royal Sun Alliance, WPA

price guide	£
Hip replacement	7050 - 8500
Cataract removal	2150

Number of beds	55
ALS staff	2
heart services	-
Cancer services	🌐 ✓ ✓

Sawbridgeworth · **Rivers Hospital**

High Wych Rd, Sawbridgeworth
Hertfordshire, CM21 0HH
Phone: 01279 600282

The Rivers Hospital is creating a new
operating theatre and 12 new patient
rooms. The Princess Alexandra Hospital
in Harlow plans to use The Rivers for
extra capacity this winter.

Capio Healthcare UK

Insurers: BUPA*, PPP*, Norwich*,
Standard Life*, Royal Sun Alliance*, WPA*

price guide	£
Hip replacement	8270-13349
Cataract removal	2190-2272

Number of beds	
ALS staff	1
heart services	-
Cancer services	🌐 ✓ ✓

Southend-on-Sea · **BUPA Wellesley Hospital**

Eastern Avenue, Southend-on-Sea
Essex, SS2 4XH
Phone: 01702 462944

The hospital offers a wide range of
medical and surgical procedures. The
outpatients department includes ten
consulting rooms, with facilities for
minor procedures to be carried out.

BUPA Hospitals

Insurers: BUPA, PPP, Norwich, Standard Life,
Royal Sun Alliance, WPA

price guide	£
Hip replacement	7722-7722
Cataract removal	2055-2393

Number of beds	51
ALS staff	2
heart services	-
Cancer services	🌐 🌓 ✓ ✓

Watford · **BUPA Hospital Bushey**

Heathbourne Road, Bushey
Herts, WD23 1RD
Phone: 020 8950 9090

BUPA Hospital Bushey offers a wide variety of services and facilities ranging from the BUPA Approved Breast Care Unit to hip and knee replacements, cataract removal and plastic surgery.

BUPA Hospitals

Insurers: BUPA, PPP, Norwich, Standard Life, Royal Sun Alliance, WPA

price guide	£
Hip replacement	7605-7605
Cataract removal	2390-2390

Number of beds	73
Doctors per beds	3
heart services	–
Cancer services	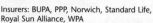

London

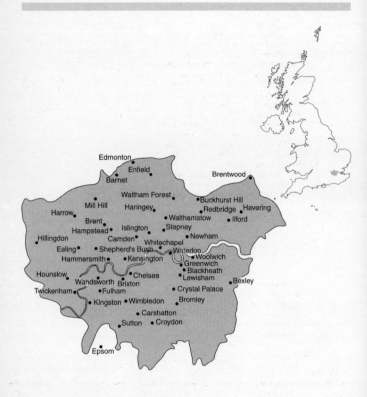

	NHS
Archway	Whittington Hospital, The
Barking	Barking Hospital
Barnet	Barnet Hospital
Bow	St Andrew's Hospital
Bromley	Bromley Hospital
Camberwell	King's College Hospital
Carshalton	St Helier Hospital
Croydon	Mayday Hospital
Edmonton	North Middlesex University Hospital, The
Enfield	Chase Farm Hospital
Epsom	Epsom General Hospital
Fulham	Chelsea and Westminster Hospital
Hackney	Homerton Hospital
Hammersmith	Charing Cross Hospital
Hampstead	Queen Mary's Hospital
Hampstead	Royal Free Hospital
Harrow	Northwick Park Hospital

Ilford	King George Hospital
Isleworth	West Middlesex University Hospital
Kingston upon Thames	Kingston Hospital
Lewisham	University Hospital Lewisham
Leytonstone	Whipps Cross University Hospital
Marylebone	Middlesex & University College Hospitals
Orpington	Farnborough Hospital
Orpington	Orpington Hospital
Paddington	St Mary's Hospital
Park Royal	Central Middlesex Hospital
Plaistow	Newham General Hospital
Romford	Harold Wood Hospital
Romford	Oldchurch Hospital
Shepherd's Bush	Hammersmith Hospital
Sidcup	Queen Mary's Hospital
Southall	Ealing Hospital
Summerstown	St George's Hospital
Uxbridge	Hillingdon Hospital
Waterloo	Guy's Hospital
Waterloo	St Thomas' Hospital
West Smithfield	St Bartholomew's Hospital
Whitechapel	Royal London Hospital
Woolwich	Queen Elizabeth Hospital

Private

Ashtead	Ashtead Hospital
Beckenham	BMI The Sloane Hospital
Bermondsey	London Bridge Hospital
Blackheath	BMI The Blackheath Hospital
Brentwood	BUPA Hartswood Hospital
Brentwood	Essex Nuffield Hospital
Brixton	Guthrie Clinic
Buckhurst Hill	Holly House Hospital
Chelsea	Lister Hospital
Croydon	BMI Shirley Oaks Hospital
Enfield	BMI The King's Oak Hospital
Enfield	North London Nuffield Hospital
Harrow	BMI The Clementine Churchill Hospital
Hendon	BMI Garden Hospital
Ilford	BUPA Roding Hospital
Kingston upon Thames	New Victoria Hospital
Marylebone	Harley Street Clinic
Marylebone	King Edward VII's Hospital Sister Agnes
Marylebone	London Clinic
Marylebone	Princess Grace Hospital
Orpington	BMI Chelsfield Park Hospital
South Kensington	Cromwell Hospital
St John's Wood	Wellington Hospital
Stepney	BMI London Independent Hospital
Sutton	St Anthony's Hospital
Wimbledon	Parkside Hospital

Archway · **Whittington Hospital**

Highgate Hill, Archway
London, N19 5NF
Phone: 020 7272 3070

Trust: Whittington Hospital NHS Trust

Construction begins early in 2002 to build a wide range of new facilities including refurbishing the A&E at the Whittington. Overall, the mortality rate for the hospital is low and waiting times are shorter than average. Multidisciplinary teams are offered for treatment of lung, breast, stomach and colorectal cancers. Government targets are met to ensure that stroke patients should be scanned within 48 hours. Paediatric surgery is offered and a paediatrician is on site round-the-clock.

Number of beds		470
✪ ⊕ ♘ ✪ ☏ ◉		
		regional
Overall mortality	90	96
Vacancy rates	0	3
Doctors per 100 beds	45	37
Nurses per 100 beds	143	107
Cancelled operations	0.5	4
Complaints	2	4
Complaints clear up	24	48
waiting times		
Inpatient	91	72
Outpatient	82	76

Barking · **Barking Hospital**

Upney Lane, Barking
Essex, IG11 9LX
Phone: 020 8983 8000

Trust: Barking, Havering and Redbridge Hospitals NHS Trust

Barking Hospital, part of the recently merged Barking, Havering and Redbridge NHS Trust, is a rehabilitation hospital. It does not have an A&E unit and provides services together with the larger King George Hospital in Ilford and the Harold Wood Hospital in Romford.

Number of beds		115
		regional
Overall mortality	106	96
Vacancy rates	-	3
Doctors per 100 beds	25	42
Nurses per 100 beds	76	117
Cancelled operations	-	4
Complaints	4	4
Complaints clear up	54	48
waiting times		
Inpatient	67	72
Outpatient	73	76

Barnet · **Barnet Hospital**

Wellhouse Lane, Barnet
Hertfordshire, EN5 3DH
Phone: 020 8216 4000

Trust: Barnet and Chase Farm Hospitals
NHS Trust

Barnet Hospital is a large facility north of London currently undergoing major building work. New wards and departments are being developed so that all outpatient services, pathology services, and medical and elderly care wards will be brought together on one site when facilities open in spring 2002. The Trust, which operates this hospital and the nearby Chase Farm site, has an average overall mortality rate.

Number of beds		459
		regional
Overall mortality	107	96
Vacancy rates	1	3
Doctors per 100 beds	38	42
Nurses per 100 beds	123	117
Cancelled operations	0	4
Complaints	4	4
Complaints clear up	64	48
waiting times		
Inpatient	64	72
Outpatient	69	76

Bow · **St Andrew's Hospital**

Devons Road, Bow
London, E3 3HT
Phone: 020 7476 4000

Trust: Newham Healthcare NHS Trust

St. Andrew's Hospital, part of Newham Healthcare Trust, is due to close in 2004, when services will be transferred to the larger Newham General Hospital. There is no A&E department at the hospital.

Number of beds		78
		regional
Overall mortality	109	96
Vacancy rates	3	3
Doctors per 100 beds	33	37
Nurses per 100 beds	99	107
Cancelled operations	-	4
Complaints	3	4
Complaints clear up	29	48
waiting times		
Inpatient	83	72
Outpatient	77	76

Bromley · **Bromley Hospital**

Cromwell Avenue, Bromley
Kent, BR2 9AJ
Phone: 020 8289 7000

Trust: Bromley Hospitals NHS Trust

Bromley is the main district general hospital for the Bromley Hospital NHS Trust. Farnborough Hospital, which is currently under construction, will shortly replace it. The Trust has a relatively high death rate for emergency hip fracture admissions but average death rates in other areas. Its A&E unit has separate children's waiting and treatment areas; however, there is not always a paediatrician on site at the hospital and there is no separate paediatric ward. The A&E unit is due to close in 2003.

Number of beds		201
○ ⊕ ⊘ ⊗ ⊕		
		regional
Overall mortality	98	96
Vacancy rates	7	3
Doctors per 100 beds	34	37
Nurses per 100 beds	81	107
Cancelled operations	5	4
Complaints	5	4
Complaints clear up	50	48
waiting times		
Inpatient	63	72
Outpatient	80	76

Camberwell · **King's College Hospital**

Denmark Hill
London, SE5 9RS
Phone: 0207 737 4000

Trust: King's Healthcare NHS Trust

King's College Hospital is a major London teaching hospital that specialises in areas such as liver disease and transplantation and neurology. Coronary angiographies are performed and the hospital meets a key national standard in this procedure. All suspected stroke patients receive CT scans within 48 hours of admission, in line with the Government target. Death rates at the hospital are average or low, with a low death rate for people requiring emergency treatment for a broken hip.

Number of beds		907
○ ⊕ ⊘ ⊕ ⊗ ⊕ ◉		
		regional
Overall mortality	95	96
Vacancy rates	4	3
Doctors per 100 beds	59	56
Nurses per 100 beds	157	154
Cancelled operations	1	4
Complaints	5	4
Complaints clear up	63	48
waiting times		
Inpatient	74	72
Outpatient	86	76

Carshalton · **St Helier Hospital**

Wrythe Lane, Carshalton
Surrey, SM5 1AA
Phone: 020 8296 2000

Trust: Epsom and St Helier NHS Trust

Following recent criticism over high death rates, St Helier has been battling to improve standards. Although death rates for emergency broken hip surgery remain high, its overall mortality rate is now no higher than most other hospitals. The hospital provides thrombolysis for heart attack patients within the target average of 30 minutes from arrival and has a 6-bed single-sex CCU. The hospital has MRI and CT scanning facilities. Multidisciplinary teams manage the treatment of lung, colorectal and stomach cancer patients.

Number of beds		600
➊ ➕ ♫ ✖ ☎ ◉		
		regional
Overall mortality	105	96
Vacancy rates	3	3
Doctors per 100 beds	43	42
Nurses per 100 beds	115	117
Cancelled operations	0	4
Complaints	3	4
Complaints clear up	57	48
waiting times		
Inpatient	73	72
Outpatient	82	76

Croydon · **Mayday Hospital**

London Road, Croydon
CR7 7YE
Phone: 0208 401 3000

Trust: Mayday Healthcare NHS Trust

Mayday University Hospital serves the population of Croydon. A key Government standard for coronary angiography is achieved with over 500 catheterisations performed each year and heart attack patients are given thrombolytic drugs within the target 30 minutes of arrival on average. However, suspected stroke patients are not guaranteed a CT scan within 48 hours of admission and death rates for emergency broken hip patients are high. Inpatient waiting times are worse than average but outpatient waiting times are good.

Number of beds		719
➊ ♫ ✖ ☎ ◉		
		regional
Overall mortality	110	96
Vacancy rates	1	3
Doctors per 100 beds	36	37
Nurses per 100 beds	101	107
Cancelled operations	4	4
Complaints	3.9	4
Complaints clear up	30	48
waiting times		
Inpatient	68	72
Outpatient	78	76

Edmonton · **North Middlesex University Hospital**

Sterling Way
London, N18 1QX
Phone: 020 8887 2000

Trust: North Middlesex Hospital NHS Trust

North Middlesex Hospital serves around 500,000 people within the London Boroughs of Enfield and Haringey and treats around 20,000 inpatients a year. This hospital offers coronary angiography and performs 500 catheterisations per year. Heart attack patients can expect to receive thrombolysis within the target average of 30 minutes of their arrival. CT scans are performed on all suspected stroke patients within 48 hours of being admitted. The A&E department also has separate child treatment and waiting areas.

Number of beds		481
➊ ⊕ ⟐ ⊕ ✖ ⊗ ◉		
		regional
Overall mortality	91	96
Vacancy rates	8	3
Doctors per 100 beds	45	37
Nurses per 100 beds	138	107
Cancelled operations	2	4
Complaints	2	4
Complaints clear up	42	48
waiting times		
Inpatient	59	72
Outpatient	64	76

Enfield · **Chase Farm Hospital**

The Ridgeway, Enfield
Middlesex, EN2 8JL
Phone: 020 8366 6600

Trust: Barnet and Chase Farm Hospitals NHS Trust

Chase Farm Hospital is an acute district general situated in North Enfield. Building and development programmes have been ongoing in recent years. A new surgical block opened in 1995 and last year the Health Secretary agreed a £41 million grant for a new diagnostic and treatment centre. The overall mortality rate for the Trust that operates this hospital and Barnet Hospital is average. Death rates following emergency admissions with hip fractures and strokes are also average.

Number of beds		469
➊ ⟐ ✖ ⊗ ◉		
		regional
Overall mortality	107	96
Vacancy rates	1	3
Doctors per 100 beds	38	42
Nurses per 100 beds	123	117
Cancelled operations	-	4
Complaints	4	4
Complaints clear up	64	48
waiting times		
Inpatient	64	72
Outpatient	69	76

Epsom · **Epsom General Hospital**

Dorking Road, Epsom
Surrey, KT18 7EG
Phone: 01372 735 735

Trust: Epsom and St Helier NHS Trust

After last year's critical government report, the hospital is currently seeing some changes and improvements. The hospital's death rate for emergency hip fracture admissions is high and only 55 per cent of A&E patients are dealt with within 4 hours. However, on other measures of mortality, the hospital performs in line with expectations. Also, inpatient and outpatient waiting times are average. Not all stroke patients receive a CT scan within the recommended 48 hours of admission.

Number of beds		300
✚ ⊕ ⚕ ✖ ☏ ◉		
		regional
Overall mortality	105	96
Vacancy rates	3	3
Doctors per 100 beds	43	42
Nurses per 100 beds	115	117
Cancelled operations	0	4
Complaints	3	4
Complaints clear up	57	48
waiting times		
Inpatient	73	72
Outpatient	82	76

Fulham · **Chelsea and Westminster Hospital**

369 Fulham Road
London, SW10 9NH
Phone: 020 8746 8000

Trust: Chelsea and Westminster
  Healthcare NHS Trust

The Chelsea and Westminster Hospital opened in 1993 and offers a range of clinical services. It is a teaching centre and part of Imperial College School of Medicine.

It has a low overall mortality rate and low death rates for patients admitted in an emergency with a stroke or fractured hip. However, heart attack patients don't always receive thrombolysis within the recommended 30 minutes of A&E arrival.

Number of beds		497
✚ ⊕ ⚕ ✖ ☏ ◉		
		regional
Overall mortality	81	96
Vacancy rates	0	3
Doctors per 100 beds	70	56
Nurses per 100 beds	155	154
Cancelled operations	4	4
Complaints	3	4
Complaints clear up	82	48
waiting times		
Inpatient	82	72
Outpatient	89	76

Hackney · **Homerton Hospital**

Homerton Row
London, E9 6SR
Phone: 020 8510 5555

Trust: Homerton Hospital NHS Trust

The Homerton Hospital provides specialist treatments for people across London. It is also a major teaching centre. Nine out of ten patients needing emergency treatment are now seen within 4 hours. Death rates, particularly following broken hip surgery, are low. The hospital has multidisciplinary cancer teams. Homerton does not yet administer thrombolysis for heart attack patients within 30 minutes.

Number of beds		482
✚ ⊕ ✿ ✖ ⬙		
		regional
Overall mortality	90	96
Vacancy rates	0	3
Doctors per 100 beds	33	40
Nurses per 100 beds	114	114
Cancelled operations	0.5	4
Complaints	2	4
Complaints clear up	56	48
waiting times		
Inpatient	99	72
Outpatient	76	76

Hammersmith · **Charing Cross Hospital**

Fulham Palace Road
London, W6 8RF
Phone: 020 8383 0000

Trust: Hammersmith Hospitals NHS Trust

Charing Cross is a large acute hospital in West London with a busy A&E department. The hospital's overall mortality rate is low, but deaths following emergency admission with a broken hip are high. Also, heart attack patients don't always receive thrombolysis within the recommended 30 minutes of arrival in A&E. Recent improvements include refurbished facilities for older people and a new call centre booking system for GPs to book appointments at a time convenient to their patient.

Number of beds		640
✚ ✿ ✖ ⬙ ◉		
		regional
Overall mortality	87	96
Vacancy rates	2	3
Doctors per 100 beds	48	56
Nurses per 100 beds	154	154
Cancelled operations	-	4
Complaints	3	4
Complaints clear up	72	48
waiting times		
Inpatient	83	72
Outpatient	87	76

Hampstead · **Queen Mary's Hospital**

124 Heath Street, Hampstead
London, NW3 1DU
Phone: 020 7794 0500

Trust: Royal Free Hampstead NHS Trust

Queen Mary's Hospital is affiliated to the Royal Free Hampstead, which has a low death rate, and multidisciplinary teams treat all major cancers. Between the two hospitals there are dedicated stroke facilities and all suspected stroke patients receive a CT scan within 24 hours of admission. There is also a coronary care unit, but the hospital does not offer angiography. The hospital has a renal unit.

Number of beds		-
		regional
Overall mortality	79	96
Vacancy rates	2	3
Doctors per 100 beds	53	56
Nurses per 100 beds	128	154
Cancelled operations	3	4
Complaints	6	4
Complaints clear up	42	48
waiting times		
Inpatient	71	72
Outpatient	72	76

Hampstead · **Royal Free Hospital**

Pond Street, Hampstead
London, NW3 2QG
Phone: 020 7794 0500

Trust: Royal Free Hampstead NHS Trust

The Royal Free is internationally regarded as a centre for excellence in a range of specialties including cancer, neurosciences, HIV, and transplantation surgery. The overall mortality rate for the hospital is low and the death rates for emergency stroke admissions is also low. The Royal Free is one of only a few hospitals to provide CT scans to all suspected stroke patients within 24 hours of admission. The hospital performs coronary angiography and meets key government standards for heart services.

Number of beds		1200
➊ ⊕ ⚕ ✖ ⚕ ☉		
		regional
Overall mortality	79	96
Vacancy rates	2	3
Doctors per 100 beds	53	56
Nurses per 100 beds	128	154
Cancelled operations	3	4
Complaints	6	4
Complaints clear up	42	48
waiting times		
Inpatient	71	72
Outpatient	72	76

Harrow · **Northwick Park Hospital**

Watford Road, Harrow
Middlesex, HA1 3UJ
Phone: 020 8864 3232

Trust: North West London Hospitals
Trust

Northwick Park Hospital has undergone major development and refurbishment in the past year. It has a low mortality rate, and the rate of deaths following emergency stroke admissions is also low. It performs CT scans on all suspected stroke patients within the recommended time of 24 hours and meets Government targets in two key areas of heart disease therapy by administering thrombolysis to heart attack patients within an average of 30 minutes of arrival and performing the recommended level of coronary angiographies.

Number of beds		850
➕ ⊕ ☣ ❌ ☎ ◉		
		regional
Overall mortality	86	96
Vacancy rates	0	3
Doctors per 100 beds	55	42
Nurses per 100 beds	132	117
Cancelled operations	2	4
Complaints	6	4
Complaints clear up	35	48
waiting times		
Inpatient	66	72
Outpatient	79	76

Ilford · **King George Hospital**

Barley Lane, Ilford
Essex, IG3 8YB
Phone: 020 8983 8000

Trust: Barking, Havering and
Redbridge Hospitals NHS Trust

The King George Hospital, Ilford, serves a population of around 230,000, drawn from the London Boroughs of Redbridge, Barking and Dagenham and Waltham Forest. The hospital has single-sex wards. The A&E department has separate child treatment and waiting areas and all suspected stroke patients receive a CT scan within 24 hours of admission. Paediatric surgery is performed at the hospital and there is a paediatrician on site 24 hours a day as recommended by the Royal College of Surgeons.

Number of beds		514
➕ ⊕ ☣ ❌ ☎ ◉		
		regional
Overall mortality	106	96
Vacancy rates	-	3
Doctors per 100 beds	25	42
Nurses per 100 beds	76	117
Cancelled operations	7	4
Complaints	4	4
Complaints clear up	54	48
waiting times		
Inpatient	67	72
Outpatient	73	76

Isleworth · **West Middlesex University Hospital**

Twickenham Road, Isleworth
Middlesex, TW7 6AF
Phone: 020 8560 2121

Trust: West Middlesex University
Hospital NHS Trust

West Middlesex Hospital is currently undergoing a £50 million development programme. Death rates for emergency broken hip surgery and stroke are high, and the overall mortality rate is slightly above average. Inpatient waiting times are worse than average. Patients suffering heart attacks are given thrombolysis within 30 minutes of entering the hospital and multidisciplinary teams are in place for treatment of breast, lung, stomach and colorectal cancers.

Number of beds		418

➕ ⊕ 🜨 ⊗ ☏ ◉

		regional
Overall mortality	110	96
Vacancy rates	0	3
Doctors per 100 beds	46	40
Nurses per 100 beds	117	114
Cancelled operations	3	4
Complaints	5	4
Complaints clear up	69	48
waiting times		
Inpatient	63	72
Outpatient	85	76

Kingston upon Thames · **Kingston Hospital**

Galsworthy Road, Kingston upon Thames,
Surrey, KT2 7QB
Phone: 020 8546 7711

Trust: Kingston Hospital NHS Trust

Kingston Hospital has just opened its new A&E department. Lung, breast, stomach and colorectal cancers are treated there, with multidisciplinary teams on hand for each. The hospital has single-sex wards and the A&E department has separate child treatment and waiting areas. There is no MRI scanner here. On both death rates and waiting times the hospital performs in line with national averages.

Number of beds		597

➕ ⊕ 🜨 ⊗ ☏

		regional
Overall mortality	101	96
Vacancy rates	0	3
Doctors per 100 beds	44	37
Nurses per 100 beds	143	107
Cancelled operations	4	4
Complaints	5	4
Complaints clear up	61	48
waiting times		
Inpatient	73	72
Outpatient	83	76

Lewisham · **University Hospital Lewisham**

University Hospital, Lewisham
London, SE13 6LH
Phone: 020 8333 3000

Trust: Lewisham Hospital NHS Trust

University Hospital Lewisham currently has slightly above average death rates for emergency broken hip surgery, although overall mortality rate is average. It has a 6-bed CCU and a rehabilitation stroke unit. Eight out of ten A&E patients are treated within 4 hours. In April 2001, this hospital opened a new on-site primary care suite in an effort to reduce waiting times for emergency minor treatment; the Government has given the hospital Beacon status for its outpatient services.

Number of beds		650
⊕ ⊕ ⚕ ⊕ ⊗ ☏ ◉		
		regional
Overall mortality	106	96
Vacancy rates	0	3
Doctors per 100 beds	39	37
Nurses per 100 beds	134	107
Cancelled operations	0.5	4
Complaints	4	4
Complaints clear up	17	48
waiting times		
Inpatient	68	72
Outpatient	73	76

Leytonstone · **Whipps Cross University Hospital**

Whipps Cross Road
London, E11 1NR
Phone: 020 8539 5522

Trust: Whipps Cross University NHS Trust

Whipps Cross University Hospital serves Waltham Forest and the surrounding boroughs. It has one of the busiest Accident & Emergency departments in London. A&E waiting times are long with many patients waiting more than 4 hours to be dealt with. However, this may now improve following completion of a £1.4 m upgrade of the casualty department. The whole hospital is due to be rebuilt in 2007. Multidisciplinary teams for cancer treatment are offered for lung, stomach, breast and colorectal cancers. Waiting lists are longer than average but have been improving.

Number of beds		785
⊕ ⊕ ⚕ ⊗ ☏ ◉		
		regional
Overall mortality	-	96
Vacancy rates	4	3
Doctors per 100 beds	-	42
Nurses per 100 beds	-	117
Cancelled operations	-	4
Complaints	3	4
Complaints clear up	59	48
waiting times		
Inpatient	63	72
Outpatient	62	76

Marylebone · **Middlesex & University College Hospitals**

Mortimer Street
London, W1T 3AA
Phone: 020 7636 8333

Trust: University College London
  Hospitals NHS Trust

The Middlesex Hospital, University College Hospital (UCH) and the Elizabeth Garret Anderson Obstetric Hospital are teaching hospitals. They currently operate from next-door sites but they are set to merge onto a single site in Euston in the near future. Overall, the mortality rate for this hospital is one of the lowest in the country. They have a good stroke care record – death rates following emergency stroke admissions are low. There is a dedicated stroke unit and suspected stroke patients are always given a CT scan within 24 hours of being admitted.

Number of beds		659
➊ ➕ ⚕ ✖ ☎ ◉		
		regional
Overall mortality	68	96
Vacancy rates	0	3
Doctors per 100 beds	60	56
Nurses per 100 beds	-	154
Cancelled operations	3	4
Complaints	1	4
Complaints clear up	64	48
waiting times		
Inpatient	78	72
Outpatient	78	76

Orpington · **Farnborough Hospital**

Farnborough Common, Orpington
Kent, BR6 8ND
Phone: 01689 814 000

Trust: Bromley Hospitals NHS Trust

Farnborough Hospital is part of Bromley Hospitals NHS Trust. A new hospital is being built on the site, due for completion in spring 2003, which will house all the Trust's inpatient services and A&E department. At present, Farnborough doesn't have an A&E department. There is a paediatric ward and a paediatrician is on site 24 hours a day.

Number of beds		198
✖		
		regional
Overall mortality	98	96
Vacancy rates	7	3
Doctors per 100 beds	34	37
Nurses per 100 beds	81	107
Cancelled operations	5	4
Complaints	5	4
Complaints clear up	50	48
waiting times		
Inpatient	63	72
Outpatient	80	76

Orpington · **Orpington Hospital**

Sevenoaks Road, Orpington
Kent, BR6 9JU
Phone: 01689 815 000

Trust: Bromley Hospitals NHS Trust

Orpington Hospital offers acute medical services and rehabilitation and therapy facilities for the elderly. There is no A&E department. It meets the Government target of providing single-sex wards and performs CT scans on all suspected stroke patients within 48 hours of being admitted. The death rate for the Trust that runs the hospital is lower than average.

Number of beds		222
✖		
		regional
Overall mortality	98	96
Vacancy rates	7	3
Doctors per 100 beds	34	37
Nurses per 100 beds	81	107
Cancelled operations	-	4
Complaints	5	4
Complaints clear up	50	48
waiting times		
Inpatient	63	72
Outpatient	80	76

Paddington · **St Mary's Hospital**

Praed Street
London, W2 1NY
Phone: 020 7886 6666

Trust: St Mary's NHS Trust

St Mary's in London, one of the UK's leading university hospitals, has a low overall mortality rate and average death rates for stroke and broken hip emergency admissions. It offers coronary angiography and meets the Government target of 500 cardiac catheterisations a year. St Mary's also offers thrombolysis to heart attack patients within the target average of 30 minutes of arrival at A&E and performs CT scans on all suspected stroke patients within 48 hours of admission.

Number of beds		593
➕ ⊕ ✪ ⊕ ✖ 🚇 ◓		
		regional
Overall mortality	88	96
Vacancy rates	3	3
Doctors per 100 beds	68	42
Nurses per 100 beds	159	117
Cancelled operations	2	4
Complaints	-	4
Complaints clear up	41	48
waiting times		
Inpatient	79	72
Outpatient	82	76

Park Royal · **Central Middlesex Hospital**

Acton Lane
Wembley, NW10 7NS
Phone: 020 8965 5733

Trust: North West London Hospitals
  Trust

Central Middlesex Hospital is currently being redeveloped. When completed, in 2005, it will have over 200 beds and will include a major elective surgery service and an urgent treatment area combining minor A&E cases. Death rates at the Trust are good with a low overall death rate and a low death rate for emergency stroke admissions. All suspected stroke patients receive a CT scan within 24 hours of admission and heart attack patients on average receive thrombolysis within 30 minutes of arriving at the hospital.

Number of beds		243
➊ ➋ ➌ ➍ ➎		
		regional
Overall mortality	86	96
Vacancy rates	0	3
Doctors per 100 beds	55	42
Nurses per 100 beds	132	117
Cancelled operations	2	4
Complaints	6	4
Complaints clear up	35	48
waiting times		
Inpatient	66	72
Outpatient	79	76

Plaistow · **Newham General Hospital**

Glen Road
London, E13 8SL
Phone: 020 7476 4000

Trust: Newham Healthcare NHS Trust

Newham General Hospital is a medium-sized district general serving East London. It looks set to take on the services of St Andrews Hospital over the next two years. Heart attack patients do not currently receive thrombolytic drugs within an average of 30 minutes of arrival. Death rates following emergency admission with broken hip or stroke are high. Waiting times are above average.

Number of beds		482
➊ ➋ ➌ ➍ ➎		
		regional
Overall mortality	109	96
Vacancy rates	3	3
Doctors per 100 beds	33	37
Nurses per 100 beds	99	107
Cancelled operations	2	4
Complaints	3	4
Complaints clear up	29	48
waiting times		
Inpatient	83	72
Outpatient	77	76

Romford · **Harold Wood Hospital**

Gubbins Lane, Romford
Essex, RM3 0BE
Phone: 01708 345 533

Trust: **Barking, Havering and Redbridge Hospitals NHS Trust**

Harold Wood Hospital has a high overall mortality rate but does better than average on its waiting time performance. It has recently merged its management with King George Hospital in Ilford. Developments at Harold Wood Hospital include a new ambulatory care unit. An 8-bed coronary care unit is available. Paediatric surgery is performed and a paediatrician is on site 24 hours a day. There is no A&E (although there is a minor injuries unit), no CT scanner and no MRI scanner here.

Number of beds		390
❌		
		regional
Overall mortality	112	96
Vacancy rates	7	3
Doctors per 100 beds	36	42
Nurses per 100 beds	99	117
Cancelled operations	9	4
Complaints	4	4
Complaints clear up	47	48
waiting times		
Inpatient	67	72
Outpatient	73	76

Romford · **Oldchurch Hospital**

Waterloo Road, Romford
Essex, RM7 0BE
Phone: 01708 345 533

Trust: **Barking, Havering and Redbridge Hospitals NHS Trust**

Oldchurch Hospital is a medium-sized district general based in Romford. It has recently improved its A&E department. The hospital meets Government recommendations by providing single-sex wards and performing CT scans on all suspected stroke patients within 24 hours of admission. It treats breast, lung, colo-rectal and stomach cancers and has multidisciplinary teams in place for each. Overall the death rate for the hospital is high and in particular there is a high death rate for people requiring emergency treatment for broken hips.

Number of beds		482
➕ ⊕ ⚕ ❌ ☎ ◉		
		regional
Overall mortality	112	96
Vacancy rates	7	3
Doctors per 100 beds	36	42
Nurses per 100 beds	99	117
Cancelled operations	9	4
Complaints	4	4
Complaints clear up	47	48
waiting times		
Inpatient	67	72
Outpatient	73	76

Shepherd's Bush · **Hammersmith Hospital**

Du Cane Road
London, W12 0HS
Phone: 020 8383 1000

Trust: Hammersmith Hospitals NHS
Trust

Hammersmith is a teaching hospital with an international reputation for work in many areas such as leukaemia where it is developing a new research and treatment centre. The hospital is still putting in place multidisciplinary teams for treatments of some cancers. Overall the mortality rate for the Trust, which also runs the Charing Cross Hospital, are low. But the death rate for heart bypass surgery, for which this hospital is a centre, is high. There is no A&E at this hospital.

Number of beds		380
		regional
Overall mortality	87	96
Vacancy rates	2	3
Doctors per 100 beds	48	56
Nurses per 100 beds	154	154
Cancelled operations	-	4
Complaints	3	4
Complaints clear up	72	48
waiting times		
Inpatient	83	72
Outpatient	87	76

Sidcup · **Queen Mary's Hospital**

Frognal Avenue, Sidcup
Kent, DA14 6LT
Phone: 020 8302 2678

Trust: Queen Mary's Sidcup NHS Trust

The hospital is a single-site acute general hospital with additional outpatient and community services based externally. It is a designated Beacon site for management of emergency and winter pressures, having introduced a number of initiatives including ensuring that all patients admitted are seen by a consultant within 24 hours. Death rates for the hospital are average. However, waiting times are worse than average. Paediatric surgery is performed but a paediatrician is not on site 24 hours a day.

Number of beds		430
		regional
Overall mortality	104	96
Vacancy rates	7	3
Doctors per 100 beds	39	56
Nurses per 100 beds	112	154
Cancelled operations	1	4
Complaints	3	4
Complaints clear up	36	48
waiting times		
Inpatient	56	72
Outpatient	70	76

Southall · **Ealing Hospital**

Uxbridge Road, Southall
Middlesex, UB1 3HW
Phone: 020 8967 5000

Trust: Ealing Hospitals NHS Trust

Ealing Hospital is a medium-sized district general serving West London and the surrounding areas. The hospital's performance on both the analysis of death rates and against waiting times targets is average. It has a coronary care unit, but does not offer angiography. Multidisciplinary teams for the treatment of cancer patients are in place for breast, lung, stomach and colorectal cancers. The A&E department, which was partly refurbished last year, has separate facilities for children. There is no stroke unit.

Number of beds		410
✛ ⊕ ⚕ ✖ ☎		
		regional
Overall mortality	103	96
Vacancy rates	4	3
Doctors per 100 beds	40	40
Nurses per 100 beds	112	114
Cancelled operations	0	4
Complaints	4	4
Complaints clear up	29	48
waiting times		
Inpatient	74	72
Outpatient	76	76

Summerstown · **St George's Hospital**

Blackshaw Road
London, SW17 0QT
Phone: 020 8672 1255

Trust: St George's Healthcare NHS Trust

St George's Hospital is an important teaching hospital, a centre for heart surgery and has one of the busiest neonatal units in the capital. Death rates for emergency hip admissions are high, but overall death rates are average. The proportion of operations cancelled for non-medical reasons is average, with nearly six out of ten operations rescheduled within the recommended 31 days. The hospital has separate treatment areas for children in A&E and a paediatric ITU.

Number of beds		937
✛ ⊕ ⚕ ⊕ ✖ ☎ ◐		
		regional
Overall mortality	92	96
Vacancy rates	0	3
Doctors per 100 beds	54	56
Nurses per 100 beds	141	154
Cancelled operations	4	4
Complaints	6	4
Complaints clear up	56	48
waiting times		
Inpatient	72	72
Outpatient	78	76

Uxbridge · **Hillingdon Hospital**

Pield Heath Road, Uxbridge
Middlesex, UB8 3NN
Phone: 01895 238 282

Trust: Hillingdon Hospital NHS Trust

Hillingdon Hospital has recently upgraded its A&E department, including the dedicated children's A&E area. The hospital's overall mortality rate is high, but the death rate for emergency hip fracture admissions is low. There is a stroke unit, but suspected stroke patients don't always receive a CT scan within 48 hours of admission. On average 4 per cent of operations are cancelled for non-medical reasons but all were rescheduled within 31 days.

Number of beds		590
⊕ ⊕ ⊘ ⊗ ⊕		
		regional
Overall mortality	112	96
Vacancy rates	0	3
Doctors per 100 beds	31	37
Nurses per 100 beds	101	107
Cancelled operations	4	4
Complaints	3	4
Complaints clear up	45	48
waiting times		
Inpatient	84	72
Outpatient	73	76

Waterloo · **Guy's Hospital**

St Thomas Street
London, SE1 9RT
Phone: 020 7955 5000

Trust: Guy's and St Thomas's NHS Trust

A well-known teaching hospital and part of Guy's and St Thomas's NHS Trust, this hospital has a low overall mortality rate. Heart bypass surgery is performed at the hospital and the death rate for the procedure is average. The Trust does less well on waiting times but the hospital and the trust are working on reducing waiting times at Guy's Hospital, particularly for cancer patients. Multidisciplinary teams are available for the treatment of the major cancers. A renal unit is also on site.

Number of beds		553
⊕ ⊕ ⊘ ⊗ ⊕ ⊙		
		regional
Overall mortality	83	96
Vacancy rates	0	3
Doctors per 100 beds	58	56
Nurses per 100 beds	-	154
Cancelled operations	-	4
Complaints	3	4
Complaints clear up	53	48
waiting times		
Inpatient	64	72
Outpatient	70	76

Waterloo · **St Thomas' Hospital**

Lambeth Palace Road
London, SE1 7EH
Phone: 020 7928 9292

Trust: Guy's and St Thomas's NHS Trust

St Thomas' Hospital, one of London's largest and best known teaching hospitals, has a low overall mortality rate. Two key heart disease treatment measures are met as the hospital offers angiographies and meets the target of 500 cardiac catheterisations a year. It is also able to administer thrombolysis to heart attack patients within 30 minutes. However, patients wait longer than average in A&E.

Number of beds		813
✪ ⊕ ♠ ✖ ⊗ ◑		
		regional
Overall mortality	83	96
Vacancy rates	0	3
Doctors per 100 beds	58	56
Nurses per 100 beds	-	154
Cancelled operations	0.6	4
Complaints	3	4
Complaints clear up	53	48
waiting times		
Inpatient	64	72
Outpatient	70	76

West Smithfield · **St Bartholomew's Hospital**

West Smithfield
London, EC1A 7BE
Phone: 020 7377 7000

Trust: Barts and The London NHS Trust

St Bartholomew's is a teaching hospital that provides general hospital services to the people of Tower Hamlets and London. The Trust, which runs this hospital and the Royal London, has a low overall death rate – one of the best in the country. It meets government targets in two key areas for heart disease. There is no A&E unit here although there is a minor injuries unit.

Number of beds		290
✪ ⊕ ♠ ✖ ⊗ ◑		
		regional
Overall mortality	68	96
Vacancy rates	3	3
Doctors per 100 beds	63	56
Nurses per 100 beds	153	154
Cancelled operations	1	4
Complaints	3	4
Complaints clear up	32	48
waiting times		
Inpatient	72	72
Outpatient	73	76

Whitechapel · **Royal London Hospital**

Whitechapel
London, E1 1BB
Phone: 020 7377 7000

Trust: Barts and The London NHS Trust

The Royal London Hospital is one of three teaching hospitals run by Barts and The London NHS Trust. Death rates for broken hip operations and stroke are low and it is one of the few sites to carry out heart bypass surgery. Overall death rates are low at the Royal London. Thrombolysis is given to heart attack patients within 30 minutes of arrival.

Number of beds		630
⊕ ⊕ ⊛ ⊗ ☏ ◒		
		regional
Overall mortality	68	96
Vacancy rates	3	3
Doctors per 100 beds	63	56
Nurses per 100 beds	153	154
Cancelled operations	1	4
Complaints	3	4
Complaints clear up	32	48
waiting times		
Inpatient	72	72
Outpatient	73	76

Woolwich · **Queen Elizabeth Hospital**

Stadium Road
London, SE18 4QH
Phone: 020 8858 8141

Trust: Queen Elizabeth Hospital NHS Trust

The new Queen Elizabeth Hospital, London, opened in 2001. It meets the Government target in a key area of heart disease therapy by administering thombolysis to heat attack patients within an average of 30 minutes of arrival. It also performs coronary angiographies and achieves the government recommended target of 500 catheterisations per year. The hospital does not perform CT scans on all suspected stroke patients within 48 hours of arrival, and the death rate following emergency stroke admissions is high.

Number of beds		583
⊕ ⊕ ⊛ ⊗ ☏ ◒		
		regional
Overall mortality	113	96
Vacancy rates	0	3
Doctors per 100 beds	27	42
Nurses per 100 beds	138	117
Cancelled operations	-	4
Complaints	4	4
Complaints clear up	25	48
waiting times		
Inpatient	87	72
Outpatient	72	76

Ashtead · **Ashtead Hospital**

The Warren, Ashtead
Surrey, KT21 2SB
Phone: 01372 276161

Ashtead Hospital offers a wide range of surgical procedures. It has extensive diagnostic and treatment facilities including a fully equipped MRI/CT imaging unit. Fixed Cost surgery is offered.

Community Hospitals Group

Insurers: BUPA*, PPP*, Norwich*, Standard Life*, Royal Sun Alliance*, WPA*

price guide	£
Hip replacement	6947-7165
Cataract removal	2604

Number of beds	
ALS staff	1
heart services	-
Cancer services	🌐 ① ⊘ ✅

Beckenham · **BMI The Sloane Hospital**

125 Albemarle Rd, Beckenham
Kent, BR3 5HS
Phone: 0208 4666911

The Sloane Hospital, Beckenham, is situated on the outskirts of London. Most rooms are single, but the hospital has double rooms to accommodate parents wishing to stay overnight with their children.

General Healthcare Group Ltd

Insurers: BUPA*, PPP*, Norwich*, Standard Life, Royal Sun Alliance*, WPA

price guide	£
Hip replacement	7870
Cataract removal	2705-2820

Number of beds	57
ALS staff	2
heart services	-
Cancer services	⊘ ✅

Bermondsey · **London Bridge Hospital**

27 Tooley Street
London, SE1 2PR
Phone: 020 7407 3100

This hospital is known for conducting pioneering treatments. Innovative American surgical treatments for facial tumours are offered and the hospital has one of the most extensive sports injury clinics in London.

HCA International Ltd

Insurers: BUPA, PPP, WPA

price guide	£
Hip replacement	8910-13000
Cataract removal	1738-2500

Number of beds	119
ALS staff	6
heart services	
Cancer services	🌐 ① ⊘ ✅

Blackheath · **BMI The Blackheath Hospital**

40-42 Lee Terrace, Blackheath
London, SE3 9UD
Phone: 0208 318 7722

A patio and garden behind the
hospital offer a pleasant environment
in which both patients and visitors can
relax. Services include a sleep clinic,
private GPs and osteoporosis
screening.

General Healthcare Group

Insurers: BUPA*, PPP*, Norwich,
Royal Sun Alliance, WPA

price guide	£
Hip replacement	7650-8800
Cataract removal	2545-2755
Number of beds	69
ALS staff	1
heart services	-
Cancer services	

Brentwood · **BUPA Hartswood Hospital**

Eagle Way, Brentwood
Essex, CM13 3LE
Phone: 01277 232 525

BUPA Hartswood Hospital's services
include a spine centre and a chronic
fatigue clinic. The hospital also has a
minor operations theatre for
procedures requiring local anaesthetic.

BUPA Hospitals

Insurers: BUPA, PPP, Norwich, Standard Life,
Royal Sun Alliance, WPA

price guide	£
Hip replacement	6952-9743
Cataract removal	2253-2662
Number of beds	58
ALS staff	1
heart services	-
Cancer services	

Brentwood · **Essex Nuffield Hospital**

Shenfield Rd, Brentwood
Essex, CM15 8EH
Phone: 01277 695695

The Essex Nuffield is a purpose built
hospital opened in 1970 and situated
on the edge of woodland. It provides
healthcare in a relaxed and
comfortable environment.

Nuffield Hospitals

Insurers: BUPA*, PPP, Norwich*,
Standard Life*, Royal Sun Alliance*, WPA

price guide	£
Hip replacement	7000-7200
Cataract removal	1950-2400
Number of beds	48
ALS staff	5
heart services	-
Cancer services	

Brixton · **Guthrie Clinic**

King's College Hospital, Denmark Hill
London, SE5 9RS
Phone: 0207 3463192/3

The hospital provides a full range of
acute services. All generated income
is used to improve and maintain
services offered by the NHS.

King's College Hospital

Insurers: BUPA, PPP, Norwich, Standard Life,
Royal Sun Alliance, WPA

price guide	£
Hip replacement	
Cataract removal	

Number of beds	21
ALS staff	0
heart services	
Cancer services	

Buckhurst Hill · **Holly House Hospital**

High Rd, Buckhurst Hill
Essex, IG9 5HX
Phone: 0208 5053311

At Holly House is a new state-of-the-art
diagnostic centre which encompasses
MRI, CT and fluroscopy facilities. High
dependency care is available and
arrangements are in place to transfer
patients requiring intensive or coronary
care.

Aspen Healthcare Ltd

price guide	£
Hip replacement	7150
Cataract removal	1850-2095

Number of beds	55
ALS staff	1
heart services	-
Cancer services	

Chelsea · **Lister Hospital**

Chelsea Bridge Road
London, SW1W 8RH
Phone: 0207 730 3417

Among its other treatments, the Lister
Hospital's IVF unit is especially
renowned as it has one of the highest
success rates in the country. The breast
care unit provides integrated care.

HCA International Ltd

Insurers: BUPA, PPP, Norwich, Standard Life,
Royal Sun Alliance, WPA

price guide	£
Hip replacement	8910-13000
Cataract removal	1738-2500

Number of beds	70
ALS staff	8
heart services	-
Cancer services	

Croydon · **BMI Shirley Oaks Hospital**

Poppy Lane, Shirley Oaks Village
Croydon, Surrey, CR9 8AB
Phone: 0208 6555500

General Healthcare Group Ltd

 A recent inspection report from the local health authority described the staff as a "committed and dynamic team". Consultants are drawn from nearby Mayday University Hospital, King's College Hospital and St George's Hospital and a range of specialties are offered, including fertility services.

price guide	£
Hip replacement	8243
Cataract removal	1950

Number of beds	50
ALS staff	1

heart services	-
Cancer services	

Enfield · **BMI The King's Oak Hospital**

Chase Farm (North Side), The Ridgeway
Enfield, Middlesex, EN2 8SD
Phone: 020 8370 9500

General Healthcare Group Ltd

Insurers: BUPA*, PPP*, Norwich*, Royal Sun Alliance*

Enfield's King's Oak Hospital works in partnership with Chase Farm NHS Hospital to offer a range of medical services. King's Oak benefits from the extensive clinical support services at Chase Farm.

price guide	£
Hip replacement	7440-7700
Cataract removal	1600-2000

Number of beds	52
ALS staff	2

heart services	
Cancer services	

Enfield · **North London Nuffield Hospital**

Cavell Drive, Uplands Park Rd
Enfield, Middlesex, EN2 7PR
Phone: 0208 3662122

Nuffield Nursing Homes Trust

Insurers: BUPA*, PPP, Norwich*, Standard Life*, Royal Sun Alliance*, WPA

The North London Nuffield Hospital based near Enfield Town centre offers clinics in a broad range of medical and surgical specialties including physiotherapy, pathology, imaging and pharmacy.

price guide	£
Hip replacement	7600
Cataract removal	1950

Number of beds	45
ALS staff	1

heart services	-
Cancer services	

Harrow · **BMI The Clementine Churchill Hospital**

Sudbury Hill, Harrow
Middlesex, HA1 3RX
Phone: 0208 872 3872

The Clementine Churchill Hospital attracts over 350 consultants who receive support from the hospital's resident medical officers. An innovative menopause clinic run by an all-women team was recently launched.

General Healthcare Group Ltd

Insurers: BUPA*, PPP*, Norwich*, Royal Sun Alliance*, WPA

price guide	£
Hip replacement	6625-9350
Cataract removal	2629-2829

Number of beds	120
ALS staff	0
heart services	-
Cancer services	

Hendon · **BMI Garden Hospital**

46-50 Sunny Gardens Rd, Hendon
London, NW4 1RP
Phone: 0208 457 4500

This is an acute medical and surgical hospital. Its main specialties include ophthalmic, orthopaedic, gynaecology, urology and vascular surgery. The outpatient department offers an extensive range of services, many on a walk-in basis or a same-day appointment.

General Healthcare Group Ltd

price guide	£
Hip replacement	
Cataract removal	

Number of beds	35
ALS staff	3
heart services	-
Cancer services	

Ilford · **BUPA Roding Hospital**

Roding Lane South, Ilford
Essex, IG4 5PZ
Phone: 020 8551 1100

Offering surgical and medical care, and a wide range of diagnostic services and facilities, the hospital is renowned for its innovative fertility investigations and treatment.

BUPA Hospitals

Insurers: BUPA, PPP, Norwich, Standard Life, Royal Sun Alliance, WPA

price guide	£
Hip replacement	7620-7620
Cataract removal	2132-2946

Number of beds	65
ALS staff	1
heart services	-
Cancer services	

Kingston upon Thames · **New Victoria Hospital**

184 Coombe Lane West
Kingston upon Thames, Surrey, KT2 7EG
Phone: 020 8949 9000

The hospital has undergone a £5m upgrade to provide state-of-the-art facilities. It is one of few hospitals in the country capable of treating endometriosis with laser surgery.

Charitable Trust

Insurers: BUPA*, PPP*, Norwich*, Standard Life*, Royal Sun Alliance*, WPA*

price guide	£
Hip replacement	8000-9000
Cataract removal	2107-3270

Number of beds	37
ALS staff	8
heart services	-
Cancer services	

Marylebone · **Harley Street Clinic**

35 Weymouth Street
London, W1G 8BJ
Phone: 0207 935 7700

This is an acute care hospital known for its cardiac surgery and oncology in both children and adults. It also deals with all forms of heart disease in children and adolescents.

HCA International Ltd

Insurers: Bupa, PPP, WPA

price guide	£
Hip replacement	8910-13000
Cataract removal	1738-2500

Number of beds	92
ALS staff	10
heart services	
Cancer services	

Marylebone · **King Edward VII's Hospital Sister Agnes**

Beaumont Street
London, W1G 6AA
Phone: 020 7486 4411

King Edward VII's Hospital Sister Agnes has state-of-the-art facilities and new consulting and minor procedures facilities. The hospital is fully accredited by the Health Quality Service scheme.

Charitable Trust

Insurers: BUPA, PPP, Norwich, Standard Life, Royal Sun Alliance, WPA

price guide	£
Hip replacement	
Cataract removal	

Number of beds	65
ALS staff	1
heart services	-
Cancer services	

Marylebone · **London Clinic**

20 Devonshire Place, London
W1G 6BW
Phone: 020 7935 4444

The Clinic is an acute general hospital, offering a range of specialties. This not-for-profit hospital re-invests all surpluses into improving the quality of patient care. Specialties include breast, spinal and vascular surgery.

Trustees of the London Clinic

Insurers: BUPA*, PPP*, Norwich*, Standard Life*, Royal Sun Alliance*, WPA*

price guide	£
Hip replacement	
Cataract removal	

Number of beds	190
ALS staff	2
heart services	
Cancer services	

Marylebone · **Princess Grace Hospital**

42-52 Nottingham Place
London, W1U 5NY
Phone: 0207 486 1234

The Princess Grace is renowned for its cardiac surgery and cardiology. The hospital also has expertise in sports medicine, hepatitis treatment and all conditions of the hand, arm and shoulder.

HCA International Ltd

Insurers: BUPA, PPP, WPA

price guide	£
Hip replacement	8910-13000
Cataract removal	1738-2500

Number of beds	120
ALS staff	3
heart services	-
Cancer services	

Orpington · **BMI Chelsfield Park Hospital**

Bucks Cross Rd, Chelsfield
Orpington, Kent, BR6 7RG
Phone: 01689 877 855

Chelsfield Park attracts consultants from a range of neighbouring NHS hospitals including Lewisham, Greenwich, Bromley and Queen Mary's Sidcup and offers a range of services including an HFCA licensed Assisted Conception Unit. Additional principal specialties include orthopaedics and neurosurgery.

General Healthcare Group

Insurers: BUPA, PPP, Norwich, Royal Sun Alliance, WPA

price guide	£
Hip replacement	7400
Cataract removal	2300-4620

Number of beds	
ALS staff	1
heart services	-
Cancer services	

South Kensington · **Cromwell Hospital**

Cromwell Rd
London, SW5 0TU
Phone: 020 7460 2000

The hospital's specialties are cancer treatment, liver disease, neurology and cardiothoracic medicine. It runs a network of fertility centres and the Well Woman Centre provides breast screening and bone density scans.

Medical Service International

Insurers: BUPA*, PPP, Norwich, Standard Life, Royal Sun Alliance, WPA

price guide	£
Hip replacement	-
Cataract removal	-

Number of beds	150
ALS staff	3
heart services	
Cancer services	

St John's Wood · **Wellington Hospital**

8a Wellington Place
London, NW8 9LE
Phone: 020 7586 5959

One of largest private hospitals in the country, the Wellington has a large cardiac centre offering a full range of services including heart surgery. Other fields of expertise include plastic surgery and neurosurgery.

HCA International Ltd

Insurers: BUPA*, PPP*, Norwich*, Standard Life*, Royal Sun Alliance*, WPA*

price guide	£
Hip replacement	8910-13000
Cataract removal	1738-2500

Number of beds	266
ALS staff	10
heart services	
Cancer services	

Stepney · **BMI London Independent Hospital**

1 Beaumont Square, Stepney Green
London, E1 4NL
Phone: 0207 780 2400

The hospital offers a range of medical procedures, including more complex operations. Last year, it received patients from the Derriford Hospital for heart surgery to cut waiting lists. Other specialties include cardiac catheterisation and a fast track breast clinic.

General Healthcare Group Ltd

Insurers: BUPA*, PPP*, Norwich, Standard Life, Royal Sun Alliance, WPA

price guide	£
Hip replacement	8500-9000
Cataract removal	2000-2500

Number of beds	80
ALS staff	3
heart services	
Cancer services	

Sutton · **St Anthony's Hospital**

801 London Rd, North Cheam
Sutton, Surrey, SM3 9DW
Phone: 020 8337 6691

The hospital is known for heart surgery, attracting patients from around the world. It also has a specialist obesity clinic, with treatments ranging from behaviourial therapy to surgical techniques.

Congregation of the Daughters of the Cross

Insurers: Bupa*, PPP*, Norwich

price guide	£
Hip replacement	-
Cataract removal	-

Number of beds	92
ALS staff	2
heart services	
Cancer services	

Wimbledon · **Parkside Hospital**

53 Parkside, Wimbledon
London, SW19 5NX
Phone: 020 8971 8000

Parkside Hospital has a new private oncology centre which houses two linear accelerators and provides chemotherapy treatment for cancer patients in south west London and Surrey.

Aspen Healthcare Ltd

price guide	£
Hip replacement	7200-7700
Cataract removal	2300-2450

Number of beds	72
ALS staff	3
heart services	-
Cancer services	

The North

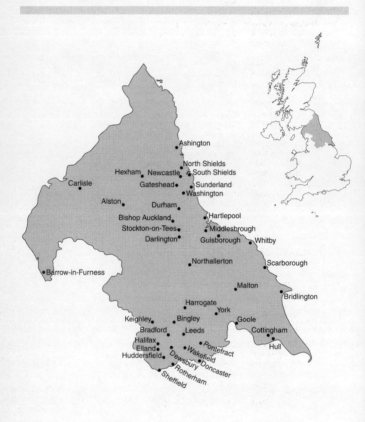

NHS

Ashington	Wansbeck General Hospital
Bishop Auckland	Bishop Auckland General Hospital
Bradford	Bradford Royal Infirmary
Bradford	St Luke's Hospital
Bridlington	Bridlington & District Hospital
Carlise	Cumberland Infirmary
Cottingham	Castle Hill Hospital
Darlington	Darlington Memorial Hospital
Dewsbury	Dewsbury & District Hospital
Dryburn	University Hospital of North Durham
Gateshead	Queen Elizabeth Hospital
Halifax	Calderdale Royal Hospital
Harrogate	Harrogate District Hospital
Hartlepool	University Hospital of Hartlepool
Hexham	Hexham General Hospital
Huddersfield	Huddersfield Royal Infirmary
Huddersfield	St Luke's Hospital
Hull	Hull Royal Infirmary
Hull	Princess Royal Hospital
Leeds	Chapel Allerton Hospital
Leeds	Leeds General Infirmary
Leeds	Seacroft Hospital
Leeds	St James's University Hospital
Leeds	Wharfdale General Hospital
Middlesbrough	James Cook University Hospital, The
Middlesbrough	Middlesbrough General Hospital
Newcastle upon Tyne	Newcastle Hospitals
North Shields	North Tyneside General Hospital
Northallerton	Friarage Hospital
Pontefract	Pontefract General Infirmary
Scarborough	Scarborough General Hospital
South Shields	South Tyneside District Hospital
Steeton	Airedale General Hospital
Stockton-on-Tees	University Hospital of North Tees
Sunderland	Ryhope Hospital
Sunderland	Sunderland Royal Hospital
Wakefield	Pinderfields General Hospital
Whitby	Whitby Hospital
Whitehaven	West Cumberland Hospital
York	York District Hospital

Private

Bingley	The Yorkshire Clinic
Carlisle	Abbey Caldew Hospital
Cottingham	Hull Nuffield Hospital
Darlington	Woodlands Hospital
Elland	BUPA Hospital Elland
Harrogate	Duchy Nuffield Hospital
Huddersfield	Huddersfield Nuffield Hospital
Hull	BUPA Hull and East Riding Hospitals
Leeds	BUPA Hospital Leeds
Leeds	BUPA Methley Park Hospital
Leeds	Mid Yorkshire Nuffield Hospital
Newcastle upon Tyne	Newcastle Nuffield Hospital
Scarborough	BUPA Beldevere Hospital
Stockton-on-Tees	Cleveland Nuffield Hospital
Washington	BUPA Hospital Washington
York	Purey Cust Nuffield Hospital

Ashington · **Wansbeck General Hospital**

Woodhorn Lane, Ashington
Northumberland, NE63 9JJ
Phone: 01670 521212

Trust: Northumbria Healthcare NHS
  Trust

Wansbeck General Hospital has recently opened a new 27-bed acute stroke unit.

It has low death rates for emergency broken hip surgery and stroke, but overall mortality rate is average. There are multidisciplinary teams for cancer treatment.

The hospital has coronary angiography facilities but does not yet carry our the volume of cardiac catheterisations to meet Government recommendations. CT scans for stroke patients are not always given within 48 hours of admission.

Number of beds		267
⊕ ⟳ ⊗ ⊕		
		regional
Overall mortality	99	97
Vacancy rates	5	4
Doctors per 100 beds	23	29
Nurses per 100 beds	92	111
Cancelled operations	0.2	1
Complaints	2	3
Complaints clear up	41	49
waiting times		
Inpatient	83	78
Outpatient	92	82

Bishop Auckland · **Bishop Auckland General Hospital**

Cockton Hill Road, Bishop Auckland
Co Durham, DL14 6AD
Phone: 01388 454000

Trust: South Durham Healthcare NHS
  Trust

Bishop Auckland General Hospital is currently a medium-sized acute hospital, however, building is under way to provide a new facility on the site and should be completed in 2002. All A&E patients are dealt with within 4 hours and there is a separate children's treatment area in the A&E. There are dedicated stroke facilities and all stroke patients receive a CT scan within 24 hours of admission. However, the hospital does not meet the recommendation that emergency heart attack admissions receive thrombolysis within 30 minutes of arriving in A&E.

Number of beds		313
⊕ ⟳ ⊗ ⊕ ⊙		
		regional
Overall mortality	103	97
Vacancy rates	3	4
Doctors per 100 beds	29	29
Nurses per 100 beds	107	111
Cancelled operations	0.1	1
Complaints	1	3
Complaints clear up	74	49
waiting times		
Inpatient	82	78
Outpatient	89	82

Bradford · **Bradford Royal Infirmary**

Duckworth Lane, Bradford
West Yorkshire, BD9 6RJ
Phone: 01274 542 200

Trust: Bradford Hospitals NHS Trust

Bradford Royal Infirmary underwent a major refit and received several awards last year. New services and facilities include a new A&E department, incorporating a specialist children's unit. The hospital has a coronary care unit and meets Government targets for rapid treatment of heart attack patients and for provision of coronary angiography. It does not have a stroke unit, but all suspected stroke patients receive a CT scan within 24 hours of admission. Death rates for emergency stroke patients are average.

Number of beds		925
⊕ ⊕ ⊛ ⊗ ⊕ ⊕		
		regional
Overall mortality	95	97
Vacancy rates	4	4
Doctors per 100 beds	37	29
Nurses per 100 beds	123	111
Cancelled operations	1	1
Complaints	1	3
Complaints clear up	29	49
waiting times		
Inpatient	78	78
Outpatient	83	82

Bradford · **St Luke's Hospital**

Little Horton Lane, Bradford
West Yorkshire, BD5 0NA
Phone: 01274 734 744

Trust: Bradford Hospitals NHS Trust

St Luke's Hospital is managed centrally along with the larger Bradford Royal Infirmary. All the facilities at both sites are available to all patients depending on their clinical needs. There is no A&E at this unit. Recent developments at St Luke's include a Digital Screening Room, housing the most up to date fluoroscopy equipment and a new CT scanning service, which has led to reduced waiting times and improved patient facilities. The hospital has facilities for stroke patients and all stroke emergency patients undergo a CT scan within 24 hours of admission.

Number of beds		309
⊗ ⊕		
		regional
Overall mortality	95	97
Vacancy rates	4	4
Doctors per 100 beds	37	29
Nurses per 100 beds	123	111
Cancelled operations	1	1
Complaints	1	3
Complaints clear up	29	49
waiting times		
Inpatient	78	78
Outpatient	83	82

Bridlington · **Bridlington & District Hospital**

Bessingby Road, Bridlington
North Yorkshire, YO16 4QP
Phone: 01262 606 666

Trust: Scarborough & North East
    Yorkshire Healthcare NHS Trust

Bridlington & District Hospital is a community hospital providing acute services as part of the Scarborough and North East Yorkshire Healthcare NHS Trust. A new dedicated Coronary Monitoring Unit is planned to improve observation of patients, ensure continuity of care, and help standardise the service across the Trust. Plans to add a rapid access outpatient clinic will improve stroke rehabilitation services.

Number of beds		117
✪		
		regional
Overall mortality	96	97
Vacancy rates	6	4
Doctors per 100 beds	26	25
Nurses per 100 beds	114	108
Cancelled operations	-	1
Complaints	2	3
Complaints clear up	38	49
waiting times		
Inpatient	82	78
Outpatient	82	82

Carlisle · **Cumberland Infirmary**

Newtown Road, Carlisle
Cumbria, CA2 7HY
Phone: 01228 523444

Trust: North Cumbria Acute Hospitals
    NHS Trust

Cumberland Infirmary opened in 2000 and is the main district general hospital for East Cumbria. The Trust has a good record on handling A&E patients quickly. Nearly 98 per cent are dealt with within 4 hours. However, 6 per cent of operations were cancelled for non-medical reasons – a higher rate than other hospitals. The hospital meets the Government target to administer thrombolytic drugs to heart attack patients within 30 minutes of admission.

Number of beds		442
✪ ✚ 🔆 ✖ 🚆 ◉		
		regional
Overall mortality	96	97
Vacancy rates	0	4
Doctors per 100 beds	34	31
Nurses per 100 beds	116	110
Cancelled operations	6	1
Complaints	4	3
Complaints clear up	79	49
waiting times		
Inpatient	72	78
Outpatient	86	82

Cottingham · **Castle Hill Hospital**

Castle Road, Cottingham
East Yorkshire, HU16 5JQ
Phone: 01482 875875

Trust: Hull and East Yorkshire Hospitals
NHS Trust

Castle Hill Hospital provides acute medical and surgical care to patients in the East Yorkshire area. Together with Hull Royal Infirmary and The Princess Royal Hospital, Castle Hill provides cancer services for 1.2 million people living in and around Hull. A new wing for outpatient urology and radiology services should be completed by early 2002. The hospital does not have an A&E unit or paediatric ward.

Number of beds		??
		regional
Overall mortality	101	97
Vacancy rates	3	4
Doctors per 100 beds	34	29
Nurses per 100 beds	124	111
Cancelled operations	-	1
Complaints	4	3
Complaints clear up	57	49
waiting times		
Inpatient	68	78
Outpatient	76	82

Darlington · **Darlington Memorial Hospital**

Hollyhurst Road, Darlington
Co Durham, DL3 6HW
Phone: 01325 380100

Trust: South Durham Healthcare NHS
Trust

Darlington Memorial Hospital provides acute healthcare services. Waiting times have recently been reduced and patient access to services have been improved with the introduction of a booked admissions scheme. The Trust that runs this hospital has average death rates and performs better than average on inpatient, outpatient and A&E waiting times. There are dedicated stroke facilities and all suspected stroke patients receive a CT scan within 24 hours of admission.

Number of beds		447
		regional
Overall mortality	103	97
Vacancy rates	3	4
Doctors per 100 beds	29	29
Nurses per 100 beds	107	111
Cancelled operations	0.1	1
Complaints	1	3
Complaints clear up	74	49
waiting times		
Inpatient	82	78
Outpatient	89	82

Dewsbury · **Dewsbury and District Hospital**

Halifax Road, Dewsbury
West Yorkshire, WF13 4HS
Phone: 01924 512 000

Trust: Dewsbury & District NHS Trust

Dewsbury and District Hospital serves the northern area of Kirklees, and parts of Leeds, Bradford and Wakefield. The death rate following emergency fractured hip admissions is low and over 93 per cent of patients in A&E are dealt with within 4 hours. Other death rates are average and the Trust does better than average against waiting time targets. It meets government targets for rapid treatment of heart attacks and for the number of cardiac catheterisations performed.

Number of beds		534
❍ ❀ ✖ ㉄		
		regional
Overall mortality	105	97
Vacancy rates	6	4
Doctors per 100 beds	30	25
Nurses per 100 beds	118	108
Cancelled operations	-	1
Complaints	3	3
Complaints clear up	75	49
waiting times		
Inpatient	85	78
Outpatient	86	82

Dryburn · **University Hospital of North Durham**

North Road, Dryburn
Co Durham, DH1 5TW
Phone: 0191 333 2333

Trust: North Durham Healthcare NHS Trust

The hospital has average death rates for emergency hip operations and stroke admissions and an average overall mortality rate. It offers multidisciplinary teams for cancer treatment. The hospital has research and education links with the major hospitals in Newcastle. It is one of just a handful of UK hospitals to use digital X-rays. Heart attack patients receive thrombolysis within 30 minutes of arriving at the hospital and all emergency stroke patients are given a CT scan within 48 hours.

Number of beds		543
❍ ⊕ ❀ ✖ ㉄ ◗		
		regional
Overall mortality	101	97
Vacancy rates	3	4
Doctors per 100 beds	28	29
Nurses per 100 beds	97	111
Cancelled operations	2	1
Complaints	3	3
Complaints clear up	41	49
waiting times		
Inpatient	73	78
Outpatient	71	82

Gateshead · **Queen Elizabeth Hospital**

Queen Elizabeth Avenue, Gateshead
Tyne & Wear, NE9 6SX
Phone: 0191 482 0000

Trust: Gateshead Health NHS Trust

Queen Elizabeth Hospital, Gateshead, is an acute district general providing a wide range of services to the local population. It meets Government targets in two key areas for heart disease by administering thrombolysis to heart attack patients within an average of 30 minutes of their arrival, and by performing the recommended minimum of 500 cardiac catheterisations per year. It ensures all suspected stroke patients receive CT scans within 48 hours of admission.

Number of beds		675
➕ ⊕ ♻ ✖ 🆑		
		regional
Overall mortality	104	97
Vacancy rates	4	4
Doctors per 100 beds	23	29
Nurses per 100 beds	97	111
Cancelled operations	0.6	1
Complaints	2	3
Complaints clear up	60	49
waiting times		
Inpatient	73	78
Outpatient	89	82

Halifax · **Calderdale Royal Hospital**

Salterhebble
Halifax, HX3 0PW
Phone: 01422 357 171

Trust: Calderdale and Huddersfield NHS Trust

The Calderdale Royal Hospital, Halifax opened in April 2001. With 557 beds, this is a large hospital offering acute services. Nearly 100 per cent of A&E patients are dealt with within 4 hours. The hospital has a coronary care unit, and provides services for heart patients. However, it does not yet meet the Government target of performing at least 500 angiographies per year. There is a dedicated stroke facility but the hospital does not give all stroke patients a CT scan within 48 hours of admission as recommended.

Number of beds		577
➕ ♻ ✖ 🆑 ◉		
		regional
Overall mortality	98	97
Vacancy rates	9	4
Doctors per 100 beds	28	29
Nurses per 100 beds	111	111
Cancelled operations	0.5	1
Complaints	3	3
Complaints clear up	36	49
waiting times		
Inpatient	89	78
Outpatient	79	82

Harrogate · **Harrogate District Hospital**

Lancaster Park Road
Harrogate, HG2 7SX
Phone: 01423 885 959

Trust: Harrogate Health Care NHS Trust

Harrogate District Hospital has benefited from a recent development programme and now includes a new cancer facility led by multidisciplinary teams and catering for breast, lung, stomach and colorectal cancers. The hospital is the main A&E services provider in the area and 99 per cent of patients leave the department within 4 hours. All suspected stroke patients receive a CT scan within 48 hours of emergency admission. Death rates are average and waiting times are better than average.

Number of beds		379
➕ ⊕ ♦ ✖ ☻		
		regional
Overall mortality	95	97
Vacancy rates	0	4
Doctors per 100 beds	24	25
Nurses per 100 beds	99	108
Cancelled operations	2	1
Complaints	3	3
Complaints clear up	72	49
waiting times		
Inpatient	86	78
Outpatient	85	82

Hartlepool · **University Hospital of Hartlepool**

Holdforth Road
Hartlepool, TS24 9AH
Phone: 01429 266654

Trust: North Tees and Hartlepool NHS
Trust

The University Hospital of Hartlepool serves the population of Stockton-on-Tees, Hartlepool, East Durham and Sedgefield. It has low death rates in emergency broken hip surgery and provides thrombolysis to heart attack patients within 30 minutes of their arrival. Emergency stroke patients receive a CT scans within 24 hours, which is better than the Government's target of doing this within 48 hours.

Number of beds		334
➕ ⊕ ♦ ✖ ☻ ◕		
		regional
Overall mortality	101	97
Vacancy rates	8	4
Doctors per 100 beds	31	29
Nurses per 100 beds	115	111
Cancelled operations	2	1
Complaints	2	3
Complaints clear up	-	49
waiting times		
Inpatient	85	78
Outpatient	85	82

Hexham · **Hexham General Hospital**

Corbridge Road, Hexham
Northumberland, NE46 1QJ
Phone: 01434 655655

Trust: Northumbria Healthcare NHS
Trust

Hexham General is a small district general and is part of Northumbria Healthcare NHS Trust which has low death rates for emergency broken hip and stroke admissions. There is an A&E and a unit for acute stroke care and post-stroke rehabilitation, but not all suspected stroke patients are given a CT scan within 48 hours of admission. Surgery is performed on children, but the hospital does not have a paediatrician on site 24 hours a day.

Number of beds		103
➕ ❌ ⒢		
		regional
Overall mortality	99	97
Vacancy rates	5	4
Doctors per 100 beds	23	29
Nurses per 100 beds	92	111
Cancelled operations	0.2	1
Complaints	2	3
Complaints clear up	41	49
waiting times		
Inpatient	83	78
Outpatient	92	82

Huddersfield · **Huddersfield Royal Infirmary**

Acre Street, Huddersfield
Yorkshire, HD3 3EA
Phone: 01484 342000

Trust: Calderdale and Huddersfield NHS
Trust

Huddersfield Royal Infirmary has low death rates for both stroke patients and people requiring emergency treatment for a broken hip. The Trust also has a better than average record on waiting times for inpatients and for urgent cancer patients who can expect to be seen within 2 weeks as recommended by the Government.

Number of beds		545
➕ ⒩ ❌ ⒢ ◉		
		regional
Overall mortality	92	97
Vacancy rates	1	4
Doctors per 100 beds	27	29
Nurses per 100 beds	112	111
Cancelled operations	-	1
Complaints	2	3
Complaints clear up	57	49
waiting times		
Inpatient	89	78
Outpatient	79	82

Huddersfield · **St Luke's Hospital**

Blackmoorfoot Road, Huddersfield
Yorkshire, HD4 5RQ
Phone: 01484 654 711

Trust: Calderdale and Huddersfield NHS
Trust

St Luke's has a strong intermediate care focus. Death rates are low. Patients are referred to larger local hospitals for coronary angiography but thrombolysis for heart attacks is given within the target average of 30 minutes from arrival. There are multidisciplinary teams treating most major forms of cancer.

Number of beds		172
		regional
Overall mortality	92	97
Vacancy rates	1	4
Doctors per 100 beds	27	29
Nurses per 100 beds	112	111
Cancelled operations	-	1
Complaints	2	3
Complaints clear up	57	49
waiting times		
Inpatient	89	78
Outpatient	79	82

Hull · **Hull Royal Infirmary**

Anlaby Road
Hull, HU3 2JZ
Phone: 01482 328541

Trust: Hull and East Yorkshire Hospitals
NHS Trust

Hull Royal Infirmary provides A&E services for around 570,000 people. It has recently built a new pathology unit and now aims to improve its stroke services. The hospital boasts low death rates for emergency broken hip and stroke admissions. It also meets a key Government standard for coronary angiography and has CT and MRI scanning facilities. The hospital performs children's surgery but there is no dedicated paediatric ITU.

Number of beds		669
➊ ➋ ➌ ➐ ➎		
		regional
Overall mortality	101	97
Vacancy rates	3	4
Doctors per 100 beds	34	29
Nurses per 100 beds	124	111
Cancelled operations	0	1
Complaints	4	3
Complaints clear up	57	49
waiting times		
Inpatient	68	78
Outpatient	76	82

Hull · **Princess Royal Hospital**

Saltshouse Road
Hull, HU8 9HE
Phone: 01482 701151

Trust: Hull and East Yorkshire Hospitals
NHS Trust

The Princess Royal hospital is a small acute hospital serving Hull and the surrounding area. The mortality rate for the Trust is average as are the levels of both doctors and nurses per 100 beds. The hospital does not have an A&E department or intensive care facilities, nor does it provide MRI scanning facilities.

Number of beds		-

		regional
Overall mortality	101	97
Vacancy rates	3	4
Doctors per 100 beds	34	29
Nurses per 100 beds	124	111
Cancelled operations	-	1
Complaints	4	3
Complaints clear up	57	49
waiting times		
Inpatient	68	78
Outpatient	76	82

Leeds · **Chapel Allerton Hospital**

Chapeltown Road, Leeds
Yorkshire, LS7 4RB
Phone: 0113 392 4595

Trust: Leeds Teaching Hospitals NHS
Trust

The new £12 m Chapel Allerton hospital mainly looks after elderly patients. It has a nationally renowned rehabilitation centre, plus rheumatology services and a prosthetics centre. Leeds Teaching Hospitals NHS Trust, which runs the hospital, has a low overall mortality rate.

Number of beds		-

		regional
Overall mortality	88	97
Vacancy rates	2	4
Doctors per 100 beds	42	45
Nurses per 100 beds	137	144
Cancelled operations	0	1
Complaints	4	3
Complaints clear up	49	49
waiting times		
Inpatient	70	78
Outpatient	78	82

Leeds · **Leeds General Infirmary**

Great George Street, Leeds
West Yorkshire, LS1 3EX
Phone: 0113 243 2799

Trust: Leeds Teaching Hospitals NHS
Trust

Leeds General Infirmary provides regional cardiothoracic and neurosurgical facilities and is part of the Leeds Teaching Hospitals NHS Trust which also runs St James's Hospital. This hospital is a centre for heart surgery and has a low death rate for patients undergoing heart bypass surgery. The Trust also has a low death rate following emergency stroke admissions. Heart attack patients are administered thrombolysis within an average of 30 minutes of their arrival at A&E.

Number of beds		1334
➕ 🔵 ➕ ❌ 🔵 🔵		
		regional
Overall mortality	88	97
Vacancy rates	2	4
Doctors per 100 beds	42	45
Nurses per 100 beds	137	144
Cancelled operations	0	1
Complaints	4	3
Complaints clear up	49	49
waiting times		
Inpatient	70	78
Outpatient	78	82

Leeds · **Seacroft Hospital**

York Road, Leeds
Yorkshire, LS14 6UH
Phone: 0113 264 8164

Trust: Leeds Teaching Hospitals NHS
Trust

Seacroft Hospital is a small acute hospital which is part of the Leeds Teaching Hospitals NHS Trust. The hospital seeks to maintain high standards and is currently aiming to send out appointments within 10 days of referral and to see all children within 6 weeks.

Number of beds		-
		regional
Overall mortality	88	97
Vacancy rates	2	4
Doctors per 100 beds	42	45
Nurses per 100 beds	137	144
Cancelled operations	0	1
Complaints	4	3
Complaints clear up	49	49
waiting times		
Inpatient	70	78
Outpatient	78	82

Leeds · **St James's University Hospital**

Beckett Street, Leeds
West Yorkshire, LS9 7TF
Phone: 0113 243 3144

Trust: Leeds Teaching Hospitals NHS
Trust

St James's University Hospital is one of the largest teaching hospitals in Europe with a low overall mortality rate. Also, death rates for emergency stroke admissions are more than 10 per cent lower than average. The hospital has MRI and CT scanning facilities.

Number of beds		1101
		regional
Overall mortality	88	97
Vacancy rates	2	4
Doctors per 100 beds	42	45
Nurses per 100 beds	137	144
Cancelled operations	0	1
Complaints	4	3
Complaints clear up	49	49
waiting times		
Inpatient	70	78
Outpatient	78	82

Leeds · **Wharfdale General Hospital**

Newall Carr Road, Leeds
Yorkshire, LS21 2LY
Phone: 0113 292 2000

Trust: Leeds Teaching Hospitals NHS
Trust

Wharfedale Hospital provides a range of health services for the population of north-west Leeds. It is a smaller hospital attached to the Leeds Teaching Hospitals NHS Trust which has low death rates. There is no A&E department at the hospital.

Number of beds		91
		regional
Overall mortality	88	97
Vacancy rates	2	4
Doctors per 100 beds	42	45
Nurses per 100 beds	137	144
Cancelled operations	0	1
Complaints	4	3
Complaints clear up	49	49
waiting times		
Inpatient	70	78
Outpatient	78	82

Middlesbrough · **James Cook University Hospital**

Marton Rd
Middlesbrough, TS4 3BW
Phone: 01642 850850

Trust: South Tees Hospitals NHS Trust

James Cook University Hospital was formerly known as the South Cleveland Hospital. The hospital does not have an A&E department and emergency services are provided at Middlesbrough General Hospital. James Cook hospital is a centre for heart surgery and here also the death rate following heart bypass operations is average. In cancer services, the hospital has multidisciplinary teams in place for major cancers including breast, lung, stomach and colorectal cancers.

Number of beds		730
		regional
Overall mortality	99	97
Vacancy rates	3	4
Doctors per 100 beds	39	29
Nurses per 100 beds	130	111
Cancelled operations	1	1
Complaints	2	3
Complaints clear up	20	49
waiting times		
Inpatient	72	78
Outpatient	78	82

Middlesbrough · **Middlesbrough General Hospital**

Ayresome Green Lane
Middlesbrough, TS5 5AZ
Phone: 01642 850850

Trust: South Tees Hospitals NHS Trust

This hospital provides A&E services for Middlesbrough as well as a range of other services. The hospital Trust has piloted pre-booked admission systems in four specialties – gynaecology, cardiology, endoscopy and ENT. The A&E has separate facilities for children and 89 per cent of patients are dealt with within 4 hours. Death rates for the Trust that runs the hospital are average. Paediatric surgery is performed at the hospital but there is not a paediatrician on site 24 hours a day as recommended by the Royal College of Surgeons.

Number of beds		291
		regional
Overall mortality	99	97
Vacancy rates	3	4
Doctors per 100 beds	39	29
Nurses per 100 beds	130	111
Cancelled operations	1	1
Complaints	2	3
Complaints clear up	20	49
waiting times		
Inpatient	72	78
Outpatient	78	82

Freeman Hospital
Newcastle upon Tyne, NE7 7DN
Phone: 0191 284 3111

Trust: Newcastle upon Tyne Hospitals
**   NHS Trust (The)**

The Freeman Hospital in Newcastle upon Tyne is a major teaching hospital and is famous for heart and lung transplants. The hospital is now operated as part of one service with the Royal Victoria Infirmary and the Newcastle General. The overall mortality rate for the service is low and deaths for emergency stroke and fractured hip admissions are also low. There are coronary care and stroke units and Government targets in key areas of heart disease treatment have been met.

Number of beds		2026
⊕ ⊕ ⊕ ⊕ ⊗ ⊞ ⊙		
		regional
Overall mortality	88	97
Vacancy rates	0	4
Doctors per 100 beds	51	45
Nurses per 100 beds	162	144
Cancelled operations	-	1
Complaints	2	3
Complaints clear up	45	49
waiting times		
Inpatient	78	78
Outpatient	82	82

North Shields · **North Tyneside General Hospital**

Rake Lane, North Shields
Tyne and Wear, NE29 8NH
Phone: 0191 259 6660

Trust: Northumbria Healthcare NHS
**   Trust**

North Tyneside General Hospital opened a new high dependency unit in 2001 to free up intensive care beds. The hospital has a dedicated stroke unit and death rates for emergency stroke admissions are low. However, CT scans are not always performed on suspected stroke patients within 48 hours of admission. Paediatric surgery is performed but a paediatrician is not available 24 hours a day as recommended by the Royal College of Surgeons.

Number of beds		340
⊕ ⊕ ⊕ ⊗ ⊞		
		regional
Overall mortality	99	97
Vacancy rates	5	4
Doctors per 100 beds	23	29
Nurses per 100 beds	92	111
Cancelled operations	0.4	1
Complaints	2	3
Complaints clear up	41	49
waiting times		
Inpatient	83	78
Outpatient	92	82

Northallerton · **Friarage Hospital**

Northallerton
North Yorkshire, DL6 1JG
Phone: 01609 779911

Trust: Northallerton Health Services
    NHS Trust

Friarage Hospital is the main hospital in Northallerton and serves the surrounding rural area in North Yorkshire. The Trust that runs the hospital has a good record on death rates. The overall mortality rate is low as are death rates for emergency stroke and fractured hip admissions. The hospital has a dedicated stroke unit although not all suspected stroke patients receive a CT scan within the recommended 48 hours of admission. The hospital operates a well-regarded spinal clinic.

Number of beds		343
⊕ ⊕ ⊕ ⊗ ⊛		
		regional
Overall mortality	88	97
Vacancy rates	0	4
Doctors per 100 beds	27	31
Nurses per 100 beds	104	110
Cancelled operations	0.5	1
Complaints	5	3
Complaints clear up	69	49
waiting times		
Inpatient	84	78
Outpatient	85	82

Pontefract · **Pontefract General Infirmary**

Friarwood Lane, Pontefract
West Yorkshire, WF8 1PL
Phone: 01977 600 600

Trust: Pinderfields & Pontefract
    Hospitals NHS Trust

The hospital – part of Pinderfields and Pontefracts Hospitals NHS Trust – is being developed as a diagnostic and treatment centre. Government funds of £2.1 m will improve inpatient maternity services and serve the entire district. Almost all A&E patients are admitted, transferred or discharged within the target 4 hours of arrival, but suspected stroke patients do not always receive a CT scan within 48 hours of admission.

Number of beds		478
⊕ ⊕ ⊕ ⊗ ⊛		
		regional
Overall mortality	96	97
Vacancy rates	2	4
Doctors per 100 beds	31	29
Nurses per 100 beds	110	111
Cancelled operations	4	1
Complaints	3	3
Complaints clear up	60	49
waiting times		
Inpatient	72	78
Outpatient	78	82

Scarborough · **Scarborough General Hospital**

Woodlands Drive, Scarborough
North Yorkshire, YO12 6QL
Phone: 01723 368 111

Trust: Scarborough & North East
    Yorkshire Healthcare NHS Trust

Scarborough General Hospital has carried out a number of improvements recently, including the addition of 49 new beds. Death rates for emergency hip admissions are high, although in other areas death rates are average. Heart attack patients are given thrombolysis treatment within the target average of 30 minutes of arrival. The hospital does not currently provide coronary angiography.

Number of beds		-
➕ 🚑 ❌ 📞		
		regional
Overall mortality	96	97
Vacancy rates	6	4
Doctors per 100 beds	26	25
Nurses per 100 beds	114	108
Cancelled operations	-	1
Complaints	2	3
Complaints clear up	38	49
waiting times		
Inpatient	82	78
Outpatient	82	82

South Shields · **South Tyneside District Hospital**

Harton Lane, South Shields
Tyne & Wear, NE34 0PL
Phone: 0191 454 8888

Trust: South Tyneside Health Care NHS
    Trust

At South Tyneside District Hospital almost all patients awaiting treatment in A&E are admitted, transferred or discharged within the recommended maximum time of 4 hours. Death rates for emergency broken hip admission are low. The hospital has multidisciplinary teams for treating breast, colorectal, stomach and lung cancers. All suspected stroke patients receive CT scans within the recommended 48 hours of admission. The hospital plans to build a new centre for care of the elderly and invest in its cardiology services.

Number of beds		612
➕ ⊕ 🚑 ❌ 📞		
		regional
Overall mortality	105	97
Vacancy rates	4	4
Doctors per 100 beds	23	25
Nurses per 100 beds	80	108
Cancelled operations	0	1
Complaints	3	3
Complaints clear up	38	49
waiting times		
Inpatient	87	78
Outpatient	80	82

Steeton · **Airedale General Hospital**

Skipton Road, Steeton
West Yorkshire, BD20 6TD
Phone: 01535 652 511

Trust: Airedale NHS Trust

Airedale General is a large hospital with a low overall mortality rate. Death rates for emergency hip fracture and stroke admission are also low. It meets Government targets in key areas of heart disease but not the target for CT scan administration within 48 hours of admission with stroke. In A&E, nearly 100 per cent of patients are dealt with within 4 hours. The hospital has a better than average performance for both inpatient and outpatient waiting times.

Number of beds		610
✚ ⚕ ✖ ☎		
		regional
Overall mortality	84	97
Vacancy rates	0	4
Doctors per 100 beds	26	25
Nurses per 100 beds	98	108
Cancelled operations	0.6	1
Complaints	2	3
Complaints clear up	34	49
waiting times		
Inpatient	80	78
Outpatient	82	82

Stockton-on-Tees · **University Hospital of North Tees**

Hardwick, Stockton-on-Tees
Cleveland, TS19 8PE
Phone: 01642 617617

Trust: North Tees and Hartlepool NHS
Trust:

The University Hospital of North Tees has recently built a new children's ward and a £7m project has been completed to include new maternity facilities as well as a breast-screening unit. Death rates for emergency broken hip surgery are currently lower than almost any other hospital in the country. Overall death rates are average.

Number of beds		446
✚ ⊕ ⚕ ✖ ☎ ◕		
		regional
Overall mortality	101	97
Vacancy rates	8	4
Doctors per 100 beds	31	29
Nurses per 100 beds	115	111
Cancelled operations	1	1
Complaints	2	3
Complaints clear up	-	49
waiting times		
Inpatient	85	78
Outpatient	85	82

Sunderland · **Ryhope Hospital**

Ryhope, Sunderland
Tyne & Wear, SR2 8AE
Phone: 0191 565 6256

Trust: City Hospitals Sunderland NHS
Trust

Sunderland-based Ryhope Hospital is in the process of being closed down and now only offers limited services. This year additional beds have been made available to cope with winter pressures. In the last year, the Trust has transferred rehabilitation and elderly medicine wards from the Ryhope Hospital into Sunderland City Hospital.

Number of beds		-

		regional
Overall mortality	100	97
Vacancy rates	7	4
Doctors per 100 beds	32	29
Nurses per 100 beds	117	111
Cancelled operations	-	1
Complaints	2	3
Complaints clear up	71	49
waiting times		
Inpatient	79	78
Outpatient	70	82

Sunderland · **Sunderland Royal Hospital**

Kayll Road, Sunderland
Tyne & Wear, SR4 7TP
Phone: 0191 565 6256

Trust: City Hospitals Sunderland NHS
Trust

Sunderland Royal is an acute hospital serving a population of around 330,000. It is part of the City Hospitals Sunderland NHS Trust. The hospital's overall mortality rate is average, as are its stroke and broken hip emergency admission mortality rates. The hospital has yet to meet Government targets for providing thrombolysis to heart attack patients within an average 30 minutes and ensuring stroke patients are given a CT scan within 48 hours of admittance. Children arriving in A&E are treated by specialist paediatricians rather than casualty officers.

Number of beds		947

		regional
Overall mortality	100	97
Vacancy rates	7	4
Doctors per 100 beds	32	29
Nurses per 100 beds	117	111
Cancelled operations	0.9	1
Complaints	2	3
Complaints clear up	71	49
waiting times		
Inpatient	79	78
Outpatient	70	82

Wakefield · **Pinderfields General Hospital**

Aberford Road, Wakefield
Yorkshire, WF1 4DG
Phone: 01924 201 688

Trust: Pinderfields & Pontefract
**   Hospitals NHS Trust**

Part of Pinderfields and Pontefract Hospitals NHS Trust, the hospital is the burns and spinal injuries centre for the north of England. The hospital has plans to build an acute specialist centre at Pinderfields and a diagnostic and treatment centre at Pontefract. Nearly all A&E patients are dealt with in 4 hours, but suspected stroke patients do not always receive a CT scan within the recommended 48 hours. The A&E department has separate waiting and treatment areas for children. Death rates and waiting times for the Trust are average.

Number of beds		596
➊ ➌ ➍ ✖ ☺ ☻		
		regional
Overall mortality	96	97
Vacancy rates	2	4
Doctors per 100 beds	31	29
Nurses per 100 beds	110	111
Cancelled operations	4	1
Complaints	3	3
Complaints clear up	60	49
waiting times		
Inpatient	72	78
Outpatient	78	82

Whitby · **Whitby Hospital**

Spring Hill, Whitby
North Yorkshire, YO21 1EE
Phone: 01947 604 851

Trust: Scarborough & North East
**   Yorkshire Healthcare NHS Trust**

Whitby Hospital has recently opened an endoscopy service and now plans to improve stroke rehabilitation facilities. Following ongoing contributions from the League of Friends, the hospital has been able to make other valuable improvements including building a conservatory and purchasing new equipment for the minor injuries unit. The Trust that runs the hospital has an average overall mortality rate.

Number of beds		-
		regional
Overall mortality	96	97
Vacancy rates	6	4
Doctors per 100 beds	26	25
Nurses per 100 beds	114	108
Cancelled operations	-	1
Complaints	2	3
Complaints clear up	38	49
waiting times		
Inpatient	82	78
Outpatient	82	82

Whitehaven · **West Cumberland Hospital**

Hensingham, Whitehaven
Cumbria, CA28 8JG
Phone: 01946 693181

Trust: North Cumbria Acute Hospitals
    NHS Trust

West Cumberland Hospital is the major acute facility in West Cumbria. It has recently opened a dedicated stroke unit and added an extra bed to its ITU. The hospital has multidisciplinary teams for lung, breast, colorectal and stomach cancers. It provides coronary angiography and meets the recommended level of 500 cardiac catheterisations per year. Outpatient waiting times for the Trust are shorter than most. The Trust that runs this hospital has a high overall mortality rate.

Number of beds		389
⊕ ⊕ ⚕ ⊗ ☏		
		regional
Overall mortality	113	97
Vacancy rates	0	4
Doctors per 100 beds	21	25
Nurses per 100 beds	122	108
Cancelled operations	3	1
Complaints	4	3
Complaints clear up	49	49
waiting times		
Inpatient	72	78
Outpatient	86	82

York · **York District Hospital**

Wigginton Road, York
Yorkshire, YO31 8HE
Phone: 01904 631 313

Trust: York Health Services NHS Trust

York District Hospital has average death rates. It offers MRI scanning, CT scans for suspected stroke patients within 24 hours, and meets the government target to ensure hospitals that perform angiography carry out at least 500 cardiac catheterisations each year. A paediatrician is on site 24 hours a day and there are separate waiting and treatment areas for children in A&E.

Number of beds		835
⊕ ⊕ ⚕ ⊗ ☏ ◉		
		regional
Overall mortality	107	97
Vacancy rates	1	4
Doctors per 100 beds	22	29
Nurses per 100 beds	97	111
Cancelled operations	0.9	1
Complaints	4	3
Complaints clear up	59	49
waiting times		
Inpatient	70	78
Outpatient	81	82

Bingley · **The Yorkshire Clinic**

Bradford Road, Bingley
West Yorkshire, BD16 1TW
Phone: 01274 560 311

The Yorkshire Clinic has dedicated one of its four operating theatres to cardiac surgery. Other services include cosmetic surgery, dental treatment, sports injury and back clinics.

Capio Healthcare UK

Insurers: BUPA*, PPP*, Norwich*, Standard Life*, Royal Sun Alliance, WPA

price guide	£
Hip replacement	5785-8090
Cataract removal	1869-2032

Number of beds	
ALS staff	4
heart services	
Cancer services	

Carlisle · **Abbey Caldew Hospital**

64 Dalston Road, Carlisle
Cumbria, CA2 5NW
Phone: 01228 531713

Abbey Caldew Hospital, situated in the city centre of Carlisle, offers specialties including cosmetic surgery, dermatology, general surgery and orthopaedics. There is a day ward for those receiving treatment that requires a stay of less than 4 hours.

Abbey Hospitals Ltd

Insurers: BUPA, PPP, Norwich, Standard Life, Royal Sun Alliance, WPA

price guide	£
Hip replacement	
Cataract removal	

Number of beds	11
ALS staff	1
heart services	-
Cancer services	

Cottingham · **Hull Nuffield Hospital**

Entrance 3, Castle Hill Hospital, Castle Rd
Cottingham, East Yorkshire, HU16 5FQ
Phone: 01482 623500

Hull Nuffield Hospital provides surgical treatment in a number of key specialties including orthopaedics, ophthalmology, cosmetic surgery, neurosurgery and urology.

Nuffield Hospitals

Insurers: BUPA*, Norwich, Standard Life, Royal Sun Alliance, WPA

price guide	£
Hip replacement	7520
Cataract removal	2220-2600

Number of beds	38
ALS staff	2
heart services	-
Cancer services	

Darlington · **Woodlands Hospital**

Morton Park, Darlington
County Durham, DL1 4PL
Phone: 01325 341 700

Woodlands Hospital is purpose built
offering modern facilities and a full
range of medical and surgical services.
It has a well-equipped operating
theatre and also focuses on pre- and
post-operative care.

Woodlands Healthcare

Insurers: BUPA, PPP, Norwich*, Standard
Life*,Royal Sun Alliance*, WPA*

price guide	£
Hip replacement	
Cataract removal	
Number of beds	34
ALS staff	2
heart services	-
Cancer services	

Elland · **BUPA Hospital Elland**

Elland Lane, Elland
West Yorkshire, HX5 9EB
Phone: 01422 324000

BUPA Elland Hospital serves Halifax,
Huddersfield and Dewsbury. Staff at
the hopsital are committed to high
standards of patient care and regularly
update their skills through training
programmes.

BUPA Hospitals

Insurers: BUPA, PPP, Norwich, Standard Life,
Royal Sun Alliance, WPA

price guide	£
Hip replacement	6900-7500
Cataract removal	2310-2570
Number of beds	41
ALS staff	1
heart services	-
Cancer services	

Harrogate · **Duchy Nuffield Hospital**

Queen's Rd, Harrogate
North Yorkshire, HG2 0HF
Phone: 01423 567136

The Duchy Nuffield Hospital is situated
in a residential area within easy reach
of Harrogate town centre. A major
refurbishment and equipment
programme has recently been
completed.

Nuffield Hospitals

Insurers: BUPA*, PPP*, Norwich*,
Standard Life*, Royal Sun Alliance*, WPA

price guide	£
Hip replacement	6499-7700
Cataract removal	2100-2300
Number of beds	26
ALS staff	0
heart services	-
Cancer services	

Huddersfield · **Huddersfield Nuffield Hospital**

Birkby Hall Rd, Huddersfield
Yorkshire, HD2 2BL
Phone: 01484 533131

Huddersfield Nuffield performs a wide range of surgery. Outpatient consulting rooms, pathology, physiotherapy, a one-stop breast clinic and X-ray departments are also available.

Nuffield Nursing Homes Trust

Insurers: BUPA*, PPP, Norwich, Standard Life*,Royal Sun Alliance, WPA

price guide	£
Hip replacement	7270-7570
Cataract removal	2000-2250

Number of beds	29
ALS staff	1
heart services	-
Cancer services	😵 ✓ ✓

Hull · **BUPA Hull And East Riding Hospital**

Lowfield Road, Anlaby, Hull
East Yorkshire, HU10 7AZ
Phone: 01482 659471

BUPA Hospital Hull and East Riding is currently undergoing major redevelopment. Special facilities offered by the hospital include a decompression chamber to treat patients suffering from smoke and carbon monoxide inhalation.

BUPA Hospitals

Insurers: BUPA, PPP, Norwich, Standard Life, Royal Sun Alliance, WPA

price guide	£
Hip replacement	9330-9330
Cataract removal	2440-2440

Number of beds	40
ALS staff	1
heart services	-
Cancer services	😵 ✓ ✓

Leeds · **BUPA Hospital Leeds**

Jackson Avenue, Roundhay, Leeds
West Yorkshire, LS8 1NT
Phone: 0113 269 3939

The BUPA Hospital Leeds offers a range of procedures from plastic surgery to cataract removal. This is a purpose-built hospital with 10 day-case beds, parent/child rooms and high dependency and intensive care units.

BUPA Hospitals

Insurers: BUPA, PPP, Norwich, Standard Life, Royal Sun Alliance, WPA

price guide	£
Hip replacement	7655-7655
Cataract removal	2421-2421

Number of beds	83
ALS staff	4
heart services	😊 ✓ 🔟
Cancer services	😵 ✓ ✓

Leeds · **BUPA Methley Park Hospital**

Methley Lane, Methley
Leeds, LS26 9HG
Phone: 01977 518518

BUPA Methley Park Hospital holds 29
beds including three parent/child
rooms. Specialties include cosmetic
surgery and other facilities are MRI
scanning, bone density screening and
laser surgery.

BUPA Hospitals

Insurers: BUPA, PPP, Norwich, Standard Life,
Royal Sun Alliance, WPA

price guide	£
Hip replacement	7028-7228
Cataract removal	2247-3507

Number of beds	29
ALS staff	2
heart services	-
Cancer services	🌐 ① ✓

Leeds · **Mid Yorkshire Nuffield Hospital**

Outwood Lane, Horsforth
Leeds, LS18 4HP
Phone: 0113 2588756

The Mid Yorkshire Nuffield Hospital has
a comprehensively equipped twin
operating theatre suite. Facilities for
out-patient consultation and treatment
are provided together with a
diagnostic X-ray department.

Nuffield Nursing Homes Trust

Insurers: BUPA*, Norwich*,
Standard Life*, Royal Sun Alliance*, WPA

price guide	£
Hip replacement	-
Cataract removal	-

Number of beds	30
ALS staff	3
heart services	-
Cancer services	🌐 ✓

Newcastle upon Tyne · **Newcastle Nuffield Hospital**

Clayton Rd, Jesmond
Newcastle upon Tyne, NE2 1JP
Phone: 0191 2816131

The Newcastle Nuffield Hospital draws
consultants from nearby hospitals
including the major teaching hospitals
in Newcastle. The hospital has a self-
contained acute psychiatry unit, The
Lindisfarne Suite.

Nuffield Nursing Homes Trust

Insurers: BUPA*, PPP*, Norwich*,
Standard Life*, Royal Sun Alliance*, WPA

price guide	£
Hip replacement	6369-7077
Cataract removal	1980

Number of beds	53
ALS staff	1
heart services	-
Cancer services	🌐 ① ✓

Scarborough · **BUPA Belvedere Hospital**

Belvedere Road, Scarborough
North Yorkshire, YO11 2UT
Phone: 01723 365363

The BUPA Belvedere hospital draws its
consultants from Scarborough and
North East Yorkshire NHS Trust. The
North Yorkshire Health Authority rates
the hospital as well equipped.

BUPA Hospitals

Insurers: BUPA, PPP, Norwich, Standard Life,
Royal Sun Alliance, WPA

price guide	£
Hip replacement	7700-7700
Cataract removal	2385-2385

Number of beds	37
ALS staff	1
heart services	-
Cancer services	☺ ✓

Stockton-on-Tees · **Cleveland Nuffield Hospital**

Junction Rd, Norton, Stockton-on-Tees
Cleveland, TS20 1PX
Phone: 01642 360100

The Cleveland Nuffield Hospital has
undergone an extension and
renovation programme over the last
ten years. Additions include a minor
procedure suite and an expanded
outpatients department.

Nuffield Nursing Homes Trust

Insurers: BUPA*, PPP*, Norwich*,
Standard Life*, Royal Sun Alliance*, WPA

price guide	£
Hip replacement	6500-8200
Cataract removal	2100-2400

Number of beds	31
ALS staff	2
heart services	☻
Cancer services	☺ ➤

Washington · **BUPA Hospital Washington**

Picktree Lane, Rickleton, Washington
Tyne & Wear, NE38 9JZ
Phone: 0191 415 1272

As well as general surgical and medical
services, the hospital offers an infertility
clinic, a cardiac surgery programme,
24-hour resident doctor cover, and
extensive laser surgery.

BUPA Hospitals

Insurers: BUPA, PPP, Norwich, Standard Life,
Royal Sun Alliance, WPA

price guide	£
Hip replacement	7375-7375
Cataract removal	2000-2310

Number of beds	53
ALS staff	3
heart services	☻
Cancer services	☺ ① ✓ ✔

York · **Purey Cust Nuffield Hospital**

Precentors Court, York
Yorkshire, YO1 7EL
Phone: 01904 641571

The Purey Cust Nuffield Hospital is modern and well equipped, offering a range of services, including pain management, outpatient physiotherapy services, and bone density scanning for osteoporosis.

Nuffield Nursing Homes Trust

Insurers: BUPA*, PPP*, Norwich*, Standard Life, Royal Sun Alliance, WPA

price guide	£
Hip replacement	7200-8800
Cataract removal	2100-2300

Number of beds	31
ALS staff	4
heart services	–
Cancer services	✈ ✓

North West

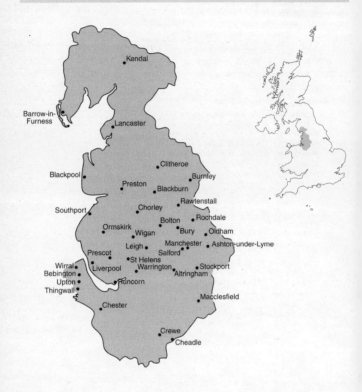

Kendal

Barrow-in-
Furness

Lancaster

Blackpool

Clitheroe

Burnley

Preston

Blackburn

Rawtenstall

Chorley

Southport

Rochdale

Bolton

Ormskirk

Bury

Oldham

Wigan

Manchester

Ashton-under-Lyme

Leigh

Salford

Prescot

St Helens

Wirral

Liverpool

Warrington

Stockport

Bebington

Altringham

Upton

Runcorn

Thingwall

Macclesfield

Chester

Crewe

Cheadle

NHS

Ashton-under-Lyme	Tameside General Hospital
Barrow-in-Furness	Furness General Hospital
Blackburn	Blackburn Royal Infirmary
Blackburn	Queen's Park Hospital
Blackpool	Blackpool Victoria Hospital
Bolton	Royal Bolton Hospital
Burnley	Burnley General Hospital
Bury	Fairfield General Hospital
Chester	Countess of Chester Hospital
Chorley	Chorley & South Ribble District Hospital
Crewe	Leighton Hospital
Kendal	Westmoreland General Hospital
Lancaster	Royal Lancaster Infirmary
Leigh	Leigh Hospital
Liverpool	Broadgreen Hospital
Liverpool	Royal Liverpool University Hospital
Liverpool	University Hospital Aintree
Macclesfield	Macclesfield District General Hospital
Manchester	Manchester Royal Infirmary
Manchester	North Manchester General Hospital
Manchester	Trafford General Hospital
Manchester	Wythenshawe Hospital
Oldham	Royal Oldham Hospital
Ormskirk	Ormskirk and District General Hospital
Prescot	Whiston Hospital
Preston	Royal Preston Hospital
Rawtenstall	Rossendale General Hospital
Rochdale	Rochdale Infirmary
Runcorn	Halton General Hospital
Salford	Hope Hospital
Southport	Southport & Formby District General Hospital
St Helens	St Helens Hospital
Stockport	Stepping Hill Hospital
Warrington	Warrington Hospital
Wigan	Billinge Hospital
Wigan	Royal Albert Edward Infirmary
Wirral	Wirral Hospital

Private

Blackburn	BMI The Beardwood Hospital
Blackpool	BUPA Fylde Coast
Bolton	BMI The Beaumont Hospital
Cheadle	BMI The Alexandra Hospital
Chester	Grovesnor Nuffield Hospital
Chorley	Euxton Hall Hospital
Clitheroe	Abbey Gisburne Park
Crewe	BMI The South Cheshire Hospital Wirral
Lancaster	Lancaster & Lakeland Nuffield Hospital
Liverpool	Abbey Sefton Hospital
Liverpool	Lourdes Hospital
Macclesfield	BUPA Regency Hospital
Manchester	BUPA Hospital Manchester
Manchester	BMI The Alexandra Hospital Victoria Park
Ormskirk	Renacres Hall Hospital
Preston	Fulwood Hall Hospital
Rochdale	BMI The Highfield Hospital
Salford	Oaklands Hospital
St Helens	Fairfield Hospital
Warrington	BUPA North Cheshire Hospital
Wirral	BUPA Murrayfield Hospital

Ashton-under-Lyne · **Tameside General Hospital**

Fountain Street, Ashton-under-Lyne
Lancashire, OL6 9RW
Phone: 0161 331 6000

Trust: Tameside & Glossop Acute
Sevices NHS Trust

In an effort to meet new standards in the Government's recent NSF for coronary heart disease, Tameside General Hospital has bought new heart monitoring equipment and an echocardiography machine. Overall, the mortality rate is average, although the death rate for emergency broken hip patients is high. The hospital has its own CCU but refers patients elsewhere for coronary angiography. Eight out of ten casualty patients are seen within 4 hours. Cancellation rates for operations are higher than average, although most are rescheduled within 31 days.

Number of beds		664
➊ ➕ ♏ ✖ 🍴		
		regional
Overall mortality	106	104
Vacancy rates	-	4
Doctors per 100 beds	35	30
Nurses per 100 beds	141	119
Cancelled operations	4	1
Complaints	3	3
Complaints clear up	47	57
waiting times		
Inpatient	88	76
Outpatient	67	76

Barrow-in-Furness · **Furness General Hospital**

Dalton Lane, Barrow-in-Furness
Cumbria, LA14 4LF
Phone: 01229 870 870

Trust: Morecambe Bay Hospitals NHS
Trust

Furness General is a medium-sized acute district general hospital. Nearly 96 per cent of A&E patients are dealt with within 4 hours. However, heart attack patients do not currently receive thrombolytic drugs within an average of 30 minutes of A&E arrival. There is no stroke unit and not all suspected stroke patients receive a CT scan within 48 hours of admission. However, the death rate for emergency stroke patients is in line with national averages as are other death rates. The A&E has separate children's waiting and treatment areas.

Number of beds		400
➊ ➕ ♏ ✖ 🍴		
		regional
Overall mortality	92	104
Vacancy rates	5	4
Doctors per 100 beds	24	28
Nurses per 100 beds	106	111
Cancelled operations	1	1
Complaints	3.3	3
Complaints clear up	51	57
waiting times		
Inpatient	74	76
Outpatient	79	76

Blackburn · **Blackburn Royal Infirmary**

Bolton Road, Blackburn
Lancashire, BB2 3LR
Phone: 01254 263 555

Trust: Blackburn, Hyndburn & Ribble
Valley Healthcare NHS Trust

Blackburn Royal Infirmary, a medium-sized acute service, is currently struggling with cramped facilities. However, the site is due to close by 2005 when services will have been centralised onto the Queen's Park Hospital site. The A&E department deals with 94 per cent of patients within 4 hours. The overall mortality rate for the Blackburn, Hyndburn and Ribble Valley Trust is 10 per cent above average and the death rate for emergency stroke admissions is also high. There is no stroke unit at this hospital.

Number of beds		318
		regional
Overall mortality	110	104
Vacancy rates	9	4
Doctors per 100 beds	28	28
Nurses per 100 beds	120	111
Cancelled operations	1	1
Complaints	2.5	3
Complaints clear up	80	57
waiting times		
Inpatient	77	76
Outpatient	81	76

Blackburn · **Queens Park Hospital**

Haslingden Road, Blackburn
Lancashire, BB2 3HH
Phone: 01245 263 555

Trust: Blackburn, Hyndburn & Ribble
Valley Healthcare NHS Trust

Queens Park Hospital, based in Blackburn, is undergoing a £70 million scheme to consolidate the Blackburn, Hyndburn and Ribble NHS Trust's services on its site by spring 2005. The trust has an above average mortality rate and a high mortality rate for emergency stroke patients. The hospital does not have an A&E department and does not have CT or MRI scanning facilities. However, it has a stroke rehabilitation unit. Breast, stomach, lung and colorectal cancers are all treated, and multidisciplinary teams are in place for most of these.

Number of beds		502
		regional
Overall mortality	110	104
Vacancy rates	9	4
Doctors per 100 beds	28	28
Nurses per 100 beds	120	111
Cancelled operations	1	1
Complaints	2.5	3
Complaints clear up	80	57
waiting times		
Inpatient	77	76
Outpatient	81	76

Blackpool · **Blackpool Victoria Hospital**

Whinney Heys Road
Blackpool, FY3 8NR
Phone: 01253 300 000

Trust: Blackpool Victoria Hospital NHS Trust

The Blackpool Victoria Hospital is a large acute hospital. A new block has been built to replace 25 per cent of the beds. Emergency hip fracture and stroke admission death rates, plus the overall mortality rate, are high. Stroke patients do not always receive a CT scan within 48 hours of admission and heart attack patients are not usually treated with thrombolysis within 30 minutes of arrival in A&E. However, waiting times figures are good and the hospital meets new targets for provision of multidisciplinary teams to treat cancer.

Number of beds		767
⊕ ⊕ 🜨 ⊗ 🜨 🜨		
		regional
Overall mortality	111	104
Vacancy rates	2	4
Doctors per 100 beds	41	28
Nurses per 100 beds	118	111
Cancelled operations	-	1
Complaints	2	3
Complaints clear up	36	57
waiting times		
Inpatient	78	76
Outpatient	82	76

Bolton · **Royal Bolton Hospital**

Farnworth, Bolton
BL4 0JR
Phone: 01204 390 390

Trust: Bolton Hospitals NHS Trust

The hospital's overall death rate is high, as are its death rates for emergency stroke and fractured hip admissions. Thrombolysis is administered to heart attack patients within the target average of 30 minutes of arrival. However, not all suspected stroke patients receive a CT scan within the recommended 48 hours after admission. There are multidisciplinary teams in place for treatment of breast, lung, stomach and colorectal cancers. The hospital's eye unit has received an award for high standards.

Number of beds		965
⊕ 🜨 ⊗ 🜨		
		regional
Overall mortality	113	104
Vacancy rates	2	4
Doctors per 100 beds	26	28
Nurses per 100 beds	108	111
Cancelled operations	3	1
Complaints	3	3
Complaints clear up	20	57
waiting times		
Inpatient	78	76
Outpatient	74	76

Burnley · **Burnley General Hospital**

Casterton Avenue, Burnley
Lancashire, BB10 2PQ
Phone: 01282 425071

Trust: Burnley Health Care NHS Trust

Burnley General Hospital is a large facility serving Burnley, Pendle and Rossendale. A £15 m programme to modernise the A&E department has recently been completed. The Burnley Healthcare Trust does not perform well on mortality measures with a high overall mortality rate and death rates for emergency hip fracture admissions above average. There are dedicated stroke facilities, but not all stroke patients receive a CT scan within 48 hours of admission.

Number of beds		657
➊ ⊕ ⚕ ✖ ⚕		
		regional
Overall mortality	112	104
Vacancy rates	6	4
Doctors per 100 beds	26	28
Nurses per 100 beds	102	111
Cancelled operations	2	1
Complaints	2	3
Complaints clear up	72	57
waiting times		
Inpatient	74	76
Outpatient	71	76

Bury · **Fairfield General Hospital**

Rochdale Old Road, Bury
Lancashire, BL9 7TD
Phone: 0161 764 6081

Trust: Bury Health Care NHS Trust

Fairfield Hospital serves Bury and the surrounding areas and has recently undergone an extensive development programme taking over services from Bury General. The overall mortality rate for the Trust is higher than average although death rates for emergency patients with broken hips or strokes are average. On waiting times the Trust does better than average. A&E has separate children's waiting and treatment areas.

Number of beds		596
➊ ⊕ ⚕ ✖ ⚕		
		regional
Overall mortality	111	104
Vacancy rates	9	4
Doctors per 100 beds	24	30
Nurses per 100 beds	93	105
Cancelled operations	0.4	1
Complaints	1.8	3
Complaints clear up	46	57
waiting times		
Inpatient	79	76
Outpatient	81	76

Chester · **Countess of Chester Hospital**

Liverpool Road, Chester
Cheshire, CH2 1UL
Phone: 01244 365 000

Trust: Countess of Chester Hospital
  NHS Trust

The Countess of Chester is a large hospital, serving Chester, Ellesmere Port and rural West Cheshire. The hospital has an A&E department which deals with over 90 per cent of patients within 4 hours. The hospital's overall mortality rate and the death rate for emergency stroke admissions are high. Although there is no dedicated stroke unit at the hospital, suspected stroke patients receive a CT scan within 48 hours of admission.

Number of beds		603
⊕ ⊕ ⊗ ⊗ ⊚ ⊚		
		regional
Overall mortality	111	104
Vacancy rates	3	4
Doctors per 100 beds	44	30
Nurses per 100 beds	133	105
Cancelled operations	4	1
Complaints	3.4	3
Complaints clear up	56	57
waiting times		
Inpatient	62	76
Outpatient	81	76

Chorley · **Chorley & South Ribble District General**

Preston Road, Chorley
Lancashire, PR7 1PP
Phone: 01257 261222

Trust: Chorley and South Ribble NHS
  Trust

Chorley and South Ribble Hospital, with the Royal Preston and Sharoe Green Hospitals, provides a range of acute services to Central Lancashire, plus specialist services to Lancashire and South Cumbria. There are separate treatment and waiting areas for children in A&E. However, emergency heart attack patients do not receive thrombolysis within 30 minutes of arrival in A&E. The Trust performs in line with national averages on analysis of mortality rates.

Number of beds		410
⊕ ⊕ ⊗ ⊗ ⊚		
		regional
Overall mortality	95	104
Vacancy rates	13	4
Doctors per 100 beds	23	28
Nurses per 100 beds	99	111
Cancelled operations	0.3	1
Complaints	2.3	3
Complaints clear up	65	57
waiting times		
Inpatient	-	76
Outpatient	-	76

Crewe · **Leighton Hospital**

Middlewich Road, Crewe
Lancashire, CW1 4QJ
Phone: 01270 255 141

Trust: Mid Cheshire Hospitals Trust

Leighton Hospital forms part of the Mid Cheshire Hospitals NHS Trust and is the District General Hospital for South Cheshire. The overall mortality rate is high although the Trust has a lower than expected death rate for patients with broken hips. It has a higher than expected death rate for emergency stroke patients, although there is a dedicated stroke unit and CT scans are performed on suspected stroke patients within 48 hours of admission.

Number of beds		700
⊕ ⊕ ⊕ ⊗ ⊕ ⊕		
		regional
Overall mortality	114	104
Vacancy rates	2	4
Doctors per 100 beds	28	30
Nurses per 100 beds	108	105
Cancelled operations	2	1
Complaints	5.2	3
Complaints clear up	92	57
waiting times		
Inpatient	69	76
Outpatient	73	76

Kendal · **Westmorland General Hospital**

Burton Road, Kendal
Cumbria, LA9 7RG
Phone: 01539 732 288

Trust: Morecambe Bay Hospitals NHS Trust

Westmorland General Hospital, part of Morecambe Bay Hospitals NHS Trust, is a small acute hospital. The overall mortality rate for the trust is average and very few operations are cancelled for non-medical reasons. Multidisciplinary teams are in place for lung, breast, stomach and colorectal cancer treatment. Although there is a dedicated four-bed coronary care unit, the hospital does not offer coronary angiography.

Number of beds		214
⊗		
		regional
Overall mortality	92	104
Vacancy rates	5	4
Doctors per 100 beds	24	28
Nurses per 100 beds	106	111
Cancelled operations	0	1
Complaints	3.3	3
Complaints clear up	51	57
waiting times		
Inpatient	74	76
Outpatient	79	76

Lancaster · **Royal Lancaster Infirmary**

Ashton Road
Lancaster, LA1 4RP
Phone: 01524 659 44

Trust: Morecambe Bay Hospitals NHS
Trust

The Royal Lancaster Infirmary has recently refurbished its women's unit and ITU in an effort to improve facilities. It is currently developing a new £800,000 combined MRI and Spiral CT Scanner. The hospital has an average mortality rate and its A&E department deals with almost all patients within 4 hours. Around 5 per cent of operations are cancelled for non-medical reasons – more than most hospitals – with one in nine rescheduled within 31 days.

Number of beds		437

○ ⊕ ⊛ ⊕ ⊗ ⊖

		regional
Overall mortality	92	104
Vacancy rates	5	4
Doctors per 100 beds	24	28
Nurses per 100 beds	106	111
Cancelled operations	5	1
Complaints	3.3	3
Complaints clear up	51	57
waiting times		
Inpatient	74	76
Outpatient	79	76

Leigh · **Leigh Infirmary**

The Avenue, Leigh
Lancashire, WN7 1HS
Phone: 01942 672 333

Trust: Wrightington, Wigan and Leigh
Health Services NHS Trust

This small acute hospital has three operating departments, which perform day surgery, as well as a comprehensive, well-equipped recovery unit. There is also a nurse-led walk-in centre, which sees approximately 33,000 patients with minor injuries each year. There is no A&E and the hospital does not have MRI or CT scanning facilities.

Number of beds		245

⊗

		regional
Overall mortality	106	104
Vacancy rates	2	4
Doctors per 100 beds	27	28
Nurses per 100 beds	112	111
Cancelled operations	-	1
Complaints	3	3
Complaints clear up	53	57
waiting times		
Inpatient	74	76
Outpatient	75	76

Liverpool · **Broadgreen Hospital**

Thomas Drive
Liverpool, L14 3LB
Phone: 0151 706 2000

Trust: Royal Liverpool & Broadgreen
University Hospitals NHS Trust

Broadgreen Hospital provides a range of services to the local population and shares the site with Liverpool's Cardiothoracic Centre. Several development programmes have improved the hospital's facilities, including a new elderly rehabilitation unit. There is a coronary care unit and the hospital provides angiography. It also meets Government targets in the provision of thrombolysis within 30 minutes. Death rates are in line with national averages but waiting times are above average.

Number of beds		235
✪ ✖ ⊕		
		regional
Overall mortality	95	104
Vacancy rates	5	4
Doctors per 100 beds	34	43
Nurses per 100 beds	112	130
Cancelled operations	-	1
Complaints	3.2	3
Complaints clear up	39	57
waiting times		
Inpatient	70	76
Outpatient	64	76

Liverpool · **Royal Liverpool University Hospital**

Prescot Street
Liverpool, L7 8XP
Phone: 0151 7062000

Trust: Royal Liverpool & Broadgreen
University Hospitals NHS Trust

Since opening in 1978, the Royal Liverpool University Hospital has grown to become the city's largest acute district general hospital. Less than half of patients awaiting treatment in A&E are dealt with within the target 4 hours. All suspected stroke patients are given a CT scan within the target 48 hours of admission. Death rates are average.

Number of beds		1280
✚ ✪ ✖ ⊕ ◉		
		regional
Overall mortality	95	104
Vacancy rates	5	4
Doctors per 100 beds	34	43
Nurses per 100 beds	112	130
Cancelled operations	0.7	1
Complaints	3.2	3
Complaints clear up	39	57
waiting times		
Inpatient	70	76
Outpatient	64	76

Liverpool · **University Hospital Aintree**

Longmoor Lane, Liverpool
Merseyside, L9 7AL
Phone: 0151 525 5980

Trust: Aintree Hospitals NHS Trust

University Hospital Aintree has low death rates for stroke but rates for emergency broken hip surgery are average. It offers multidisciplinary teams for lung, breast, stomach and colorectal cancer and has MRI and CT scanning facilities. The hospital has a stroke unit but currently does not scan stroke patients within the Government recommended time of 48 hours. Thrombolysis treatment for heart attack patients is administered within the recommended 30 minutes. Few operations are cancelled for non-medical reasons.

Number of beds		896
➊ ➋ ➌ ➍ ➎		
		regional
Overall mortality	97	104
Vacancy rates	6	4
Doctors per 100 beds	28	28
Nurses per 100 beds	86	111
Cancelled operations	0.7	1
Complaints	3	3
Complaints clear up	54	57
waiting times		
Inpatient	79	76
Outpatient	77	76

Macclesfield · **Macclesfield District General**

Victoria Road, Macclesfield
Cheshire, SK10 3BL
Phone: 01625 421 000

Trust: East Cheshire NHS Trust

Macclesfield District General Hospital serves the population of Macclesfield, Bollington, Poynton and the surrounding areas. It meets Government guidelines by ensuring that all suspected stroke patients are given a CT scan within 48 hours of admission. It also has a stroke rehabilitation unit. However, heart attack patients do not receive thrombolysis within an average of 30 minutes of arriving at A&E. Surgery on children is performed but a paediatrician is not on site 24 hours a day.

Number of beds		576
➊ ➋ ➌ ➍ ➎ ➏		
		regional
Overall mortality	102	104
Vacancy rates	0	4
Doctors per 100 beds	26	30
Nurses per 100 beds	109	105
Cancelled operations	1	1
Complaints	3.1	3
Complaints clear up	55	57
waiting times		
Inpatient	86	76
Outpatient	77	76

Manchester · **Manchester Royal Infirmary**

Oxford Road
Manchester, M13 9WL
Phone: 0161 276 1234

Trust: Central Manchester/Manchester
Childrens University Hospital NHS
Trust

The Manchester Royal Infirmary teaching hospital provides acute services to central Manchester. The hospital meets government targets in two key areas for heart disease: thrombolysis is give to heart attack patients within an average of 30 minutes of admission and its coronary angiography service performs at least 500 catheterisations per year. Despite performing CT scans on all suspected stroke patients within 48 hours of admission, the hospital has an above average mortality rate for stroke patients admitted as emergencies.

Number of beds		519
✚ ⊕ ⚙ ✖ 🚑 ◑		
		regional
Overall mortality	102	104
Vacancy rates	1	4
Doctors per 100 beds	59	43
Nurses per 100 beds	168	130
Cancelled operations	-	1
Complaints	2	3
Complaints clear up	60	57
waiting times		
Inpatient	-	76
Outpatient	-	76

Manchester · **North Manchester General Hospital**

Crumpsall
Manchester, M8 5RL
Phone: 0161 795 4567

Trust: North Manchester Healthcare
NHS Trust

North Manchester General Hospital serves a population of 250,000. It has a dedicated stroke unit and ensures that all suspected stroke patients are given a CT scan within 48 hours of admission. Government recommendations on single-sex wards are met. On average, heart attack patients receive thrombolytic drugs within the target 30 minutes of arrival. Overall the mortality rate for the hospital is above average although the death rates for emergency stroke patients and those with broken hips is average.

Number of beds		702
✚ ⚙ ✖ 🚑 ◑		
		regional
Overall mortality	110	104
Vacancy rates	5	4
Doctors per 100 beds	39	28
Nurses per 100 beds	118	111
Cancelled operations	2	1
Complaints	3	3
Complaints clear up	46	57
waiting times		
Inpatient	88	76
Outpatient	73	76

Manchester · **Trafford General Hospital**

Moorside Road
Manchester, M41 5SL
Phone: 0161 748 4022

Trust: Trafford Healthcare NHS Trust

Trafford General Hospital is undergoing redevelopment which will bring new departments for audiology and A&E. Hip and stroke mortality death rates at the hospital are above average. The hospital does not meet the recommended 30 minute door-to-needle time for thrombolysis for heart attack patients. Also, it does not offer patients CT scans within 48 hours.

Number of beds		497
✪ ⊕ 🅰 ✖ 🚆		
		regional
Overall mortality	105	104
Vacancy rates	0	4
Doctors per 100 beds	26	30
Nurses per 100 beds	95	105
Cancelled operations	0.9	1
Complaints	2	3
Complaints clear up	61	57
waiting times		
Inpatient	79	76
Outpatient	82	76

Manchester · **Wythenshawe Hospital**

Southmoor Road
Manchester, M23 9LT
Phone: 0161 998 7070

Trust: South Manchester University Hospitals NHS Trust

Wythenshawe has 16 CCU beds and has dedicated stroke units for acute treatment and rehabilitation. It has both MRI and CT scanning facilities, but does not perform scans for stroke patients within 48 hours. Nor are heart attack patients guaranteed thrombolysis within half an hour. However, the hospital's angiography service does meet Government targets to carry out 500 cardiac catheterisations each year. Death rates and waiting times are average.

Number of beds		720
✪ ⊕ 🅰 ✖ 🚆 ◐		
		regional
Overall mortality	95	104
Vacancy rates	1	4
Doctors per 100 beds	43	43
Nurses per 100 beds	129	130
Cancelled operations	2	1
Complaints	2.2	3
Complaints clear up	62	57
waiting times		
Inpatient	73	76
Outpatient	82	76

Oldham · **Royal Oldham Hospital**

Rochdale Road
Oldham, OL1 2JH
Phone: 0161 624 0420

Trust: Oldham NHS Trust

The Royal Oldham Hospital has recently added an 8-bed observation ward and an additional resuscitation bay to its A&E department. Eight out of 10 patients awaiting treatment in A&E are currently dealt with within the recommended time of 4 hours. The death rate for emergency broken hip admissions is lower than average, but the overall mortality rate is higher than average. Waiting times are better then most hospitals.

Number of beds		829
➕ ⊕ ⚕ ❌ ⚕ ⚕		
		regional
Overall mortality	111	104
Vacancy rates	10	4
Doctors per 100 beds	28	28
Nurses per 100 beds	120	111
Cancelled operations	0.5	1
Complaints	1.1	3
Complaints clear up	71	57
waiting times		
Inpatient	82	76
Outpatient	81	76

Ormskirk · **Ormskirk and District General Hospital**

Wigan Road, Ormskirk
Lancashire, L39 2AZ
Phone: 01695 577 111

Trust: Southport & Ormskirk Hospital
NHS Trust

Ormskirk and District Hospital added a 2-bed observation ward to its casualty department in 2001. The hospital provides single -sex wards and gives heart attack patients thrombolysis within an average of 30 minutes of being admitted. All suspected stroke patients receive a CT scan within 24 hours of arriving in A&E – better than the Government's recommended target of ensuring that stroke patients get a scan within 48 hours. The hospital has a rehabilitation stroke unit and the death rate following emergency stroke admission is below average.

Number of beds		273
➕ ⊕ ⚕ ❌ ⚕		
		regional
Overall mortality	99	104
Vacancy rates	4	4
Doctors per 100 beds	33	30
Nurses per 100 beds	102	105
Cancelled operations	1	1
Complaints	3.8	3
Complaints clear up	93	57
waiting times		
Inpatient	70	76
Outpatient	63	76

Prescot · **Whiston Hospital**

Whiston, Prescot
Merseyside, L35 5DR
Phone: 0151 426 1600

Trust: St Helens and Knowsley
   Hospitals NHS Trust

Whiston Hospital serves around
330,000 people in the northwestern
Merseyside area and is also a regional
centre for plastic surgery and burns.
Whiston has a high overall mortality
rate and high death rates for
emergency broken hip operations and
emergency stroke patients. It has a 6-
bed CCU but does not offer coronary
angiography. Stroke patients are not
always given a CT scan within the
Government's recommended time of
48 hours. Multidisciplinary teams for
cancer treatment are in place.

Number of beds		829
✚ ⊕ ♫ ✖ ☺ ◉		
		regional
Overall mortality	111	104
Vacancy rates	6	4
Doctors per 100 beds	21	28
Nurses per 100 beds	100	111
Cancelled operations	5	1
Complaints	2	3
Complaints clear up	45	57
waiting times		
Inpatient	79	76
Outpatient	80	76

Preston · **Royal Preston Hospital**

Sharoe Green Lane North
Preston, PR2 9HT
Phone: 01772 716 565

Trust: Preston Acute Hospitals NHS
   Trust

The Royal Preston Hospital works in
partnership with the Sharoe Green and
Chorley & South Ribble Hospital
providing outpatient and inpatient
services to more than 300,000
patients a year. It has a low overall
mortality rate and provides
multidisciplinary teams for cancer. It
does not perform coronary
angiography and heart attack patients
are not given thrombolysis within the
target average of 30 minutes from
their arrival in A&E.

Number of beds		822
✚ ⊕ ♫ ✖ ☺ ◉		
		regional
Overall mortality	92	104
Vacancy rates	3	4
Doctors per 100 beds	43	28
Nurses per 100 beds	126	111
Cancelled operations	1	1
Complaints	2.3	3
Complaints clear up	65	57
waiting times		
Inpatient	82	76
Outpatient	76	76

Rawtenstall · **Rossendale General Hospital**

Haslingden Road, Rawtenstall
Lancashire, BB4 6NE
Phone: 01706 215 151

Trust: Burnley Health Care NHS Trust

Rossendale Hospital is a small hospital which provides a wide range of outpatient and day case services. The hospital provides treatment for colorectal cancer and has a multi-disciplinary team in place. In line with Government recommendations, wards are single-sex.

Number of beds		79
✗		
		regional
Overall mortality	112	104
Vacancy rates	6	4
Doctors per 100 beds	26	28
Nurses per 100 beds	102	111
Cancelled operations	0.7	1
Complaints	2	3
Complaints clear up	72	57
waiting times		
Inpatient	74	76
Outpatient	71	76

Rochdale · **Rochdale Infirmary**

Whitehall Street, Rochdale
Lancashire, OL12 0NB
Phone: 01706 377 777

Trust: Rochdale Healthcare NHS Trust

Rochdale Infirmary meets Government guidelines by providing single-sex wards and ensuring all suspected stroke patients receive CT scans within 48 hours of admission. The hospital meets government recommendations on coronary angiographies by performing at least 500 catheterisations each year. However, on average thrombolysis is not administered to heart attack patients within the target 30 minutes of arrival. Casualty is child friendly with separate child treatment and waiting areas. Death rates and waiting times are in line with national averages.

Number of beds		272
➕ ⊕ ⚕ ✗ ☺		
		regional
Overall mortality	108	104
Vacancy rates	8	4
Doctors per 100 beds	25	30
Nurses per 100 beds	102	105
Cancelled operations	0.6	1
Complaints	3.4	3
Complaints clear up	59	57
waiting times		
Inpatient	75	76
Outpatient	78	76

Runcorn · **Halton General Hospital**

Hospital Way, Runcorn
Cheshire, WA7 2DA
Phone: 01928 714 567

Trust: North Cheshire Hospitals NHS
Trust

Halton General Hospital merged with Warrington Hospital in April 2001 and forms part of North Cheshire Hospitals NHS Trust. Halton treats most major cancer types and, except for cancers of the upper gastrointestinal tract, care is delivered by multidisciplinary teams. Services for heart patients include a coronary care unit, but angiography is not offered. The hospital performs surgery on children, but does not have either a paediatric ward or a paediatrician on site 24 hours a day.

Number of beds		242
✢ ⊗ ☏		
		regional
Overall mortality	101	104
Vacancy rates	-	4
Doctors per 100 beds	25	30
Nurses per 100 beds	97	119
Cancelled operations	1.7	1
Complaints	-	3
Complaints clear up	-	57
waiting times		
Inpatient	64	76
Outpatient	88	76

Salford · **Hope Hospital**

Stott Lane
Salford, M6 8WH
Phone: 0161 789 7373

Trust: Salford Royal Hospitals NHS
Trust

Following a £750,000 cash boost, the A&E department at Hope Hospital now has four new bays in the resuscitation area. It has also expanded its ITU to 16 beds. The overall mortality rate is average but the waiting times performance could be improved. The hospital has multidisciplinary teams for major cancer treatment as recommended and provides thrombolysis to heart attack patients within 30 minutes. Wards are single-sex throughout the hospital, including the ITU and CCU.

Number of beds		800
✚ ✢ ⊗ ☏ ◉		
		regional
Overall mortality	99	104
Vacancy rates	0	4
Doctors per 100 beds	46	43
Nurses per 100 beds	129	130
Cancelled operations	1	1
Complaints	2.9	3
Complaints clear up	52	57
waiting times		
Inpatient	66	76
Outpatient	68	76

Southport · **Southport & Formby District General**

Town Lane, Southport
Merseyside, PR8 6PN
Phone: 01704 547 471

Trust: Southport & Ormskirk Hospital
  NHS Trust

Southport and Formby District General Hospital is one of only a few to have a helipad for emergency admissions and a decontamination suite. The Trust has an average death rate for emergency broken hip admissions but the death rate for emergency stroke admissions is lower than average. The overall mortality figure is in line with the national average. The A&E department sees 8 out of 10 patients within the recommended maximum of 4 hours and the hospital has multidisciplinary teams for treating most cancers.

Number of beds		357
⊕ ⊕ ⊕ ⊗ ☏ ◉		
		regional
Overall mortality	99	104
Vacancy rates	4	4
Doctors per 100 beds	33	30
Nurses per 100 beds	102	105
Cancelled operations	0.3	1
Complaints	3.8	3
Complaints clear up	93	57
waiting times		
Inpatient	70	76
Outpatient	63	76

St Helens · **St Helens Hospital**

Marshalls Cross Road, St Helens
Merseyside, WA9 3EA
Phone: 01744 266 633

Trust: St Helens and Knowsley
  Hospitals NHS Trust

St Helens Hospital, Merseyside, is a small acute hospital within the St Helens and Knowsley Hospitals NHS Trust. It does not have an A&E department but has some acute facilities. Breast, lung, stomach and colorectal cancers are treated here and multidisciplinary teams are in place for each. The overall mortality rate for the Trust is higher than average.

Number of beds		288
⊗		
		regional
Overall mortality	111	104
Vacancy rates	6	4
Doctors per 100 beds	21	28
Nurses per 100 beds	100	111
Cancelled operations	1	1
Complaints	2	3
Complaints clear up	45	57
waiting times		
Inpatient	79	76
Outpatient	80	76

Stockport · **Stepping Hill Hospital**

Poplar Grove, Stockport
Cheshire, SK2 7JE
Phone: 0161 483 1010

Trust: Stockport NHS Trust

In response to the Government's drive to improve standards in coronary care, the hospital has created a rapid-access chest pain clinic and installed new heart-monitoring equipment. There is a rehabilitation unit for stroke victims and the hospital provide CT scans within 48 hours. Patients needing coronary angiography are currently referred elsewhere. Stepping Hill has high death rates for emergency admissions of both hip surgery and stroke patients, yet the overall mortality rate is average.

Number of beds		753
✛ ⊕ ✿ ⊕ ✖ ☎ ◕		
		regional
Overall mortality	103	104
Vacancy rates	0	4
Doctors per 100 beds	25	28
Nurses per 100 beds	123	111
Cancelled operations	1	1
Complaints	1.6	3
Complaints clear up	87	57
waiting times		
Inpatient	71	76
Outpatient	76	76

Warrington · **Warrington Hospital**

Lovely Lane, Warrington
Cheshire, WA5 1QG
Phone: 01925 635 911

Trust: North Cheshire Hospitals NHS
Trust

Warrington hospital has multidisciplinary teams for the major cancers, and meets Government targets on administering thrombolysis to heart attack patients within 30 minutes. The overall mortality rate is average, although the rate for emergency broken hip patients is low. The hospital does not offer coronary angiography and cannot guarantee scans for stroke patients within 48 hours. The hospital recently upgraded its radiology department and has a new medical admissions unit to ease admissions pressures on A&E staff.

Number of beds		642
✛ ✿ ✖ ☎ ◕		
		regional
Overall mortality	103	104
Vacancy rates	6	4
Doctors per 100 beds	32	30
Nurses per 100 beds	108	105
Cancelled operations	0.8	1
Complaints	-	3
Complaints clear up	-	57
waiting times		
Inpatient	64	76
Outpatient	88	76

Wigan · **Billinge Hospital**

Upholland Road, Wigan
Lancashire, WN5 7ET
Phone: 01942 244 000

Trust: Wrightington, Wigan and Leigh
Health Services NHS Trust

Billinge Hospital provides maternity and gynaecology services to the local population.

Number of beds		133

		regional
Overall mortality	106	104
Vacancy rates	2	4
Doctors per 100 beds	27	28
Nurses per 100 beds	112	111
Cancelled operations	-	1
Complaints	-	3
Complaints clear up	-	57
waiting times		
Inpatient	74	76
Outpatient	75	76

Wigan · **Royal Albert Edward Infirmary**

Wigan Lane, Wigan
Lancashire, WN1 2NN
Phone: 01942 244 000

Trust: Wrightington, Wigan and Leigh
Health Services NHS Trust

This hospital has a busy A&E dealing with around 80,000 patients each year. Death rates for emergency patients with broken hips and strokes are high. However, the overall mortality rate for the hospital is average. There are major development plans to upgrade emergency and X-ray services. Although it does not have a children's ITU, a paediatrician is onsite 24 hours and there are separate treatment and waiting areas for children in A&E. Thrombolysis for heart attack patients is administered within 30 minutes.

Number of beds		480

		regional
Overall mortality	106	104
Vacancy rates	2	4
Doctors per 100 beds	27	28
Nurses per 100 beds	112	111
Cancelled operations	-	1
Complaints	-	3
Complaints clear up	-	57
waiting times		
Inpatient	74	76
Outpatient	75	76

Wirral · **Wirral Hospital**

Arrowe Park Road, Wirral
Merseyside, CH49 5PE
Phone: 0151 678 5111

Trust: Wirral Hospital NHS Trust

Wirral Hospital (Arrowe Park and Clatterbridge) serves all the major cancers and multidisciplinary teams are available for most of these. The hospital's death rate for broken hip is average, but death rates for emergency stroke admissions are higher than average. The hospital provides thrombolysis to heart attack patients within 30 minutes of arrival. The hospital also has a coronary care unit and a coronary angiography service which performs 500 catheterisations a year.

Number of beds		1253
✚ ⚕ ✖ 🚑		
		regional
Overall mortality	101	104
Vacancy rates	2	4
Doctors per 100 beds	26	28
Nurses per 100 beds	115	111
Cancelled operations	0.8	1
Complaints	2.1	3
Complaints clear up	41	57
waiting times		
Inpatient	81	76
Outpatient	79	76

Blackburn · **BMI The Beardwood Hospital**

Preston New Rd, Blackburn
Lancashire, BB2 7AE
Phone: 01254 507607

In an unusual partnership, the
Beardwood Hospital works with the
neighbouring Blackburn, Hyndburn
and Ribble Valley Healthcare Trust to
keep NHS waiting lists down. Services
include dietary advice, an erectile
dysfunction clinic and osteoporosis
screening.

General Healthcare Group

Insurers: Bupa*, PPP*, Norwich*,
Royal Sun Alliance*, WPA

price guide	£
Hip replacement	6841-6916
Cataract removal	1850-1986

Number of beds	31
ALS staff	1
heart services	-
Cancer services	✅ ✅

Blackpool · **BUPA Fylde Coast Hospital**

St Walburgas Road, Blackpool
Lancashire, FY3 8BP
Phone: 01253 394188

BUPA Fylde Coast Hospital draws its
consultants from hospitals in the
Blackpool and Preston NHS Trusts.
The hospital carries out a wide range
of diagnostic and surgical procedures.

BUPA Hospitals

Insurers: Bupa, PPP, Norwich, Standard Life,
Royal Sun Alliance, WPA

price guide	£
Hip replacement	7037-7643
Cataract removal	1725-2255

Number of beds	37
ALS staff	1
heart services	-
Cancer services	🌐 🔵

Bolton · **BMI The Beaumont Hospital**

Old Hall Clough, Chorley New Rd
Lostock, Bolton, Lancashire, BL6 4LA
Phone: 01204 404 404

The physiotherapy department provides
hydrotherapy and supports a strong
orthopaedic specialty, facilities for which
also include an operating suite designed
specifically for orthapaedic surgery.
Other facilities include osteoporosis
screening and an allergy clinic.

General Healthcare Group

Insurers: Bupa*, PPP*, Norwich*,
Royal Sun Alliance*, WPA

price guide	£
Hip replacement	7057-9057
Cataract removal	1850-2000

Number of beds	34
ALS staff	2
heart services	🟢
Cancer services	🌐 🔵 ✅ ✅

Cheadle · **BMI The Alexandra Hospital**

Mill Lane, Cheadle
Cheshire, SK8 2PX
Phone: 0161 428 3656

Spread across two sites, the hospital offers a full range of services, including heart and neurosurgery. It has a large critical care unit with six intensive care beds and seven high dependency beds.

General Healthcare Group

Insurers: Bupa*, PPP*, Norwich*, Standard Life, Royal Sun Alliance*, WPA

price guide	£
Hip replacement	7165
Cataract removal	1985

Number of beds	170
ALS staff	6
heart services	
Cancer services	

Chester · **Grosvenor Nuffield Hospital**

Wrexham Rd, Chester
Cheshire, CH4 7QP
Phone: 01244 680444

The Grosvenor Nuffield has over 80 admitting consultants drawn largely from the local Countess of Chester Hospital NHS Trust. Major surgery can be carried out on site.

Nuffield Hospitals

Insurers: Bupa*, PPP*, Norwich*, Standard Life*, Royal Sun Alliance*, WPA

price guide	£
Hip replacement	7395-8895
Cataract removal	2050-2700

Number of beds	35
ALS staff	1
heart services	-
Cancer services	

Chorley · **Euxton Hall Hospital**

Wigan Rd, Euxton, Chorley
Lancashire, PR7 6DY
Phone: 01257 276261

Euxton Hall is an Accredited Centre of Excellence for Hip and Knee replacement surgery and is a Bupa Accredited Breastcare Centre of Excellence.

Capio Healthcare UK

Insurers: Bupa*, PPP*, Norwich*, Standard Life*, Royal Sun Alliance*, WPA

price guide	£
Hip replacement	7150-8150
Cataract removal	2235-2325

Number of beds	
ALS staff	1
heart services	-
Cancer services	

Clitheroe · **Abbey Gisburne Park**

Gisburn, Clitheroe
Lancashire, BB7 4HX
Phone: 01200 445 693

Abbey Hospitals Limited

The hospital offers speciliased programmes including alcohol and drug detoxification and counselling. Short-term rehabilitation is also available for patients needing an active therapy programme including pain management, physiotherapy and occupational therapy.

price guide	£
Hip replacement	6700
Cataract removal	1820

Number of beds	35
ALS staff	1
heart services	-
Cancer services	-

Crewe · **BMI The South Cheshire Private Hospital**

Leighton, Crewe
Cheshire, CW1 4PQ
Phone: 01270 500411

General Healthcare Group

Insurers: Bupa*, PPP*, Norwich, Standard Life, Royal Sun Alliance, WPA

The South Cheshire Private Hospital has an endoscopy suite, two operating theatres, a minor procedures suite and access to an extensive range of facilities due to its NHS partnership with Leighton Hospital.

price guide	£
Hip replacement	8262
Cataract removal	2075

Number of beds	32
ALS staff	4
heart services	-
Cancer services	🌐 ⓘ ✅

Lancaster · **Lancaster and Lakeland Nuffield**

Meadowside, Lancaster
Lancashire, LA1 3RH
Phone: 01524 62345

Nuffield Nursing Homes Trust

Insurers: Bupa*, PPP*, Norwich*, Standard Life*, Royal Sun Alliance*, WPA*

The Lancaster and Lakeland Nuffield Hospital provides a wide range of specialities. Diagnostic facilities include X-ray, mammography and ultrasound. Pathology and pharmacy services are available.

price guide	£
Hip replacement	6499-7700
Cataract removal	2129-2600

Number of beds	32
ALS staff	1
heart services	-
Cancer services	✅

Liverpool · **Abbey Sefton Hospital**

Park Road, Waterloo
Liverpool L22 3XE
Phone: 0151 2576700

Abbey Sefton Hospital offers a wide range of facilities and services to its patients including keyhole surgery. Most medical and surgical specialities are offered and there is a pharmacy on site.

Abbey Hospitals Ltd

Insurers: Bupa, PPP*, Norwich*, Standard Life*, Royal Sun Alliance*, WPA*

price guide	£
Hip replacement	6900
Cataract removal	1795

Number of beds	24
ALS staff	2
heart services	-
Cancer services	-

Liverpool · **Lourdes Hospital**

57 Greenbank Road
Liverpool, L18 1HQ
Phone: 0151 733 7123

Lourdes Hospital offers a broad range of medical and surgical specialties. Facilities and services at the site include endoscopy and key-hole surgery. The hospital also has an on-site surgery.

Poor Servants of the Mother of God

Insurers: Bupa*, PPP*, Norwich, Standard Life, Royal Sun Alliance, WPA

price guide	£
Hip replacement	7120-8415
Cataract removal	2300-2500

Number of beds	58
ALS staff	2
heart services	
Cancer services	☺ ❶ ✓

Macclesfield · **BUPA Regency Hospital**

West Street, Macclesfield
Cheshire, SK11 8DW
Phone: 01625 501150

The hospital provides a wide range of services including psychiatry and psychotherapy. The hospital carries out hip replacement operations on NHS patients to help reduce NHS waiting lists.

BUPA Hospitals

Insurers: Bupa, PPP, Norwich, Standard Life, Royal Sun Alliance, WPA

price guide	£
Hip replacement	7535-7535
Cataract removal	1720-1945

Number of beds	31
ALS staff	1
heart services	-
Cancer services	✓

Manchester · **BMI The Alexandra Hospital**

108-112 Daisy Bank Road, Victoria Park
Manchester, M14 5QH
Phone: 0161 2572233

This smaller hospital complements the BMI Alexandra Hospital in Cheadle and services include assisted conception and refractive eye surgery. There are 25 beds, including one high dependency bed, two theatres, X-ray facilities and physiotherapy facilities.

BMI Healthcare

Insurers: Bupa*, PPP*, Norwich*, Royal Sun Alliance*, WPA

price guide	£
Hip replacement	7165
Cataract removal	1985

Number of beds	25
ALS staff	0
heart services	-
Cancer services	-

Manchester · **BUPA Hospital Manchester**

Russell Road, Whalley Range
Manchester, M16 8AJ
Phone: 0161 226 0112

This modern hospital uses up-to-date technology and has an ongoing development programme. Leading specialists in a range of medical fields are available at the hospital.

BUPA Hospitals

Insurers: Bupa, PPP, Norwich, Standard Life, Royal Sun Alliance, WPA

price guide	£
Hip replacement	7497-7497
Cataract removal	2421-2421

Number of beds	86
ALS staff	1
heart services	-
Cancer services	✪ ⊘

Ormskirk · **Renacres Hall Hospital**

Renacres Lane, Halsall, Ormskirk
Lancashire, L39 8SE
Phone: 01704 841133

Renacres Hall is situated between Ormskirk and Southport. The hospital offers a wide range of surgical and medical procedures, plus extensive diagnostic and treatment facilities.

Capio Healthcare UK

Insurers: Bupa*, PPP*, Norwich*, Standard Life*, Royal Sun Alliance*, WPA*

price guide	£
Hip replacement	7173-8858
Cataract removal	1700-1995

Number of beds	-
ALS staff	1
heart services	-
Cancer services	✪ ⊘ ⊘

Preston · **Fulwood Hall Hospital**

Midgery Lane, Fulwood, Preston
Lancashire, PR2 9SZ
Phone: 01772 704111

Fulwood Hospital offers a full range of medical and surgical specialities including physiotherapy and sports injury clinics and cosmetic surgery.

Capio Healthcare UK

Insurers: Bupa*, PPP*, Norwich*, Standard Life*, Royal Sun Alliance*, WPA*

price guide	£
Hip replacement	6857
Cataract removal	2010-2170

Number of beds	-
ALS staff	1
heart services	
Cancer services	😊 ➀ ✅ ✅

Rochdale · **BMI The Highfield Hospital**

Manchester Rd, Rochdale
Lancashire, OL11 4LZ
Phone: 01706 655121

Rochdale's Highfield Hospital draws consultants from local NHS hospitals. A ten-bedded day care wing, enlarged physiotherapy and X-ray units, and the development of an in-hospital pharmacy are recent additions to the hospital.

BMI Healthcare

Insurers: Bupa*, PPP*, Norwich*, Standard Life*, Royal Sun Alliance*, WPA

price guide	£
Hip replacement	-
Cataract removal	-

Number of beds	57
ALS staff	2
heart services	-
Cancer services	😊 ✅

Salford · **Oaklands Hospital**

19 Lancaster Rd,
Salford, M6 8AQ
Phone: 0161 7877700

Oaklands Hospital provides a wide range of medical and surgical specialities including services keyhole surgery, speech therapy and an extensive range of cosmetic surgery options

Community Hospitals Group

Insurers: Bupa, PPP*, Norwich*, Standard Life*, Royal Sun Alliance*, WPA*

price guide	£
Hip replacement	6940-7760
Cataract removal	1650-1750

Number of beds	28
ALS staff	1
heart services	-
Cancer services	-

St Helens · **Fairfield Independent Hospital**

Crank Road, Crank, St Helens
Merseyside, WA11 7RS
Phone: 01744 739 311

Fairfield Hospital is an independent registered charity. Services include speech therapy and a menopause clinic. The physiotherapy department provides facilities for the treatment of sports injuries.

Independent

Insurers: Bupa*, PPP*, Norwich*, Standard Life*, Royal Sun Alliance*, WPA*

price guide	£
Hip replacement	6980-7680
Cataract removal	1600-1690
Number of beds	52
ALS staff	3
heart services	
Cancer services	

Warrington · **BUPA North Cheshire Hospital**

Fir Tree Close, Stretton, Warrington
Cheshire, WA4 4LU
Phone: 01925 265000

The hospital's specialities include allergies, pre-menstrual syndrome, stress and depression, and venereology; it also offers complementary therapies. There is a gymnasium, pharmacy, and sports injury clinic onsite.

BUPA Hospitals

Insurers: Bupa, PPP, Norwich, Standard Life, Royal Sun Alliance, WPA

price guide	£
Hip replacement	7625
Cataract removal	1890-2395
Number of beds	40
ALS staff	1
heart services	-
Cancer services	

Wirral · **BUPA Murrayfield Hospital Wirral**

Holmwood Drive, Thingwall, Wirral
Merseyside, CH61 1AU
Phone: 0151 648 7000

The hospital conducts all types of surgery, including orthopaedic surgery, colorectal surgery, and plastic surgery. On-site services include a multidisciplinary pathology laboratory, X-ray department and physiotherapy department.

BUPA Hospitals

Insurers: Bupa, PPP, Norwich, Standard Life, Royal Sun Alliance, WPA

price guide	£
Hip replacement	7751
Cataract removal	1960
Number of beds	63
ALS staff	2
heart services	-
Cancer services	

South East

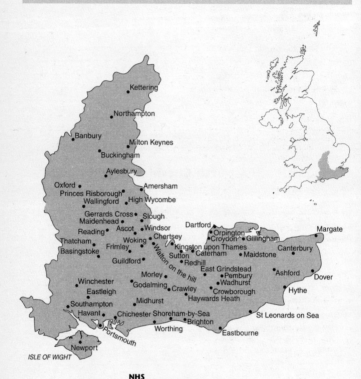

	NHS
Amersham	Amersham Hospital
Ascot	Heatherwood Hospital
Ashford	Ashford Hospital
Ashford	William Harvey Hospital
Aylesbury	Stoke Mandeville Hospital
Banbury	Horton Hospital, The
Basingstoke	North Hampshire Hospital
Brighton	Royal Sussex County Hospital
Canterbury	Kent & Canterbury Hospital
Chertsey	St Peter's Hospital
Chichester	St Richard's Hospital
Crawley	Crawley Hospital
Dartford	Darent Valley Hospital
Dover	Buckland Hospital
East Grinstead	Queen Victoria Hospital
Eastbourne	Eastbourne District General Hospital
Frimley	Frimley Park Hospital
Gillingham	Medway Maritime Hospital
Guildford	Royal Surrey County Hospital
Haywards Heath	Princess Royal Hospital
Headington	Churchill Hospital

Headington	John Radcliffe Hospital
High Wycombe	Wycombe Hospital
Kettering	Kettering General Hospital
Maidstone	Maidstone Hospital
Margate	Queen Elizabeth The Queen Mother Hospital
Milton Keynes	Milton Keynes General NHS Hospital
Newport	St Mary's Hospital
Northampton	Northampton General Hospital
Oxford	Radcliffe Infirmary
Pembury	Pembury Hospital
Portsmouth	Queen Alexandra Hospital
Portsmouth	St Mary's Hospital
Reading	Royal Berkshire & Battle Hospitals
Redhill	East Surrey & Crawley Hospitals
Shoreham by Sea	Southlands Hospital
Slough	Wexham Park Hospital
Southampton	Royal South Hants Hospital
Southampton	Southampton General Hospital
St Leonards on Sea	Conquest Hospital
Tunbridge Wells	Kent and Sussex Hospital
Winchester	Royal Hampshire County Hospital
Worthing	Worthing Hospital

Private

Basingstoke	BMI The Hampshire Clinic
Brighton	Sussex Nuffield Hospital
Canterbury	BMI The Chaucer Hospital
Caterham	North Downs Hospital
Chertsey	BMI Runnymede Hospital
Chichester	Chichester Nuffield Hospital
Crowborough	Horder Centre for Arthritis
East Grinstead	Mcindoe Surgical Centre
Eastbourne	BMI Esperance Private Hospital
Eastleigh	Wessex Nuffield Hospital
Farnham	BUPA Hospital Clare Park
Great Missenden	BMI The Chiltern Hospital
Guildford	Guildford Nuffield Hospital
Guildford	Mount Alvernia Hospital
Havant	BUPA Hospital Portsmouth
Haywards Heath	Ashdown Nuffield Hospital
High Wycombe	BMI Shelburne Hospital
Horley	BUPA Gatwick Hospital
Hythe	BUPA St Saviour's Hospital
Kettering	Woodland Hospital
Longfield	BMI Fawkham Manor Hospital
Maidstone	BMI Somerfield Hospital
Milton Keynes	BMI Saxon Clinic
Northampton	Three Shires Hospital
Oxford	Acland Nuffield Hospital
Princes Risborough	BMI Paddocks Hospital
Reading	Berkshire Independent Hospital
Reading	BUPA Dunedin Hospital
Redhill	BUPA Redwood Hospital
Slough	Thames Valley Nuffield Hospital
Southampton	BUPA Chalybeate Hospital
St Leonards on Sea	BUPA Hospital Hastings
Tunbridge Wells	BUPA Hospital Tunbridge Wells
Tunbridge Wells	Tunbridge Wells Nuffield Hospital
Walderslade	BUPA Alexandra Hospital
Winchester	BMI Sarum Road Hospital
Windsor	BMI The Princess Margaret Hospital
Windsor	HRH Princess Christian's Hospital
Woking	Woking Nuffield Hospital
Worthing	BMI Goring Hall Hospital

Amersham · **Amersham Hospital**

Whielden Street, Amersham
Buckinghamshire, HP7 0JD
Phone: 01494 434 411

Trust: South Buckinghamshire NHS
Trust

Amersham hospital has been radically
rebuilt as part of a Private Finance
Initiative. There is no A&E department
or coronary care unit and the hospital
does not provide most cancer services.
Facilities and services include three
wards, a day hospital, outpatient
department, X-ray and physiotherapy.
A specialist dermatology unit serves
the local population and patients from
further afield. Waiting times are in line
with national averages.

Number of beds		64

		regional
Overall mortality	105	99
Vacancy rates	1	2
Doctors per 100 beds	33	37
Nurses per 100 beds	106	120
Cancelled operations	-	3
Complaints	2.4	4
Complaints clear up	59	52
waiting times		
Inpatient	76	69
Outpatient	82	76

Ascot · **Heatherwood Hospital**

London Road, Ascot
Berkshire, SL5 8AA
Phone: 01344 623 333

Trust: Heatherwood and Wexham Park
Hospitals NHS Trust

Heatherwood Hospital is equipped to
carry out major surgery, including
large volumes of complex orthopaedic
surgery. The development of an
ambulatory and diagnostics unit is
under way. There is no full A&E
service, but a 24-hour minor injuries
unit is available. There is an acute
stroke unit and an 8-bed coronary care
unit. Paediatric surgery is available,
but there is no 24-hour cover by a
paediatrician and no paediatric ITU
available. The overall death rate is
high.

Number of beds		220
✗		

		regional
Overall mortality	117	99
Vacancy rates	0	2
Doctors per 100 beds	34	37
Nurses per 100 beds	114	120
Cancelled operations	1.1	3
Complaints	3.2	4
Complaints clear up	42	52
waiting times		
Inpatient	83	69
Outpatient	86	76

Ashford · **Ashford Hospital**

London Road, Ashford
Middlesex, TW15 3AA
Phone: 01784 884 488

Trust: Ashford and St Peter's Hospital
NHS Trust

Ashford Hospital is a small site situated to the west of London. Facilities include both a renal unit and a stroke unit, however, there is no A&E department. Despite performing children's surgery, the hospital has no paediatric ward or paediatrician on site 24 hours a day. The Critical Care Unit has been recently refurbished and offers 3 coronary care beds and 3 high dependency beds and is able to ventilate emergency patients for up to 24 hours.

Number of beds		222
⊗ ⊕ ⊙		
		regional
Overall mortality	97	99
Vacancy rates	0	2
Doctors per 100 beds	45	37
Nurses per 100 beds	131	120
Cancelled operations	2	3
Complaints	-	4
Complaints clear up	54	52
waiting times		
Inpatient	65	69
Outpatient	74	76

Ashford · **William Harvey Hospital**

Kennington Road, Ashford
Kent, TN24 0LZ
Phone: 01233 633331

Trust: East Kent Hospitals NHS Trust

Based in Ashford, Kent, the William Harvey Hospital has recently opened a new 2-ward block and expanded the critical care unit. There are MRI and CT scanning services but stroke services are provided at the Royal Victoria Hospital in Folkestone. Coronary angiography is also not currently offered. The hospital has multidisciplinary teams for breast, lung and colorectal cancer but not for stomach cancer.

Number of beds		547
⊕ ⊗ ⊗ ⊕ ⊙		
		regional
Overall mortality	101	99
Vacancy rates	4	2
Doctors per 100 beds	31	37
Nurses per 100 beds	108	120
Cancelled operations	0.2	3
Complaints	5	4
Complaints clear up	27	52
waiting times		
Inpatient	67	69
Outpatient	74	76

Aylesbury · **Stoke Mandeville Hospital**

Mandeville Road, Aylesbury
Buckinghamshire, HP21 8AL
Phone: 01296 315 000

Trust: Stoke Mandeville Hospital NHS
    Trust

The hospital has low mortality figures for emergency stroke admissions and average death rates for broken hip surgery. Heart attack patients receive thrombolysis within an average of 30 minutes following admission. CT scans for stroke are performed within a day. Wards at the hospital are mixed contrary to government recommendations regarding single-sex wards.

Number of beds		520
➊ ➕ ✛ ✖ 🆖 ◒		
		regional
Overall mortality	94	99
Vacancy rates	0	2
Doctors per 100 beds	41	35
Nurses per 100 beds	114	121
Cancelled operations	0	3
Complaints	2.8	4
Complaints clear up	40	52
waiting times		
Inpatient	72	69
Outpatient	80	76

Banbury · **Horton Hospital**

Oxford Road, Banbury
Oxfordshire, OX16 9AL
Phone: 01295 275 500

Trust: Oxford Radcliffe Hospitals NHS
    Trust

The Horton Hospital, part of the Oxford Radcliffe Hospitals NHS Trust, Banbury, has strong services for younger patients, with both a maternity and special care baby unit on site. Paediatric surgery is performed at the hospital and there is a paediatrician on site 24 hours a day. The A&E has separate child treatment and waiting areas. The Trust has an average mortality rate overall although deaths following emergency treatment for a broken hip are higher than average.

Number of beds		243
➊ ➕ ✛ ✖ 🆖		
		regional
Overall mortality	97	99
Vacancy rates	0	2
Doctors per 100 beds	66	63
Nurses per 100 beds	160	153
Cancelled operations	3	3
Complaints	4.4	4
Complaints clear up	54	52
waiting times		
Inpatient	76	69
Outpatient	81	76

Basingstoke · **North Hampshire Hospital**

Aldermaston Road, Basingstoke
Hampshire, RG24 9NA
Phone: 01256 473202

Trust: North Hampshire Hospitals NHS
Trust

The North Hampshire hospital is a medium-sized district general hospital serving Basingstoke and the surrounding areas. The death rate for the hospital is significantly better than average. The hospital treats stomach, breast, lung and colorectal cancers, with multidisciplinary teams in place for each. North Hampshire recently became a national centre for the treatment of a rare form of pelvic cancer. Not all suspected stroke patients receive a CT scan within 48 hours of being admitted.

Number of beds		400
✚ ⊕ � ✖ ☎ ☀		
		regional
Overall mortality	89	99
Vacancy rates	2	2
Doctors per 100 beds	20	35
Nurses per 100 beds	127	121
Cancelled operations	0.1	3
Complaints	4.3	4
Complaints clear up	63	52
waiting times		
Inpatient	76	69
Outpatient	82	76

Brighton · **Royal Sussex County Hospital**

Eastern Rd, Brighton
East Sussex, BN2 5BE
Phone: 01273 696955

Trust: Brighton Health Care NHS Trust

The Royal Sussex County Hospital has a notably low death rate for emergency broken hip admissions. Death rates are average for heart bypass surgery. The Royal Sussex County offers coronary angiography and performs the Government-recommended number of 500 catheterisations per year. Heart attack patients receive thrombolytic drugs within the target average time of 30 minutes. However, suspected stroke patients are not guaranteed CT scans within the recommended 48 hours from admission.

Number of beds		750
✚ ⊕ � ✖ ☎ ☀		
		regional
Overall mortality	97	99
Vacancy rates	1	2
Doctors per 100 beds	46	37
Nurses per 100 beds	158	120
Cancelled operations	2	3
Complaints	5.1	4
Complaints clear up	37	52
waiting times		
Inpatient	63	69
Outpatient	70	76

Canterbury · **Kent & Canterbury Hospital**

Ethelbert Road, Canterbury
Kent, CT1 3NG
Phone: 01227 766 877

Trust: East Kent Hospitals NHS Trust

The Kent and Canterbury Hospital has recently undergone a £3m development project. The future of the hospital has been under review and several services are now transferring to the newer Queen Elizabeth the Queen Mother Hospital in Margate. There is an A&E department with separate child treatment and waiting areas. However, it does not meet the recommended target of administering thrombolysis to heart attack patients within an average of 30 minutes of arrival, nor do stroke patients receive a CT scan within 48 hours.

Number of beds		425
⊕ ⊕ ⊕ ⊗ ☎ ◖		
		regional
Overall mortality	101	99
Vacancy rates	4	2
Doctors per 100 beds	31	37
Nurses per 100 beds	108	120
Cancelled operations	0.7	3
Complaints	5	4
Complaints clear up	27	52
waiting times		
Inpatient	67	69
Outpatient	74	76

Chertsey · **St Peter's Hospital**

Guildford Road, Chertsey
Surrey, KT16 0PZ
Phone: 01932 872 000

Trust: Ashford and St Peter's Hospital
NHS Trust

Located in the south west of London, St Peter's was originally opened to serve casualties in the Second World War. The hospital has recently expanded its ITU to 8 beds and opened a high dependency unit. The overall death rate is high and an above average number of operations are cancelled for non-medical reasons. The hospital has multidisciplinary teams in breast, lung, colorectal and stomach cancer. It offers coronary angiography but doesn't perform the recommended number of 500 cardiac catheterisations per year.

Number of beds		377
⊕ ⊕ ⊕ ⊗ ☎ ◖		
		regional
Overall mortality	97	99
Vacancy rates	0	2
Doctors per 100 beds	45	37
Nurses per 100 beds	131	120
Cancelled operations	8	3
Complaints	-	4
Complaints clear up	54	52
waiting times		
Inpatient	65	69
Outpatient	74	76

Chichester · **St Richard's Hospital**

Chichester
West Sussex, PO19 4SE
Phone: 01243 788122

Trust: Royal West Sussex NHS Trust

This hospital has recently refurbished its A&E department and recruited 53 nurses in an effort to improve standards. Mortality rates are low, particularly for hip surgery, and the hospital has single-sex wards throughout. Although there is no MRI scanner, St Richard's carries out CT scans within 48 hours for suspected stroke patients. Three-quarters of patients needing emergency treatment are dealt with within 4 hours.

Number of beds		405
✚ ⊕ ⚕ ✖ ⚕		
		regional
Overall mortality	82	99
Vacancy rates	5	2
Doctors per 100 beds	38	35
Nurses per 100 beds	110	121
Cancelled operations	2	3
Complaints	3.8	4
Complaints clear up	61	52
waiting times		
Inpatient	68	69
Outpatient	80	76

Crawley · **Crawley Hospital**

West Green Drive, Crawley
West Sussex, RH11 7DH
Phone: 01293 600300

Trust: Surrey and Sussex Healthcare
NHS Trust

Crawley Hospital is a medium-sized acute hospital serving the West Sussex area. The A&E was recently refurbished and has separate children's waiting and treatment areas. Surrey and Sussex Healthcare NHS Trust, which also runs the hospital at Redhill, has a high death rate for people brought to the hospital needing emergency treatment for a broken hip. Overall death rates for the Trust are also high. Crawley has dedicated stroke facilities and all suspected stroke patients receive CT scans within the recommended 48 hours of admission.

Number of beds		254
✚ ⚕ ✖ ⚕		
		regional
Overall mortality	106	99
Vacancy rates	2	2
Doctors per 100 beds	34	37
Nurses per 100 beds	92	120
Cancelled operations	2	3
Complaints	3.5	4
Complaints clear up	52	52
waiting times		
Inpatient	58	69
Outpatient	76	76

Dartford · **Darent Valley Hospital**

Darenth Wood Road, Dartford
Kent, DA2 8DA
Phone: 01322 428100

Trust: Dartford & Gravesham NHS Trust

Darent Valley Hospital opened last year, replacing three hospitals in Dartford and Gravesend. THE A&E department has separate children's waiting and treatment areas. The hospital has a wide range of facilities, including an ITU, and MRI scanner and 24-hour X-ray and CT scanning facilities. Multidisciplinary teams are in place to treat breast, lung and colorectal cancers. Outpatient waiting times are longer than average.

Number of beds		403
● ⊕ ⚕ ⊗ ☎ ◓		
		regional
Overall mortality	110	99
Vacancy rates	2	2
Doctors per 100 beds	33	32
Nurses per 100 beds	121	113
Cancelled operations	-	3
Complaints	4	4
Complaints clear up	53	52
waiting times		
Inpatient	69	69
Outpatient	69	76

Dover · **Buckland Hospital**

Coombe Valley Road, Dover
Kent, CT17 0HD
Phone: 01304 201 624

Trust: East Kent Hospitals NHS Trust

This small hospital in Dover was founded around 100 years ago. Services include surgical, rehabilitation and minor injuries units, plus women and children's health services and an outpatient centre. A new neuro-rehabilitation unit recently opened. The hospital does perform surgery on children although it does not currently ensure that there is a paediatrician on the hospital site 24 hours a day.

Number of beds		101
		regional
Overall mortality	101	99
Vacancy rates	4	2
Doctors per 100 beds	31	37
Nurses per 100 beds	108	120
Cancelled operations	-	3
Complaints	5	4
Complaints clear up	27	52
waiting times		
Inpatient	67	69
Outpatient	74	76

East Grinstead · **Queen Victoria Hospital**

Holtye Road, East Grinstead
West Sussex, RH19 3DZ
Phone: 01342 410 210

Trust: Queen Victoria Hospital NHS
Trust

The Queen Victoria Hospital, East Grinstead, met its waiting list targets last year and introduced a booked admissions system. The hospital does not have an A&E department, coronary care or stroke unit. Neither does it treat major cancers. Paediatric surgery is performed and a paediatrician is on site 24 hours a day as recommended by the Royal College of Surgeons.

Number of beds		120
✖		
		regional
Overall mortality	-	99
Vacancy rates	-	2
Doctors per 100 beds	37	32
Nurses per 100 beds	136	113
Cancelled operations	1	3
Complaints	2.9	4
Complaints clear up	87	52
waiting times		
Inpatient	76	69
Outpatient	77	76

Eastbourne · **Eastbourne District General Hospital**

Kings Drive, Eastbourne
East Sussex, BN21 2UD
Phone: 01323 417400

Trust: Eastbourne Hospitals NHS Trust

Eastbourne District General Hospital is a medium-sized district general serving the East Sussex area. The hospital's death rate for emergency hip fracture admissions is low, but deaths following emergency stroke admissions are more frequent than expected. There are dedicated stroke facilities, but despite a new MRI & CT suite, not all suspected stroke patients receive a CT scan within the recommended 48 hours of admission. The hospital does meet Government targets in emergency treatment of heart attacks.

Number of beds		538
➕ ⚕ ✖ ☎ ◉		
		regional
Overall mortality	96	99
Vacancy rates	0	2
Doctors per 100 beds	26	32
Nurses per 100 beds	104	113
Cancelled operations	2	3
Complaints	4	4
Complaints clear up	57	52
waiting times		
Inpatient	64	69
Outpatient	76	76

Frimley · **Frimley Park Hospital**

Portsmouth Road, Frimley
Surrey, GU16 7UJ
Phone: 01276 604 604

Trust: Frimley Park Hospital NHS Trust

Frimley Park is a large district general. The hospital's NHS Trust has recently spent more than £2m on developments. Almost all patients urgently referred to the hospital with suspected cancer are seen by a specialist within 2 weeks. However, named multidisciplinary teams do not currently deliver care to cancer patients as recommended by the government. Only 40 per cent of A&E patients are dealt with within 4 hours and 4 per cent of scheduled operations are cancelled for non-medical reasons.

Number of beds		690
✚ ♠ ✖ ☎ ◉		
		regional
Overall mortality	101	99
Vacancy rates	0	2
Doctors per 100 beds	33	32
Nurses per 100 beds	105	113
Cancelled operations	4	3
Complaints	3.1	4
Complaints clear up	62	52
waiting times		
Inpatient	79	69
Outpatient	80	76

Gillingham · **Medway Maritime Hospital**

Windmill Road, Gillingham
Kent, ME7 5NY
Phone: 01634 830000

Trust: The Medway NHS Trust

The Medway Maritime Hospital serves a population of 360,000 people in the Kent area. The A&E department has separate child treatment area and 84 per cent of patients in A&E are dealt with within 4 hours. However, both inpatient and outpatient waiting times are longer than average. Thrombolysis is administered to heart attack patients within an average of 30 minutes of arrival. Mortality rates for emergency broken hip patients are above average.

Number of beds		633
✚ ♠ ✖ ☎ ◉		
		regional
Overall mortality	109	99
Vacancy rates	2	2
Doctors per 100 beds	33	32
Nurses per 100 beds	111	113
Cancelled operations	1	3
Complaints	3	4
Complaints clear up	41	52
waiting times		
Inpatient	62	69
Outpatient	67	76

Guildford · **Royal Surrey County Hospital**

Egerton Road, Guildford
Surrey, GU2 7XX
Phone: 01483 571 122

Trust: Royal Surrey County Hospital
   NHS Trust

The Royal Surrey County Hospital recently opened a 14-bed assessment unit in its A&E department to provide rapid access for patients needing emergency treatment. A relatively high proportion of operations are cancelled for non-medical reasons and a significant number of these are not rescheduled within the recommended time of 31 days. The hospital performs the suggested number of 500 cardiac catheterisations and provides all suspected stroke patients with CT scans within 48 hours of admission.

Number of beds		515
➕ ⊕ ⚕ ✖ 🖅 😊		
		regional
Overall mortality	91	99
Vacancy rates	1	2
Doctors per 100 beds	45	32
Nurses per 100 beds	141	113
Cancelled operations	5	3
Complaints	5.2	4
Complaints clear up	100	52
waiting times		
Inpatient	54	69
Outpatient	80	76

Haywards Heath · **Princess Royal Hospital**

Lewes Road, Haywards Heath
West Sussex, RH16 4EX
Phone: 01444 441 881

Trust: Mid Sussex NHS Trust

The Princess Royal Hospital, Haywards Heath, is a modern acute unit. The hospital meets a key Government target by ensuring that all suspected stroke patients receive a CT scan within 48 hours of being admitted. Paediatric surgery is performed but a paediatrician is not available on site 24 hours a day as recommended by the Royal College of Surgeons. Heart attack patients do not currently receive thrombolysis within the target average of 30 minutes of arrival. Overall the death rates at the Trust are average. However, inpatient waiting times are longer than average.

Number of beds		400
➕ ⊕ ⚕ ✖ 🖅 😊		
		regional
Overall mortality	93	99
Vacancy rates	2	2
Doctors per 100 beds	33	35
Nurses per 100 beds	116	121
Cancelled operations	-	3
Complaints	6.7	4
Complaints clear up	61	52
waiting times		
Inpatient	55	69
Outpatient	70	76

Headington · **Churchill Hospital**

Old Road, Headington
Oxfordshire, OX3 7LJ
Phone: 01865 741 841

Trust: Oxford Radcliffe Hospitals NHS
Trust

The Churchill Hospital is a centre for cancer services, specialist medicine, and research. Many of the Radcliffe Infirmary's services will move there over the next 10 years. Its new Cancer Centre covers major cancers and, except for upper gastrointestinal tract cancers, multidisciplinary teams treat them all. Next year a diabetes, endocrinology and metabolism centre will open. There is also a renal unit.

Number of beds		296
✖ ☎		
		regional
Overall mortality	97	99
Vacancy rates	0	2
Doctors per 100 beds	66	63
Nurses per 100 beds	160	153
Cancelled operations	4	3
Complaints	4.4	4
Complaints clear up	54	52
waiting times		
Inpatient	76	69
Outpatient	81	76

Headington · **John Radcliffe Hospital**

Headley Way, Headington
Oxfordshire, OX3 9DU
Phone: 01865 741 166

Trust: Oxford Radcliffe Hospitals NHS
Trust

John Radcliffe hospital is a large teaching hospital linked to Oxford University. In 2001 it started a £9.5 million A&E development and started work on providing additional beds for the intensive care and high dependency units. It has a dedicated stroke unit and all suspected stroke patients receive a CT scan within 24 hours of being admitted. There is a separate child treatment area in the A&E department. However, A&E waiting times could be improved with only 57 per cent of patients dealt with within 4 hours.

Number of beds		666
✚ ⚕ ⊕ ✖ ☎ ◔		
		regional
Overall mortality	97	99
Vacancy rates	0	2
Doctors per 100 beds	66	63
Nurses per 100 beds	160	153
Cancelled operations	3	3
Complaints	4.4	4
Complaints clear up	54	52
waiting times		
Inpatient	76	69
Outpatient	81	76

High Wycombe · **Wycombe Hospital**

**Queen Alexandra Road, High Wycombe
Buckinghamshire, HP11 2TT
Phone: 01494 526 161**

**Trust: South Buckinghamshire NHS
Trust**

Wycombe Hospital has recently upgraded its A&E department as part of a £600,000 modernisation programme. The hospital does not yet offer coronary angiography; however, it plans to build a catheterisation laboratory later this year. The X-ray department provides MRI, CT and gamma camera facilities, and can perform CT scans within 24 hours. The hospital has a children's ward and a paediatrician is available on site 24 hours a day.

Number of beds		365
⊕ ⊕ ⊕ ⊗ ⊕ ⊕		
		regional
Overall mortality	105	99
Vacancy rates	1	2
Doctors per 100 beds	33	37
Nurses per 100 beds	106	120
Cancelled operations	-	3
Complaints	2.4	4
Complaints clear up	59	52
waiting times		
Inpatient	76	69
Outpatient	82	76

Kettering · **Kettering General Hospital**

**Rothwell Road, Kettering
Northamptonshire, NN16 8UZ
Phone: 01536 492 000**

**Trust: Kettering General Hospital NHS
Trust**

Kettering General Hospital is a medium-sized district general serving Kettering and the surrounding area. The A&E department also has a separate child treatment and waiting areas and a paediatrician is on site at all times. On both death rates and waiting times the hospital performs in line with national averages. However, the hospital has an above average number of cancelled operations.

Number of beds		532
⊕ ⊕ ⊕ ⊗ ⊕		
		regional
Overall mortality	104	99
Vacancy rates	0	2
Doctors per 100 beds	33	32
Nurses per 100 beds	127	113
Cancelled operations	6	3
Complaints	2.4	4
Complaints clear up	25	52
waiting times		
Inpatient	78	69
Outpatient	75	76

Maidstone · **Maidstone Hospital**

Hermitage Lane, Maidstone
Kent, ME16 9QQ
Phone: 01622 729 000

Trust: Maidstone and Tunbridge Wells
   NHS Trust

Maidstone Hospital has recently started a development project to move the Kent and County Ophthalmic and Aural Hospital onto its site. Breast, lung, stomach and colorectal cancers are treated here and multidisciplinary teams are in place for each. Also, there are MRI and CT scanning facilities. On average, thrombolytic drugs are administered to heart attack patients within the target 30 minutes of arrival at A&E. There is no dedicated stroke unit. Death rates for the trust are average.

Number of beds		381
➊ ➕ ⚕ ✖ ☎ ◉		
		regional
Overall mortality	100	99
Vacancy rates	2	2
Doctors per 100 beds	41	37
Nurses per 100 beds	124	120
Cancelled operations	2	3
Complaints	3.7	4
Complaints clear up	35	52
waiting times		
Inpatient	70	69
Outpatient	78	76

Margate · **Queen Elizabeth The Queen Mother**

St Peters Road, Margate
Kent, CT9 4AN
Phone: 01843 225544

Trust: East Kent Hospitals NHS Trust

The Queen Elizabeth The Queen Mother Hospital's A&E department is undergoing a £1.1 million refurbishment. There are separate child treatment and waiting areas. Paediatric surgery is performed; however, a paediatrician is not on site 24 hours a day as recommended by the Royal College of Surgeons. Heart attack patients receive thrombolysis within the target average of 30 minutes of arrival, but coronary angiography is not performed. Mortality rates for the trust are average.

Number of beds		499
➊ ➕ ⚕ ✖ ☎ ◉		
		regional
Overall mortality	101	99
Vacancy rates	4	2
Doctors per 100 beds	31	37
Nurses per 100 beds	108	120
Cancelled operations	0.8	3
Complaints	5	4
Complaints clear up	27	52
waiting times		
Inpatient	67	69
Outpatient	74	76

Milton Keynes · **Milton Keynes General Hospital**

Standing Way, Milton Keynes
Buckinghamshire, MK6 5LD
Phone: 01908 660 033

Trust: Milton Keynes General NHS Trust

Milton Keynes General has recently opened a new coronary care and cardiology unit, as well as a new MRI department. The hospital has a dedicated stroke unit and performs CT scans on all suspected stroke patients within 48 hours of admission. However, the death rate following emergency stroke admission is high. Only half of patients are dealt with within 4 hours of arrival at A&E. The cancer services department treats breast, lung, stomach and colorectal cancers and multidisciplinary teams are in place for all of these.

Number of beds		410
⊕ ⊕ ⊗ ⊗ ⊛ ⊙		
		regional
Overall mortality	103	99
Vacancy rates	0	2
Doctors per 100 beds	43	35
Nurses per 100 beds	139	121
Cancelled operations	9	3
Complaints	4	4
Complaints clear up	59	52
waiting times		
Inpatient	67	69
Outpatient	66	76

Newport · **St Mary's Hospital**

Newport
Isle of Wight, PO30 5TG
Phone: 01983 524 081

Trust: Isle of Wight Healthcare NHS Trust

St Mary's Hospital caters for the people of the Isle of Wight, specialising in urology, cardiology, gastroenterology, and paediatrics. Facilities include MRI and CT scanning, a 6-bed high dependency unit and 4 operating theatres. It has recently built a new children's unit in an effort to improve its paediatric services. Deaths following broken hip emergency admissions are less frequent than expected and, on average, heart attack patients receive thrombolysis within the target 30 minutes of arrival.

Number of beds		392
⊕ ⊗ ⊗ ⊛ ⊙		
		regional
Overall mortality	95	99
Vacancy rates	8	2
Doctors per 100 beds	28	37
Nurses per 100 beds	120	120
Cancelled operations	4	3
Complaints	5.7	4
Complaints clear up	89	52
waiting times		
Inpatient	71	69
Outpatient	88	76

Northampton · **Northampton General Hospital**

**Cliftonville, Northampton
Northamptonshire, NN1 5BD
Phone: 01604 634 700**

**Trust: Northamptonshire General
  Hospital NHS Trust**

Death rates at Northampton General Hospital are in line with national averages but waiting times could be improved. Heart patients can benefit from a new rapid access chest pain clinic in March 2001. The hospital does perform coronary angiographies, but does not yet meet NSF levels of 500 cardiac catheterisations per year. The hospital has a paediatric ITU and a paediatrician is available 24 hours a day.

Number of beds		700
✚ ✿ ✤ ✖ 🚑 ◉		
		regional
Overall mortality	95	99
Vacancy rates	1	2
Doctors per 100 beds	39	37
Nurses per 100 beds	149	120
Cancelled operations	-	3
Complaints	3.1	4
Complaints clear up	90	52
waiting times		
Inpatient	65	69
Outpatient	68	76

Oxford · **Radcliffe Infirmary**

**Woodstock Road, Oxford
Oxfordshire, OX2 6HE
Phone: 01865 311 188**

**Trust: Oxford Radcliffe Hospitals NHS
  Trust**

The Radcliffe Infirmary provides specialist healthcare services to patients across the region. The hospital has an A&E department, which is able to deal with the majority of patients within 4 hours. The Trust, which runs the larger John Radcliffe Hospital as well as the Radcliffe Infirmary, has below average overall mortality rates, but the number of deaths following emergency fractured hip admissions is higher than expected. A dedicated children's area in A&E is being created as part of a new development.

Number of beds		279
✚ ✿ ✖ 🚑 ◉		
		regional
Overall mortality	97	99
Vacancy rates	0	2
Doctors per 100 beds	66	63
Nurses per 100 beds	160	153
Cancelled operations	3	3
Complaints	4.4	4
Complaints clear up	54	52
waiting times		
Inpatient	76	69
Outpatient	81	76

Pembury · **Pembury Hospital**

Tonbridge Road, Pembury
Kent, TN2 4QJ
Phone: 01892 823 535

Trust: Maidstone and Tunbridge Wells
NHS Trust

Maidstone and Tunbridge Wells NHS Trust has announced plans to spend £200 million on a new 500-bed hospital for Tunbridge Wells to replace the ageing Kent and Sussex and Pembury Hospitals. The hospital has plans to improve the Ophthalmic Department's accommodation which will provide a day care unit with dedicated theatre facilities, laser treatment rooms and an outpatient department with waiting areas for adults and children.

Number of beds		224
✖ ⊛ ◓		
		regional
Overall mortality	100	99
Vacancy rates	2	2
Doctors per 100 beds	41	37
Nurses per 100 beds	124	120
Cancelled operations	-	3
Complaints	3.7	4
Complaints clear up	35	52
waiting times		
Inpatient	70	69
Outpatient	78	76

Portsmouth · **Queen Alexandra Hospital**

Southwick Hill Road, Portsmouth
Hampshire, PO6 3LY
Phone: 02392 286 000

Trust: Portsmouth Hospitals NHS Trust

The Queen Alexandra, Portsmouth, has below average mortality rates for emergency hip admissions. The overall hospital mortality rate is also below average. Paediatric surgery is performed at the hospital but a paediatrician is not on site 24 hours a day as recommended by the Royal College of Surgeons. Breast, lung, stomach and colorectal cancers are all treated but multidisciplinary teams are not currently used in cancer care as recommended by the Government.

Number of beds		550
➕ ⊕ ⚛ ✖ ⊛ ◓		
		regional
Overall mortality	90	99
Vacancy rates	2	2
Doctors per 100 beds	41	37
Nurses per 100 beds	125	120
Cancelled operations	-	3
Complaints	2.3	4
Complaints clear up	54	52
waiting times		
Inpatient	74	69
Outpatient	75	76

Portsmouth · St Mary's Hospital

Milton Road, Portsmouth
Hampshire, PO3 6AD
Phone: 02392 286 000

Trust: Portsmouth Hospitals NHS Trust

This hospital has built a new cancer support centre and installed new equipment to reduce side effects in radiotherapy. There is no A&E at this hospital, a service which is provided by the Queen Alexandra Hospital run by the same Trust. The hospital offers coronary angiography, and meets Government targets for cardiac catheterisations, but heart attack patients do not, on average, receive thrombolysis within the target 30 minutes of entering the hospital. There is no dedicated stroke unit. A paediatrician is on site 24 hours a day.

Number of beds		550
❌		
		regional
Overall mortality	90	99
Vacancy rates	2	2
Doctors per 100 beds	41	37
Nurses per 100 beds	125	120
Cancelled operations	-	3
Complaints	2.3	4
Complaints clear up	54	52
waiting times		
Inpatient	74	69
Outpatient	75	76

Reading · Royal Berkshire & Battle Hospitals

London Road, Reading
Berkshire, RG1 5AN
Phone: 0118 987 5111

Trust: Royal Berkshire & Battle
Hospitals NHS Trust

Royal Berkshire & Battle Hospitals is run as one service from two sites, with the main site at the Royal Berkshire hospital in Reading. Battle Hospital is due to be closed in 2005 at which point all services will move to the Royal Berkshire site. The hospital has an A&E department and its death rates for emergency stroke and fractured hip admissions are average. The overall death rate is also close to average. In 2001 a stroke unit opened with a permanent CT scanner. Two falls clinics were introduced and new equipment for the cardiology clinic was purchased.

Number of beds		810
➕ ⊕ ⊛ ⊕ ❌ ⊜ ◉		
		regional
Overall mortality	98	99
Vacancy rates	2	2
Doctors per 100 beds	40	37
Nurses per 100 beds	148	120
Cancelled operations	2	3
Complaints	2.9	4
Complaints clear up	73	52
waiting times		
Inpatient	65	69
Outpatient	65	76

Redhill · **East Surrey and Crawley Hospitals**

Canada Avenue, Redhill
Surrey, RH1 5RH
Phone: 01737 768511

Trust: Surrey and Sussex Healthcare
NHS Trust

East Surrey and Crawley Hospitals provide a full range of inpatient, outpatient and emergency services. East Surrey's A&E department is the main receiving centre for incidents at Gatwick. The death rate for emergency hip fracture admissions is high but within expected levels for emergency stroke patients. There is also a stroke unit and all suspected stroke patients receive a CT scan within 24 hours of admission.

Number of beds		652

		regional
Overall mortality	106	99
Vacancy rates	2	2
Doctors per 100 beds	34	37
Nurses per 100 beds	92	120
Cancelled operations	2	3
Complaints	3.5	4
Complaints clear up	52	52
waiting times		
Inpatient	58	69
Outpatient	76	76

Shoreham by Sea · **Southlands Hospital**

Upper Shoreham Rd, Shoreham by Sea
West Sussex, BN43 6TQ
Phone: 01273 455622

Trust: Worthing and Southlands
Hospitals NHS Trust

Southlands Hospital is a small acute hospital serving the West Sussex area. It provides day surgery and elderly and orthopaedic services and treats more than 350,000 outpatients each year. However, there are plans to move these services to Worthing Hospital over the next few years. A new 15-bed discharge-planning unit has recently been opened. There is no A&E department here. A&E services are available at Worthing Hospital.

Number of beds		-

		regional
Overall mortality	96	99
Vacancy rates	0	2
Doctors per 100 beds	31	32
Nurses per 100 beds	106	113
Cancelled operations	0	3
Complaints	2.4	4
Complaints clear up	41	52
waiting times		
Inpatient	63	69
Outpatient	69	76

Slough · **Wexham Park Hospital**

Wexham Street, Slough
Berkshire, SL2 4HL
Phone: 01753 633 000

Trust: Heatherwood and Wexham Park
Hospitals NHS Trust

Wexham Park Hospital has high overall mortality rates, although mortality figures are average for emergency patients with broken hips or suffering strokes. Waiting times for the Trust are better than average. The hospital does not currently provide thrombolysis within the recommended 30 minutes. Multidisciplinary teams are in place to treat lung, stomach, colorectal and breast cancers.

Number of beds		499
⊕ ⊕ ⊗ ⊗ ☺		
		regional
Overall mortality	117	99
Vacancy rates	0	2
Doctors per 100 beds	34	37
Nurses per 100 beds	114	120
Cancelled operations	1	3
Complaints	3.2	4
Complaints clear up	42	52
waiting times		
Inpatient	83	69
Outpatient	86	76

Southampton · **Royal South Hants Hospital**

Brintons Terrace
Southampton, SO14 0YG
Phone: 02380 634 288

Trust: Southampton University
Hospitals NHS Trust

The Royal South Hants Hospital is a small acute hospital within Southampton University Hospitals NHS Trust. Cancer treatment for the trust is currently based at the hospital, but a new centre being built at Southampton General Hospital will see many of these services move there. The hospital's facilities include CT scanning and ultrasound rooms containing Doppler facilities.

Number of beds		138
		regional
Overall mortality	104	99
Vacancy rates	1	2
Doctors per 100 beds	56	63
Nurses per 100 beds	138	153
Cancelled operations	0	3
Complaints	5.4	4
Complaints clear up	41	52
waiting times		
Inpatient	72	69
Outpatient	81	76

Southampton · **Southampton General Hospital**

Tremona Road
Southampton, SO16 6YD
Phone: 02380 777 222

Trust: Southampton University
Hospitals NHS Trust

Southampton General Hospital aims to create a new cancer centre as part of a £50 million improvement programme. Hospital death rates are low for heart bypass operations – the hospital is a centre for heart surgery. Coronary angiographies are available and the hospital meets a key government standard in this procedure of performing at least 500 catheterisations a year. The A&E department has a separate treatment area for children and there is a dedicated paediatric ITU with a paediatrician on site 24 hours a day.

Number of beds		1065
⊕ ⊕ ⊕ ⊗ ⊕ ⊕		
		regional
Overall mortality	104	99
Vacancy rates	1	2
Doctors per 100 beds	56	63
Nurses per 100 beds	138	153
Cancelled operations	-	3
Complaints	5.4	4
Complaints clear up	41	52
waiting times		
Inpatient	72	69
Outpatient	81	76

St Leonards on Sea · **Conquest Hospital**

The Ridge, St Leonards on Sea
East Sussex, TN37 7RD
Phone: 01424 755255

Trust: Hastings and Rother NHS Trust

Conquest Hospital is a modern acute hospital serving the East Sussex area. It has a cardiac care unit and meets Government targets in providing rapid treatment for heart attack patients and in providing angiography for people with heart disease. It also has dedicated stroke facilities and all suspected stroke patients receive a CT scan within 48 hours of admission. There is an A&E department which has separate children's waiting and treatment areas. Multidisciplinary teams are in place for treatment of people with breast, lung and colorectal cancers.

Number of beds		521
⊕ ⊕ ⊕ ⊗ ⊕ ⊕		
		regional
Overall mortality	97	99
Vacancy rates	5	2
Doctors per 100 beds	31	37
Nurses per 100 beds	95	120
Cancelled operations	3	3
Complaints	5.7	4
Complaints clear up	45	52
waiting times		
Inpatient	75	69
Outpatient	73	76

Tunbridge Wells · **Kent and Sussex Hospital**

Mount Ephraim, Tunbridge Wells
Kent, TN2 4AT
Phone: 01892 526 111

Trust: Maidstone and Tunbridge Wells
NHS Trust

The Kent and Sussex Hospital looks set to move to a new site in Tunbridge Wells at a cost of £200 million. There is an A&E department and the hospital meets the Government target of performing CT scans on all suspected stroke patients within 48 hours of admission. Also thrombolytic drugs are administered to heart attack patients within an average of 30 minutes of arrival in A&E. Death rates for the Trust that runs the hospital are average.

Number of beds		260
⊕ ⊕ ⊗ ⊗ ⊙ ⊙		
		regional
Overall mortality	100	99
Vacancy rates	2	2
Doctors per 100 beds	41	37
Nurses per 100 beds	124	120
Cancelled operations	2	3
Complaints	3.7	4
Complaints clear up	35	52
waiting times		
Inpatient	70	69
Outpatient	78	76

Winchester · **Royal Hampshire County Hospital**

Romsey Rd, Winchester
Hampshire, SO22 5DG
Phone: 01962 863535

Trust: Winchester and Eastleigh
Healthcare NHS Trust

The Royal Hampshire's 20-bed emergency medical assessment unit has helped reduce cancellations due to bed shortages. The hospital has low death rates for emergency broken hip admissions. The overall mortality rate and the death rate for stroke patients are average. Its A&E department ensures that almost all patients are dealt with within 4 hours.

Number of beds		356
⊕ ⊗ ⊗ ⊙ ⊙		
		regional
Overall mortality	95	99
Vacancy rates	1	2
Doctors per 100 beds	29	32
Nurses per 100 beds	104	113
Cancelled operations	-	3
Complaints	3.1	4
Complaints clear up	58	52
waiting times		
Inpatient	71	69
Outpatient	78	76

Worthing · **Worthing Hospital**

Lyndhurst Road, Worthing
West Sussex, BN43 6TQ
Phone: 01903 205111

Trust: Worthing and Southlands
Hospitals NHS Trust

Worthing Hospital is one of only two hospitals in West Sussex to have its own helipad. It recently opened a new £1.4 million children's centre, bringing together all paediatric services around the district. There is a paediatrician on site 24 hours a day and single-sex wards throughout the site. 5 per cent of scheduled operations are cancelled for non-medical reasons at the hospital – more than at most hospitals.

Number of beds		501

◉ ⊕ ⊛ ⊗ ☻ ◔

		regional
Overall mortality	96	99
Vacancy rates	0	2
Doctors per 100 beds	31	32
Nurses per 100 beds	106	113
Cancelled operations	5	3
Complaints	2.4	4
Complaints clear up	41	52
waiting times		
Inpatient	63	69
Outpatient	69	76

Basingstoke · **BMI The Hampshire Clinic**

Basing Road, Old Basing, Basingstoke
Hampshire, RG24 7AL
Phone: 01256 357 111

The Hampshire Clinic is a purpose-built private hospital, and has grown from 34 beds to 55, with a £7 m extension providing an extra operating theatre, consulting rooms and physiotherapy and hydrotherapy facilities.

General Healthcare Group Ltd

Insurers: Bupa*, PPP*, Norwich*, Standard Life, Royal Sun Alliance*, WPA

price guide	£
Hip replacement	7380-8729
Cataract removal	1814-2190

Number of beds	55
ALS staff	1
heart services	-
Cancer services	🌐 ✓ ✓

Brighton · **Sussex Nuffield Hospital**

Warren Rd, Woodingdean
Brighton, Sussex, BN2 6DX
Phone: 01273 624488

The Sussex Nuffield Hospital is based across two sites at Woodingdean and Hove. Amenities include 3 operating theatres and extensive outpatient and diagnostic facilities.

Nuffield Nursing Homes Trust

price guide	£
Hip replacement	6900-9900
Cataract removal	1975-2300

Number of beds	65
ALS staff	1
heart services	-
Cancer services	◑ ✓ ✓

Canterbury · **BMI The Chaucer Hospital**

Nackington Rd, Canterbury
Kent, CT4 7AR
Phone: 01227 825 100

The Chaucer hospital has over 120 consultants covering a range of specialties. The high dependency unit has recently been upgraded to intensive care and critical care units.

General Healthcare Ltd

Insurers: Bupa*, PPP, Norwich, Royal Sun Alliance, WPA

price guide	£
Hip replacement	7335
Cataract removal	2275

Number of beds	60
ALS staff	6
heart services	🔄
Cancer services	🌐 ◑ ✓ ✓

Caterham · **North Downs Hospital**

46 Tupwood Lane, Caterham
Surrey, CR3 6DP
Phone: 01883 348 981

North Downs Hospital offers a broad range of medical and surgical specialties including treatment for colorectal cancer. Other services at the hospital are complementary therapy treatment and physiotherapy.

Capio Healthcare UK

Insurers: Bupa, PPP*, Norwich*, Standard Life*, Royal Sun Alliance*, WPA

price guide	£
Hip replacement	6610-9400
Cataract removal	1620-1860

Number of beds	20
ALS staff	2
heart services	–
Cancer services	–

Chertsey · **BMI The Runnymede Hospital**

Guildford Rd, Ottershaw, Chertsey
Surrey, KT16 0RQ
Phone: 01932 877800

The Runnymeade Hospital leases land and buys facilities for its private patients from St Peter's NHS Hospital. A paediatric allergy clinic which operates on Saturday afternoons was recently opened.

General Healthcare Group

Insurers: Bupa*, PPP*, Norwich, Royal Sun Alliance, WPA

price guide	£
Hip replacement	9895
Cataract removal	2830

Number of beds	52
ALS staff	4
heart services	☺
Cancer services	

Chichester · **Chichester Nuffield Hospital**

78 Broyle Road, Chichester
West Sussex, PO19 4BE
Phone: 01243 530600

The Chichester Nuffield Hospital was purpose built in 1992. It offers a full range of services and specialist clinics including cosmetic surgery, breast reconstructive surgery and chemotherapy.

Nuffield Nursing Homes Trust

Insurers: Bupa*, PPP*, Norwich*, Standard Life*, Royal Sun Alliance*, WPA

price guide	£
Hip replacement	–
Cataract removal	–

Number of beds	39
ALS staff	1
heart services	–
Cancer services	

Crowborough · **The Horder Centre for Arthritis**

St John's Rd, Crowborough
East Sussex, TN6 1XP
Phone: 01892 665577

The Centre provides specialist and individual treatment for patients with joint and muscle problems; it is recognised for its specialist orthopaedic surgery, medical care of arthritis and intensive rehabilitation.

Charitable Trust

Insurers: Bupa, PPP, Norwich, Standard Life, Royal Sun Alliance, WPA

price guide	£
Hip replacement	5200-7000
Cataract removal	-

Number of beds	60
ALS staff	3
heart services	-
Cancer services	-

East Grinstead · **Mcindoe Surgical Centre**

Holtye Road, East Grinstead
West Sussex, RH19 3EB
Phone: 01342 330 300

The McIndoe Surgical Centre, built in the grounds of the Queen Victoria NHS Hospital, shares its consultants with the hospital. It specialises in cosmetic and reconstructive surgery but also offers other types of surgery, including ear, nose and throat, dental surgery and eye surgery.

Mcindoe Surgical Centre Ltd

Insurers: Bupa, PPP*, Norwich*, Standard Life*, Royal Sun Alliance, WPA

price guide	£
Hip replacement	-
Cataract removal	1750

Number of beds	22
ALS staff	1
heart services	-
Cancer services	-

Eastbourne · **BMI Esperance Private Hospital**

Hartington Place, Eastbourne
East Sussex, BN21 3BG
Phone: 01323 411188

The hospital was founded by the Order of the Sisters of Bordeaux, who turned the current building into a hospital. In addition to its principal specialties, which include urology, gynaecology, orthopaedics and ophthalmology, the hospital also offers acupuncture for pain management.

BMI Healthcare

Insurers: Bupa*, PPP*, Norwich, Royal Sun Alliance, WPA

price guide	£
Hip replacement	6000-6500
Cataract removal	2200-2300

Number of beds	50
ALS staff	2
heart services	-
Cancer services	◗◖

Eastleigh · **Wessex Nuffield Hospital**

Winchester Rd, Chandler's Ford,
Eastleigh, Hampshire, SO53 2DW
Phone: 02380 266377

The Wessex Nuffield has been
involved in pioneering medical
developments with Southampton
University Hospital including a test to
identify which breast cancer patients
would benefit from hormone drug
treatment.

Nuffield Hospitals

Insurers: Bupa*, PPP, Norwich*,
Standard Life*, Royal Sun Alliance*, WPA

price guide	£
Hip replacement	7100-9200
Cataract removal	2125-2125

Number of beds	44
ALS staff	1
heart services	-
Cancer services	

Farnham · **BUPA Hospital Clare Park**

Crondall Lane, Farnham
Surrey, GU10 5XX
Phone: 01252 850216

BUPA Hospital Clare Park offers a wide
range of services including a sports
injuries clinic and back pain clinic. The
closest intensive care facility is at
Frimley Park NHS Hospital.

BUPA Hospitals

Insurers: Bupa, Norwich, Standard Life,
Royal Sun Alliance, WPA

price guide	£
Hip replacement	7550-7550
Cataract removal	1750-1750

Number of beds	34
ALS staff	1
heart services	-
Cancer services	

Great Missenden · **BMI The Chiltern Hospital**

London Road, Great Missenden
Buckinghamshire, HP16 0EN
Phone: 01494 890890

The Chiltern Hospital in Great
Missenden draws many of its
consultants from the nearby Stoke
Mandeville and South Buckinghamshire
NHS Trusts. Treatment is offered from a
broad range of specialties.

General Healthcare Group

Insurers: Bupa*, PPP*, Norwich*,
Standard Life, Royal Sun Alliance*, WPA

price guide	£
Hip replacement	7800-8450
Cataract removal	2540-2540

Number of beds	75
ALS staff	2
heart services	-
Cancer services	

Guildford · **Mount Alvernia Hospital**

Harvey Rd, Guildford
Surrey, GU1 3LX
Phone: 01483 570 122

A registered charity, this hospital is administered by Catholic Franciscan Sisters and allocates surplus funds to improve hospital services and to support the sisters' heathcare missions.

Charitable Trust

Insurers: Bupa, PPP, Norwich, Standard Life, Royal Sun Alliance, WPA

price guide	£
Hip replacement	-
Cataract removal	-
Number of beds	90
ALS staff	3
heart services	
Cancer services	

Guildford · **Guildford Nuffield Hospital**

Stirling Road, Guildford
Surrey, GU2 7RF
Phone: 01483 555800

The Guildford Nuffield Hospital draws consultants from the Royal Surrey County Hospital. The hospital has a high dependency unit catering for acutely ill patients.

Nuffield Nursing Homes Trust

Insurers: Bupa*, PPP*, Norwich*, Standard Life*, Royal Sun Alliance*, WPA

price guide	£
Hip replacement	8700-9300
Cataract removal	2538-2700
Number of beds	54
ALS staff	4
heart services	
Cancer services	

Havant · **BUPA Hospital Portsmouth**

Bartons Road, Havant
Hampshire, PO9 5NP
Phone: 023 9245 6000

This hospital offers a wide range of services including a vasectomy clinic, an impotence clinic, and laser surgery for short sightedness and skin blemishes. Health screening services are available.

BUPA Hospitals

Insurers: Bupa, PPP, Norwich, Standard Life, Royal Sun Alliance, WPA

price guide	£
Hip replacement	7545-7545
Cataract removal	2433-2583
Number of beds	49
ALS staff	1
heart services	
Cancer services	

Haywards Heath · **Ashdown Nuffield Hospital**

Burrell Road, Haywards Heath
West Sussex, RH16 1UD
Phone: 01444 456999

The Ashdown Nuffield Hospital offers a
range of diagnostic and acute care
services from health screening to major
surgery across most specialties
including fertility treatment, sex-
change surgery and cosmetic surgery.

Nuffield Hospitals

price guide	£
Hip replacement	5590-7900
Cataract removal	1975-2275

Number of beds	42
ALS staff	0
heart services	-
Cancer services	-

High Wycombe · **BMI Shelburne Hospital**

Queen Alexandra Road, High Wycombe
Buckinghamshire, HP14 2TR
Phone: 01494 888700

The BMI Shelburne Hospital offers
most medical and surgical specialties
including cancer services. Other
facilities include diagnostic testing and
hydrotherapy.

General Healthcare Group

Insurers: Bupa, PPP, Norwich*, Standard Life,
Royal Sun Alliance*, WPA

price guide	£
Hip replacement	8690-7690
Cataract removal	2620

Number of beds	31
ALS staff	1
heart services	-
Cancer services	

Horley · **BUPA Gatwick Park Hospital**

Povey Cross Road, Horley
Surrey, RH6 0BB
Phone: 01293 785511

BUPA Gatwick Park Hospital offers
treatment from most specialties and is
known for its breast and colorectal
cancer treatment. The local Health
Authority describes the hospital as
busy and efficient.

BUPA Hospitals

Insurers: Bupa, PPP, Norwich, Standard Life,
Royal Sun Alliance, WPA

price guide	£
Hip replacement	7574-7574
Cataract removal	1800-2375

Number of beds	54
ALS staff	3
heart services	-
Cancer services	

Hythe · **BUPA St Saviour's Hospital**

73 Seabrook Road, Hythe
Kent, CT21 5BU
Phone: 01303 265581

The hospital offers a range of medical
and surgical services including
vasectomy, prostate assessment and
orthopaedics. Fixed price treatment is
available for uninsured patients.

BUPA Hospitals

Insurers: Bupa, PPP, Norwich, Standard Life,
Royal Sun Alliance

price guide	£
Hip replacement	7213-9181
Cataract removal	2357-2357

Number of beds	37
ALS staff	3
heart services	-
Cancer services	✿ ① ✓

Kettering · **Woodland Hospital**

Rothwell Rd, Kettering
Northamptonshire, NN16 8XF
Phone: 01536 414515

Woodland Hospital, situated outside
Kettering, offers a wide range of
services including a sports injury clinic
and health screening. Consultants are
largely drawn from the nearby
Kettering General NHS Hospital.

Community Hospitals Group

Insurers: Bupa*, PPP*, Norwich*,
Standard Life*, Royal Sun Alliance*, WPA*

price guide	£
Hip replacement	6850-8510
Cataract removal	1675

Number of beds	-
ALS staff	2
heart services	-
Cancer services	① ✓ ✓

Longfield · **BMI Fawkham Manor Hospital**

Manor Lane, Fawkham, Longfield
Kent, DA3 8ND
Phone: 01474 879 900

Fawkham Manor has 10 designated
children's rooms and one high
dependency room; it is liaising with
the Trust to treat NHS patients in an
attempt to reduce waiting lists.
Sevenoaks District Council has granted
a 'clean food' award to the hospital.

General Healthcare Group Ltd

Insurers: Bupa*, PPP*, Norwich*,
Royal Sun Alliance*, WPA

price guide	£
Hip replacement	-
Cataract removal	-

Number of beds	39
ALS staff	2
heart services	-
Cancer services	① ✓ ✓

Maidstone · **BMI Somerfield Hospital**

63-77 London Rd, Maidstone
Kent, ME16 0DU
Phone: 01622 208000

Somerfield Hospital undertakes a wide
range of surgery, including orthopaedic,
ophthalmic, ENT, urological, maxillofacial surgery and gynaecological
surgery. The physiotherapy department
has recently been extended to cope
with increasing demand. Alternative
therapies are also available.

General Healthcare Group

Insurers: Bupa*, PPP*, Norwich,
Royal Sun Alliance*, WPA

price guide	£
Hip replacement	6680-7680
Cataract removal	2360

Number of beds	48
ALS staff	10
heart services	-
Cancer services	✅ ✅

Milton Keynes · **BMI Saxon Clinic**

Chadwick Drive, Saxon Street
Milton Keynes, Buckinghamshire
MK6 5LR
Phone: 01908 665533

The hospital provides a range of
diagnostic and surgical treatment,
some in conjunction with the nearby
Milton Keynes General Hospital. The
hospital has its own dedicated
endoscopy suite, and an outpatient
extension is planned for 2002 to create
an additional 6 consulting rooms.

General Healthcare Group

Insurers: Bupa*, PPP*, Norwich,
Royal Sun Alliance, WPA

price guide	£
Hip replacement	7400-8600
Cataract removal	1961-2061

Number of beds	40
ALS staff	2
heart services	-
Cancer services	🌐 ① ✅ ✅

Northampton · **BMI Three Shires Hospital**

The Avenue, Cliftonville
Northampton, NN1 5DR
Phone: 01604 620311
Fax: 01604 629066

Three Shires Hospital opened in May
1982 following an appeal by local
businessmen and consultants to
expand the private health facilites in
Northampton. Consultants are drawn
largely from Northampton General
Hospital.

General Healthcare Group Ltd

Insurers: Bupa*, PPP*, Norwich*,
Standard Life*, Royal Sun Alliance*, WPA

price guide	£
Hip replacement	6995
Cataract removal	1995-2495

Number of beds	49
ALS staff	0
heart services	-
Cancer services	🌐 ✅ ✅

Oxford · **Acland Nuffield Hospital**

Banbury Road, Oxford
Oxfordshire, OX2 6PD
Phone: 01865 404142

The majority of the hospital's admitting consultants come from the local Oxford Radcliffe Hospitals NHS Trust, with full 24-hour medical cover provided by resident medical officers.

Nuffield Nursing Homes Trust

Insurers: Bupa*, PPP*, Norwich*, Standard Life, Royal Sun Alliance, WPA

price guide	£
Hip replacement	9100-9500
Cataract removal	2675-2885

Number of beds	37
ALS staff	1

heart services	-
Cancer services	

Princes Risborough · **BMI Paddocks Hospital**

Ayelsbury Rd, Princes Risborough
Buckinghamshire, HP27 0JS
Phone: 01844 346 951

The Paddocks Hospital in Buckinghamshire works closely with its sister site, The Chiltern Hospital. The Paddocks offers a range of services and facilities, however all pathology is referred to the Chiltern.

General Healthcare Group Ltd

Insurers: Bupa*, PPP*, Norwich*, Standard Life, Royal Sun Alliance*, WPA

price guide	£
Hip replacement	7800-8450
Cataract removal	2540-2540

Number of beds	30
ALS staff	2

heart services	-
Cancer services	

Reading · **Berkshire Independent Hospital**

Wensley Road, Coley Park, Reading
Berkshire, RG1 6UZ
Phone: 0118 902 8000

The Berkshire Independent Hospital has been recently expanded, with the addition of an operating theatre, 21 beds and an outpatient centre offering radiography and physiotherapy. The hospital houses the Reading Shoulder Unit.

Capio Healthcare UK

Insurers: Bupa, PPP*, Norwich, Standard Life, Royal Sun Alliance, WPA

price guide	£
Hip replacement	6300
Cataract removal	2180

Number of beds	72
ALS staff	0

heart services	-
Cancer services	

Reading · **BUPA Dunedin Hospital**

16 Bath Road, Reading
Berkshire, RG1 6NB
Phone: 0118 958 7676

BUPA Dunedin Hospital specialises in general surgery, orthopaedics, gynaecology and medical oncology. The nearby NHS Royal Berkshire and Battle Hospital has A&E and intensive care facilities.

BUPA Hospitals

Insurers: Bupa, PPP, Norwich, Standard Life, Royal Sun Alliance, WPA

price guide	£
Hip replacement	7800-7800
Cataract removal	2450-2450

Number of beds	50
ALS staff	1
heart services	-
Cancer services	

Redhill · **BUPA Redwood Hospital**

Canada Drive, Redhill
Surrey, RH1 5BY
Phone: 01737 277277

The hospital's specialties include cardiology and dietetics. Consultants are drawns largely from the local Surrey and Sussex Healthcare NHS Trust and the nearest ITC unit is at East Sussex and Crawley Hospital.

BUPA Hospitals

Insurers: Bupa, PPP, Norwich, Standard Life, Royal Sun Alliance, WPA

price guide	£
Hip replacement	7574-7574
Cataract removal	1800-2375

Number of beds	36
ALS staff	5
heart services	-
Cancer services	

Slough · **Thames Valley Nuffield Hospital**

Wexham St, Wexham, Slough
Berkshire, SL3 6NH
Phone: 01753 662241

Thames Valley Nuffield Hospital is located near Slough town centre. In addition to general medical and surgical services, the hospital offers complementary therapies including acupuncture and reflexology.

Nuffield Nursing Homes Trust

Insurers: Bupa, Norwich, Standard Life, Royal Sun Alliance, WPA

price guide	£
Hip replacement	5200-6200
Cataract removal	1950-2650

Number of beds	48
ALS staff	3
heart services	-
Cancer services	

Southampton · **BUPA Chalybeate Hospital**

Chalybeate Close, Tremona Road, Southampton, Hampshire, SO16 6UY
Phone: 023 8077 5544

BUPA Chalybeate hospital has been contracted to provide heart surgery for the nearby Southampton General NHS Hospital to help cut waiting lists. Parts of the hospital have recently been refurbished.

BUPA Hospitals

Insurers: Bupa, PPP, Norwich, Standard Life, Royal Sun Alliance, WPA

price guide	£
Hip replacement	7575-7575
Cataract removal	2115-2115

Number of beds	78
ALS staff	2
heart services	
Cancer services	

St Leonards on Sea · **BUPA Hospital Hastings**

The Ridge, St Leonards on Sea
East Sussex, TN37 7RE
Phone: 01424 757400

BUPA Hospital Hastings offers a range of specialties including specialist services for hip revision and spinal surgery and is a satellite centre for assisted conception.

BUPA Hospitals

Insurers: Bupa, PPP, Norwich, Standard Life, Royal Sun Alliance, WPA

price guide	£
Hip replacement	6967-8592
Cataract removal	2375-2625

Number of beds	29
ALS staff	2
heart services	-
Cancer services	

Tunbridge Wells · **Tunbridge Wells Nuffield Hospital**

Kingswood Rd, Tunbridge Wells
Kent, TN2 4UL
Phone: 01892 531111

Tunbridge Wells Nuffield Hospital recently opened the new Park House wing to house a new physiotherapy department, together with a gynaecology and IVF suite.

Nuffield Nursing Homes Trust

Insurers: Bupa*, PPP*, Norwich*, Standard Life*, Royal Sun Alliance*, WPA

price guide	£
Hip replacement	6200-7700
Cataract removal	2135-2600

Number of beds	56
ALS staff	1
heart services	-
Cancer services	

Tunbridge Wells · **BUPA Hospital Tunbridge Wells**

Fordcombe Road, Fordcombe
Tunbridge Wells, Kent, TN3 0RD
Phone: 01892 740047

The BUPA Hospital Tunbridge Wells
offers a range of services including
plastic surgery, laser surgery and
psychosexual medicine. Most
consultants are drawn from Maidstone
and Tunbridge Wells NHS Trust.

BUPA Hospitals

Insurers: Bupa, PPP, Norwich, Standard Life,
Royal Sun Alliance, WPA

price guide	£
Hip replacement	10975-10975
Cataract removal	2545-2545

Number of beds	38
ALS staff	2
heart services	-
Cancer services	⊘

Walderslade · **BUPA Alexandra Hospital**

Impton Lane, Walderslade
Kent, ME5 9PG
Phone: 01634 687166

BUPA Alexandra Hospital provides a
range of specialist procedures
including varicose vein removal, hernia
repair and cosmetic surgery. The
hospital has a strong clinical pathology
department.

BUPA Hospitals

Insurers: Bupa, PPP

price guide	£
Hip replacement	7579-8099
Cataract removal	2444-2444

Number of beds	44
ALS staff	2
heart services	-
Cancer services	

Winchester · **BMI Sarum Road Hospital**

Sarum Rd, Winchester
Hampshire, SO22 5HA
Phone: 01962 841555

This hospital provides services from
routine investigations to complex
surgery. The most recent inspection by
the Local Health Authority reported
that facilities for patients were very
good.

General Healthcare Group

Insurers: Bupa, PPP*, Norwich, Standard Life,
Royal Sun Alliance, WPA

price guide	£
Hip replacement	7541
Cataract removal	2200

Number of beds	44
ALS staff	1
heart services	-
Cancer services	

Windsor · **BMI The Princess Margaret Hospital**

Osborne Rd, Windsor
Berkshire, SL4 3SJ
Phone: 01753 743434

The Princess Margaret Hospital has a
broad range of specialist facilities
including a dedicated oncology suite,
gynaecology and orthopaedics
treatment rooms, endoscopy theatre,
physiotherapy & sports injury clinic
and antenatal services.

General Healthcare Group

Insurers: Bupa*, PPP*, Norwich*,
Royal Sun Alliance*, WPA

price guide	£
Hip replacement	7665-9520
Cataract removal	2115-2345

Number of beds	80
ALS staff	1
heart services	-
Cancer services	🌐 ⓘ ✅ ✅

Windsor · **HRH Princess Christian's Hospital**

12 Clarence Road, Windsor
Berkshire, SL4 5AG
Phone: 01753 853121

Facilities at the HRH Princess Christian's
Hospital include a back pain service by
a consultant radiologist, a specialist
breast clinic and private GP service.

Nuffield Nursing Homes Trust

Insurers: Bupa*, Norwich*,
Standard Life*, Royal Sun Alliance*, WPA

price guide	£
Hip replacement	6000-8500
Cataract removal	2500-2750

Number of beds	26
ALS staff	1
heart services	-
Cancer services	🌐 ⓘ ✅

Woking · **Woking Nuffield Hospital**

Shores Rd, Woking
Surrey, GU21 4BY
Phone: 01483 227800

The Woking Nuffield Hospital, situated
about 1 mile north of Woking town
centre, is modern and well equipped
with a successful assisted conception
unit.

Nuffield Nursing Homes Trust

Insurers: Bupa*, Norwich*, Standard Life*,
Royal Sun Alliance*, WPA

price guide	£
Hip replacement	7500-9500
Cataract removal	2500-2820

Number of beds	47
ALS staff	1
heart services	-
Cancer services	✅ ✅

Worthing · **BMI Goring Hall Hospital**

Bodiam Avenue, Goring-by-Sea
Worthing, West Sussex, BN14 0UE
Phone: 01903 506 699

With a 4-bed high dependency unit, and 24-hour on-site medical cover, Goring Hall offers a range of facilities and specialties ranging from general surgery to orthopaedics. Consultants are drawn from the nearby Worthing and Southlands NHS Hospitals.

General Healthcare Group Ltd

Insurers: Bupa*, PPP*, Norwich*, Standard Life, Royal Sun Alliance*, WPA

price guide	£
Hip replacement	-
Cataract removal	-
Number of beds	52
ALS staff	2
heart services	-
Cancer services	⊕ ⊘

South West

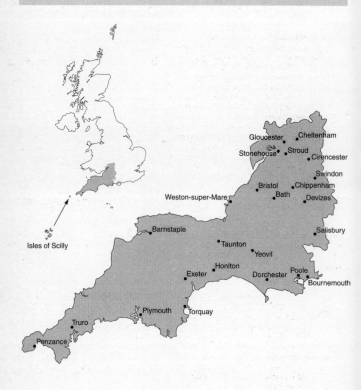

Gloucester
Cheltenham
Stonehouse Stroud
Cirencester
Swindon
Bristol Chippenham
Weston-super-Mare Bath Devizes

Barnstaple Salisbury

Taunton
Yeovil
Honiton Poole
Exeter Dorchester Bournemouth
Torquay
Plymouth
Truro
Penzance

Isles of Scilly

NHS

Barnstaple	North Devon District Hospital
Bath	Royal United Hospital
Bournemouth	Royal Bournemouth Hospital
Bristol	Bristol General Hospital
Bristol	Bristol Royal Infirmary
Bristol	Frenchay Hospital
Bristol	Southmead Hospital
Bristol	St Michael's Hospital
Cheltenham	Cheltenham General Hospital
Cirencester	Cirencester Hospital
Dorchester	Dorset County Hospital
Exeter	Royal Devon & Exeter Hospital
Gloucester	Gloucestershire Royal Hospital
Penzance	West Cornwall Hospital
Plymouth	Derriford Hospital
Poole	Poole Hospital
Salisbury	Salisbury District Hospital
Stonehouse	Standish Hospital
Stroud	Stroud General Hospital
Swindon	Princess Margaret Hospital
Taunton	Taunton & Somerset Hospital
Torquay	Torbay District General Hospital
Truro	Royal Cornwall Hospital
Weston-super-Mare	Weston General Hospital
Yeovil	Yeovil District Hospital

Private

Bath	BMI Bath Clinic
Bournemouth	Bournemouth Nuffield Hospital
Bristol	Bristol Nuffield at The Chesterfield and St Mary's
Cheltenham	Cheltenham & Gloucester Nuffield Hospital
Dorchester	BMI Winterbourne Hospital
Durdham Down	BUPA Hospital Bristol
Exeter	Exeter Nuffield Hospital
Gloucester	Winfield Hospital
Plymouth	Plymouth Nuffield Hospital
Poole	BMI The Harbour Hospital
Salisbury	New Hall Hospital
Swindon	BMI The Ridgeway Hospital
Taunton	Somerset Nuffield Hospital
Torquay	Mount Stuart Hospital
Truro	Duchy Hospital

Barnstaple · **North Devon District Hospital**

Raleigh Park, Barnstaple
Devon, EX31 4JB
Phone: 01271 322 577

Trust: Northern Devon Healthcare NHS
Trust

The North Devon District Hospital serves a population of 150,000 and has 21 wards. It boasts an efficient A&E department, which is able to see the majority of patients within 4 hours of being admitted. Government targets on providing single-sex wards and performing CT scans on stroke patients within 48 hours of being admitted are met. Paediatric surgery is carried out, but a paediatrician is not on site 24 hours a day as recommended by the Royal College of Surgeons. Death rates for the hospital are in line with the national average.

Number of beds		350
➊ ⊕ ♫ ✖ ☎		
		regional
Overall mortality	99	97
Vacancy rates	0	1
Doctors per 100 beds	19	34
Nurses per 100 beds	93	112
Cancelled operations	0.2	3
Complaints	2.1	3
Complaints clear up	55	46
waiting times		
Inpatient	71	77
Outpatient	84	80

Bath · **Royal United Hospital**

Combe Park, Bath
Somerset, BA1 3NG
Phone: 01225 428 331

Trust: Royal United Hospital Bath NHS
Trust

The Royal United Hospital Bath serves a population of around 500,000 people drawn mainly from Bath, north-east Somerset, and west and north Wiltshire. The death rate for emergency stroke admissions is low compared to other hospitals, as is the overall mortality rate. The hospital performs coronary angiography and meets the government standard for this procedure of performing at least 500 catheterisations per year. It also administers thrombolytic drugs to heart attack patients within the target average of 30 minutes.

Number of beds		566
➊ ⊕ ♫ ✖ ☎ ●		
		regional
Overall mortality	85	97
Vacancy rates	0	1
Doctors per 100 beds	53	34
Nurses per 100 beds	136	112
Cancelled operations	1	3
Complaints	4	3
Complaints clear up	55	46
waiting times		
Inpatient	61	77
Outpatient	91	80

Bournemouth · **The Royal Bournemouth Hospital**

Castle Lane East, Bournemouth
Dorset, BH7 7DW
Phone: 01202 303 626

Trust: The Royal Bournemouth and
Christchurch Hospitals NHS Trust

Royal Bournemouth currently has a good stroke care service and is noted for its rapid assessment procedures. The death rate for patients needing emergency treatment for a stroke is lower than average. Three quarters of A&E patients are seen within 4 hours. Inpatient and outpatient waiting times are better than average. Although child surgery is performed at the hospital there is currently no paediatrician on site 24 hours a day. The hospital does not have designated waiting or treatment areas for children in A&E.

Number of beds		654
✚ ♿ ✖ 🚻 ☺		
		regional
Overall mortality	100	97
Vacancy rates	3	1
Doctors per 100 beds	26	31
Nurses per 100 beds	99	113
Cancelled operations	0.6	3
Complaints	1.8	3
Complaints clear up	42	46
waiting times		
Inpatient	100	77
Outpatient	81	80

Bristol · **Bristol General Hospital**

Guinea Street,
Bristol, BS1 6SY
Phone: 0117 923 0000

Trust: United Bristol Healthcare NHS
Trust

Bristol General Hospital is a community hospital run by the United Bristol Healthcare NHS Trust, which also operates the Bristol Royal Infirmary. The Trust performs well on analysis of death rates, with a low death ratio for emergency stroke admissions. The hospital's main focus is on second stage care and rehabilitation. It specialises in falls, diabetes and muscular-skeletal diseases in the elderly and has a stroke rehabilitation unit.

Number of beds		86
♿		
		regional
Overall mortality	97	97
Vacancy rates	0	1
Doctors per 100 beds	57	57
Nurses per 100 beds	159	159
Cancelled operations	-	3
Complaints	3.3	3
Complaints clear up	62	46
waiting times		
Inpatient	79	77
Outpatient	71	80

Bristol · **Bristol Royal Infirmary**

Marlborough Street
Bristol, BS2 8HW
Phone: 0117 923 0000

Trust: United Bristol Healthcare NHS Trust

The Bristol Royal Infirmary is a major teaching hospital and the principal provider of adult acute surgical and medical services to south Bristol and specialist services throughout South West England. The Royal Infirmary is a regional centre for heart surgery and has one of the lowest death rates for heart bypass surgery in the country. The hospital was criticised for past failures in heart surgery services for children; however, as a result of changes the hospital now has a good record in this area.

Number of beds		478
➕ ⊕ 🝱 ⊕ ❌ 🝢 ◉		
		regional
Overall mortality	97	97
Vacancy rates	0	1
Doctors per 100 beds	57	57
Nurses per 100 beds	159	159
Cancelled operations	-	3
Complaints	3.3	3
Complaints clear up	62	46
waiting times		
Inpatient	79	77
Outpatient	71	80

Bristol · **Frenchay Hospital**

Beckspool Road, Bristol
South Gloucestershire, BS16 1JE
Phone: 0117 970 1070

Trust: North Bristol NHS Trust

Frenchay Hospital is a large district general serving Bristol and the surrounding areas. Death rates are in line with expectations for the Trust although inpatient waiting times are worse than average. There is a coronary care unit and angiography is offered, but the hospital does not yet meet the Government target of performing at least 500 catheterisations per year. It also does not yet manage to adminster thrombolytic drugs to heart attack patients within an average 30 minutes of their arrival in A&E.

Number of beds		610
➕ ⊕ 🝱 ⊕ ❌ 🝢 ◉		
		regional
Overall mortality	101	97
Vacancy rates	4	1
Doctors per 100 beds	32	31
Nurses per 100 beds	114	113
Cancelled operations	3	3
Complaints	4.6	3
Complaints clear up	49	46
waiting times		
Inpatient	63	77
Outpatient	78	80

Bristol · **Southmead Hospital**

Westbury on Trym
Bristol, BS10 5NB
Phone: 0117 950 5050

Trust: North Bristol NHS Trust

Southmead Hospital has a range of specialist services including urology, renal medicine and infectious diseases. The North Bristol NHS Trust which runs it has average death rates. A paediatrician is on site 24 hours a day and there is a designated children's ITU. The hospital has an A&E department but heart attack patients do not receive thrombolysis within the target average of 30 minutes of their arrival. Most patients awaiting treatment in A&E are dealt with within the recommended maximum of 4 hours.

Number of beds		693
➊ ⊕ ⚕ ⊕ ✖ ☎ ◉		
		regional
Overall mortality	101	97
Vacancy rates	4	1
Doctors per 100 beds	32	31
Nurses per 100 beds	114	113
Cancelled operations	3	3
Complaints	4.6	3
Complaints clear up	49	46
waiting times		
Inpatient	63	77
Outpatient	78	80

Bristol · **St Michael's Hospital**

Southwell St
Bristol, BS2 8EG
Phone: 0117 921 5411

Trust: United Bristol Healthcare NHS
Trust

St Michael's is part of United Bristol Healthcare Services NHS Trust and works with the Bristol Royal Infirmary and some specialist hospitals to provide services to Bristol and the surrounding area. ENT, obstetrics and gynaecology are among the services offered by St Michael's. In 2000, the hospital took part in a trial involving alternative therapy for babies suffering from colic by giving free cranial osteopathic sessions.

Number of beds		146
✖		
		regional
Overall mortality	97	97
Vacancy rates	0	1
Doctors per 100 beds	57	57
Nurses per 100 beds	159	159
Cancelled operations	-	3
Complaints	3.3	3
Complaints clear up	62	46
waiting times		
Inpatient	79	77
Outpatient	71	80

Cheltenham · **Cheltenham General Hospital**

Sandford Road, Cheltenham
Gloucestershire, GL53 7AN
Phone: 01242 222 222

Trust: East Gloucestershire NHS Trust

Cheltenham General is a large acute hospital and its recent £6.3 million development programme resulted in Cheltenham General gaining more beds, plus modern wards and facilities. The hospital meets recommended targets on two measures of treatment of heart disease patients – rapid treatment of heart attacks with thrombolytic drugs and performing more than 500 angiographies per year. However, stroke patients don't always receive a CT scan within the recommended 48 hours of admission.

Number of beds		506
⊕ ⊗ ✕ ⊡ ◉		
		regional
Overall mortality	95	97
Vacancy rates	1	1
Doctors per 100 beds	27	31
Nurses per 100 beds	107	113
Cancelled operations	2	3
Complaints	1.5	3
Complaints clear up	34	46
waiting times		
Inpatient	90	77
Outpatient	78	80

Cirencester · **Cirencester Hospital**

The Querns, Cirencester
Gloucestershire, GL7 1RR
Phone: 01285 655 711

Trust: East Gloucestershire NHS Trust

Cirencester is a small associate district hospital serving East Gloucestershire and is part of East Gloucestershire NHS Trust. Volunteers at the hospital run activities for patients undergoing rehabilitation. Within the community, collaboration between the hospital, local social services and Cotswold Primary Care Group has led to the development of rehabilitation assistants who aid patients in their own homes.

Number of beds		-
⊕ ⊕ ⊗		
		regional
Overall mortality	95	97
Vacancy rates	1	1
Doctors per 100 beds	27	31
Nurses per 100 beds	107	113
Cancelled operations	-	3
Complaints	1.5	3
Complaints clear up	34	46
waiting times		
Inpatient	90	77
Outpatient	78	80

Dorchester · **Dorset County Hospital**

Williams Avenue, Dorchester
Dorset, DT1 2JY
Phone: 01305 251 150

Trust: West Dorset General Hospitals
 NHS Trust

Dorset County Hospital is a recently built hospital that has achieved an overall mortality rate significantly below what would be expected. The hospital also has an exceptionally good record on waiting times. There is an A&E department which has separate children's waiting and treatment area and a paediatrician on site 24 hours a day. However, the hospital is yet to put in place multidisciplinary teams to treat cancer patients as recommended by the Government.

Number of beds		508
✚ ⊕ ⚕ ✖ ☎ ◉		
		regional
Overall mortality	87	97
Vacancy rates	2	1
Doctors per 100 beds	35	32
Nurses per 100 beds	116	106
Cancelled operations	2	3
Complaints	3.8	3
Complaints clear up	58	46
waiting times		
Inpatient	100	77
Outpatient	88	80

Exeter · **Royal Devon & Exeter Hospital**

Barrack Road, Exeter
Devon, EX2 5DW
Phone: 01392 411 611

Trust: Royal Devon & Exeter Healthcare
 NHS Trust

This hospital has opened two new wards in an effort to tackle waiting times for emergency admissions and elective surgery. The hospital has notably low death rates for emergency hip admissions as well as a low overall mortality rate. Over 90 per cent of patients are dealt with in A&E within 4 hours, but suspected stroke patients do not always receive a CT scan within 48 hours of admission. Coronary angiography is available, but the hospital does not perform the recommended 500 catheterisations a year.

Number of beds		858
✚ ⊕ ⚕ ⊕ ✖ ☎ ◉		
		regional
Overall mortality	87	97
Vacancy rates	0	1
Doctors per 100 beds	37	31
Nurses per 100 beds	113	113
Cancelled operations	3	3
Complaints	1.6	3
Complaints clear up	70	46
waiting times		
Inpatient	69	77
Outpatient	81	80

Gloucester · **Gloucestershire Royal Hospital**

Great Western Road, Gloucester
Gloucestershire, GL1 3NN
Phone: 01452 528 555

Trust: Gloucestershire Royal NHS Trust

The Gloucestershire Royal Hospital is undergoing a £30 m development, which will provide a new A&E department and children's unit. Paediatric surgery is performed at the hospital. The hospital has a dedicated stroke unit and all suspected stroke patients receive CT scans within 48 hours of being admitted; however, stroke death rates are above average. Other death rates are in line with national averages and the hospital does better than average on waiting times. The hospital has a renal unit.

Number of beds		823
➕ ⊕ ⊛ ✖ ☏		
		regional
Overall mortality	101	97
Vacancy rates	2	1
Doctors per 100 beds	28	34
Nurses per 100 beds	108	112
Cancelled operations	-	3
Complaints	2.9	3
Complaints clear up	27	46
waiting times		
Inpatient	81	77
Outpatient	82	80

Penzance · **West Cornwall Hospital**

Penzance
Cornwall, TR18 2PF
Phone: 01736 874 000

Trust: Royal Cornwall Hospitals Trust

The West Cornwall Hospital has recently benefited from a £10 m cash boost that has helped improve services and facilities. This is a small hospital and the A&E unit is staffed by nurses overnight between 11p.m. and 9a.m. Death rates are in line with the national average.

Number of beds		100
➕ ⊛		
		regional
Overall mortality	89	97
Vacancy rates	1	1
Doctors per 100 beds	34	31
Nurses per 100 beds	125	113
Cancelled operations	-	3
Complaints	2.3	3
Complaints clear up	69	46
waiting times		
Inpatient	72	77
Outpatient	76	80

Plymouth · **Derriford Hospital**

Plymouth
Devon, PL6 8DH
Phone: 01752 777 111

Trust: Plymouth Hospitals NHS Trust

Derriford Hospital is the main hospital in Plymouth and provides general hospital services to Plymouth, West Devon, South Hams, and East Cornwall. The hospital is a centre for heart surgery and has one of the best records for lower than expected deaths following heart bypass operations. However, thrombolysis is not administered to heart attack patients within an average of 30 minutes of their arrival in A&E. Other death rates are average.

Number of beds		941
⊕ ❖ ✖ ☎ ◉		
		regional
Overall mortality	90	97
Vacancy rates	-	1
Doctors per 100 beds	47	31
Nurses per 100 beds	146	113
Cancelled operations	1.2	3
Complaints	3.2	3
Complaints clear up	59	46
waiting times		
Inpatient	61	77
Outpatient	68	80

Poole · **Poole Hospital**

Longfleet Road, Poole
Dorset, BH15 2JB
Phone: 01202 665 511

Trust: Poole Hospitals NHS Trust

Poole Hospital is currently constructing a dedicated breast care unit, a new coronary care and cardiac rehabilitation unit and is in the process of refurbishing its operating theatres. The hospital has a below average death rate for emergency stroke admissions but does not offer all suspected stroke patients a CT scan within 48 hours of being admitted. It has two stroke units, one of which provides acute care. Breast, stomach, colorectal and lung cancers are all treated at the hospital and multidisciplinary teams are in place.

Number of beds		771
⊕ ⊕ ❖ ✖ ☎ ◉		
		regional
Overall mortality	102	97
Vacancy rates	1	1
Doctors per 100 beds	34	34
Nurses per 100 beds	106	112
Cancelled operations	1	3
Complaints	2.9	3
Complaints clear up	64	46
waiting times		
Inpatient	100	77
Outpatient	87	80

Salisbury · **Salisbury District Hospital**

Salisbury
Wiltshire, SP2 8BJ
Phone: 01722 336 262

Trust: Salisbury Health Care NHS Trust

Salisbury District Hospital has recently developed a new orthopaedic clinic and a dedicated obstetric theatre. It has low death rates for emergency broken hip admissions. In the A&E department, around three-quarters of patients awaiting treatment are dealt with within the recommended maximum time of 4 hours. There are separate child treatment and waiting areas in A&E.

Number of beds		546
➕ ⊕ ⚕ ❌ ☎ ☺		
		regional
Overall mortality	105	97
Vacancy rates	0	1
Doctors per 100 beds	29	31
Nurses per 100 beds	103	113
Cancelled operations	9	3
Complaints	2.4	3
Complaints clear up	38	46
waiting times		
Inpatient	78	77
Outpatient	84	80

Stonehouse · **Standish Hospital**

Stonehouse
Gloucestershire, GL10 3DB
Phone: 01453 822 481

Trust: Gloucestershire Royal NHS Trust

Standish Hospital, Gloucestershire, is a small hospital serving the local population. The hospital's services are due to be transferred to the larger Gloucestershire Royal. The Trust that runs both this and the Gloucestershire Royal has an average death rate overall.

Number of beds		123
❌		
		regional
Overall mortality	101	97
Vacancy rates	2	1
Doctors per 100 beds	28	34
Nurses per 100 beds	108	112
Cancelled operations	0	3
Complaints	2.9	3
Complaints clear up	27	46
waiting times		
Inpatient	81	77
Outpatient	82	80

Stroud · **Stroud General Hospital**

Trinity Road, Stroud
Gloucestershire, GL5 2HY
Phone: 01453 562 200

Trust: Severn NHS Trust

Stroud General Hospital is a small GP-led associate district general managed by the Severn NHS Trust. There is an A&E department at the hospital and an X-ray service available 24 hours a day. The staffing level for nurses per 100 beds is around average. As well as inpatient beds for medical and surgical problems, there are outpatient clinics in all main specialties. These clinics are headed up by consultants and specialists from local Acute Trusts supported by GPs from practices around the area.

Number of beds		62
✚ ✖		
		regional
Overall mortality	-	97
Vacancy rates	3	1
Doctors per 100 beds	-	31
Nurses per 100 beds	137	113
Cancelled operations	-	3
Complaints	-	3
Complaints clear up	77	46
waiting times		
Inpatient	63	77
Outpatient	83	80

Swindon · **Princess Margaret Hospital**

Okus Road, Swindon
Wiltshire, SN1 4JU
Phone: 01793 536 231

Trust: Swindon and Marlborough NHS Trust

Princess Margaret Hospital currently serves a population of 300,000 drawn from Swindon and its surrounding area. Its services will be transferred in November 2002 to a new hospital in Commonhead, Swindon. Death rates and waiting times for the hospital are in line with national averages.
Coronary angiographies are available but the hospital but does not meet the Government recommended level of 500 catheterisations per year.
Children's surgery is performed but a paediatrician is not on site 24 hours a day.

Number of beds		618
✚ ⚕ ✖ 🕾 ◕		
		regional
Overall mortality	102	97
Vacancy rates	2	1
Doctors per 100 beds	40	34
Nurses per 100 beds	118	112
Cancelled operations	-	3
Complaints	2.9	3
Complaints clear up	45	46
waiting times		
Inpatient	73	77
Outpatient	74	80

Taunton · **Taunton & Somerset Hospital**

**Musgrove Park, Taunton
Somerset, TA1 5DA
Phone: 01823 333 444**

Trust: Taunton and Somerset NHS Trust

Taunton & Somerset Hospital has lower than average death rates for stroke and figures are average for emergency broken hip surgery. The hospital provides coronary angiography and performs the recommended number of 500 catheterisations a year. It has an acute stroke unit. There are separate children's treatment and waiting areas. A paediatrician is available 24 hours a day. Recent developments have included a new catheterisation laboratory as well as additional ITU nurses.

Number of beds		764
✪ ⊕ ⚕ ✖ 🜨 ◉		
		regional
Overall mortality	105	97
Vacancy rates	1	1
Doctors per 100 beds	29	31
Nurses per 100 beds	109	113
Cancelled operations	3	3
Complaints	3.7	3
Complaints clear up	43	46
waiting times		
Inpatient	76	77
Outpatient	77	80

Torquay · **Torbay Hospital**

**Lawes Bridge, Torquay
Devon, TQ2 7AA
Phone: 01803 614 567**

Trust: South Devon Healthcare NHS Trust

The hospital's cancer service was recently expanded as part of a £5 m modernisation programme, and the hospital has spent £800,000 upgrading its A&E department. Torbay Hospital has coronary angiography facilities and performs sufficient numbers of catheterisations to meet Government targets. All wards, except CCU and ITU, are single-sex. The lower than average number of doctors per 100 beds reflects the range of community and mental health services offered, which require fewer doctors per bed.

Number of beds		600
✪ ⊕ ⚕ ✖ 🜨 ◉		
		regional
Overall mortality	97	97
Vacancy rates	-	1
Doctors per 100 beds	23	31
Nurses per 100 beds	101	113
Cancelled operations	3	3
Complaints	3.2	3
Complaints clear up	56	46
waiting times		
Inpatient	80	77
Outpatient	85	80

Truro · **Royal Cornwall Hospital**

Truro
Cornwall, TR1 3LJ
Phone: 01872 250 000

Trust: Royal Cornwall Hospitals Trust

The Royal Cornwall has a low overall mortality rate. The hospital has a 10-bed coronary care unit and provides a coronary angiography service that meets the recommended level of performing 500 catheterisations a year. There is also a designated stroke unit, but suspected stroke patients may have to wait more than 2 days for a CT scan. Cancer patients will soon benefit from a new £5 m cancer unit, which is due for completion later this year. The unit will offer the latest technology in targeting cancer tumours.

Number of beds		850
⊕ ⊕ ⊗ ⊕ ⊗ ⊕ ⊙		
		regional
Overall mortality	89	97
Vacancy rates	1	1
Doctors per 100 beds	34	31
Nurses per 100 beds	125	113
Cancelled operations	-	3
Complaints	2.3	3
Complaints clear up	69	46
waiting times		
Inpatient	72	77
Outpatient	76	80

Weston-super-Mare · **Weston General Hospital**

Grange Road, Weston-super-Mare
Somerset, BS23 4TQ
Phone: 01934 636363

Trust: Weston Area Health NHS Trust

Weston General Hospital has a notably low overall mortality rate. Death rates for emergency hip surgery and emergency stroke patients are also significantly lower than at other hospitals. The hospital has multidisciplinary teams to treat lung, breast, stomach and colorectal cancer and heart attack patients are administered thrombolysis within an average of 30 minutes of arrival. A relatively high 7 per cent of Weston General's operations are cancelled for non-medical reasons

Number of beds		330
⊕ ⊗ ⊗ ⊕		
		regional
Overall mortality	88	97
Vacancy rates	0	1
Doctors per 100 beds	33	32
Nurses per 100 beds	96	106
Cancelled operations	7	3
Complaints	4.2	3
Complaints clear up	62	46
waiting times		
Inpatient	69	77
Outpatient	77	80

Yeovil · **Yeovil District Hospital**

Higher Kingston, Yeovil
Somerset, BA21 4AT
Phone: 01935 475122

Trust: East Somerset NHS Trust

Yeovil District hospital meets targets to give heart attack patients emergency thrombolysis within 30 minutes of arrival. It does not yet provide coronary angiography and there are no dedicated stroke units. However, all suspected stroke patients receive a CT scan within 48 hours. The hospital has a higher than average overall mortality rate. There is an efficient A&E department that is able to deal with most patients within 4 hours.

Number of beds		299
⊕ ⊕ ⊕ ⊗ ⊕ ⊙		
		regional
Overall mortality	111	97
Vacancy rates	2	1
Doctors per 100 beds	28	32
Nurses per 100 beds	106	106
Cancelled operations	0.8	3
Complaints	2.4	3
Complaints clear up	34	46
waiting times		
Inpatient	77	77
Outpatient	83	80

Bath · **BMI Bath Clinic**

Claverton Down Rd, Combe Down
Bath, Avon, BA2 7BR
Phone: 01225 835 555

The Princess Margaret NHS Hospital in Swindon has sent a number of patients to the Bath Clinic to help cut its waiting lists. Infertility treatment is available through the Bath Assisted Conception Clinic, a joint project between the Clinic and the nearby Royal United Hospital Bath NHS Trust.

General Healthcare Group

Insurers: Bupa*, PPP*, Norwich*, Standard Life*, Royal Sun Alliance*, WPA*

price guide	£
Hip replacement	6175-6925
Cataract removal	1840-2500
Number of beds	75
ALS staff	1
heart services	-
Cancer services	

Bournemouth · **Bournemouth Nuffield Hospital**

67 Lansdowne Rd, Bournemouth
Dorset, BH1 1RW
Phone: 01202 291866

As the largest private hospital in the south of England, The Bournemouth Nuffield Hospital offers a range of specialist procedures, both surgical and diagnostic. In addition it also has a hydrotherapy pool for rehabilitation therapy.

Nuffield Nursing Homes Trust

price guide	£
Hip replacement	8042-9042
Cataract removal	2160-2245
Number of beds	98
ALS staff	4
heart services	-
Cancer services	

Bristol · **Bristol Nuffield Hospital**

Upper Byron Place, 3 Clifton Hill
Clifton, Bristol, BS8 1BP
Phone: 0117 9730391

Bristol Nuffield Hospital (at Chesterfield and St Mary's) is a twin site acute hospital carrying out a wide range of surgical and medical procedures.

Nuffield Nursing Homes Trust

Insurers: Bupa*, Norwich*, Standard Life*, Royal Sun Alliance*, WPA

price guide	£
Hip replacement	7500-8000
Cataract removal	2250-2500
Number of beds	63
ALS staff	2
heart services	-
Cancer services	

Cheltenham · **Cheltenham and Gloucester Nuffield**

Hatherly Lane, Cheltenham
Gloucestershire, GL51 6SY
Phone: 01242 246500

The Cheltenham and Gloucester
Nuffield hospital, which was opened in
December 2000, offers a full range of
acute medical, surgical and diagnostic
facilities. In addition, the hospital also
offers hydrotherapy and acupuncture.

Nuffield Nursing Homes Trust

Insurers: Bupa*, PPP*, Norwich*,
Standard Life*, Royal Sun Alliance*, WPA

price guide	£
Hip replacement	7260-7760
Cataract removal	1980-2200

Number of beds	38
ALS staff	1
heart services	-
Cancer services	⊘ ⊘

Dorchester · **BMI Winterbourne Hospital**

Herringston Rd, Dorchester
Dorset, DT1 2DR
Phone: 01305 263252

The BMI Winterbourne Hospital is
renowned for its infertility treatment.
The unit was recently ranked fourth in
the country with a success rate of 26.6
per cent live births per treatment
cycle.

General Healthcare Group

Insurers: Bupa*, PPP*, Norwich,
Standard Life, Royal Sun Alliance, WPA

price guide	£
Hip replacement	7000-7950
Cataract removal	2195-2200

Number of beds	38
ALS staff	1
heart services	-
Cancer services	⊕ ① ⊘ ⊘

Durdham Down · **BUPA Hospital Bristol**

Redland Hill, Durdham Down
Bristol, BS6 6UT
Phone: 0117 973 2562

BUPA Hospital Bristol is contracted to
carry out heart bypass operations and
coronary angiograms for the Bristol
Royal Infirmary. The hospital's breast
care unit practices advanced
techniques.

BUPA Hospitals

Insurers: Bupa, PPP, Norwich, Standard Life,
Royal Sun Alliance, WPA

price guide	£
Hip replacement	2322
Cataract removal	8199

Number of beds	72
ALS staff	1
heart services	⊖ ⊘ ⊛
Cancer services	⊘

Exeter · **Exeter Nuffield Hospital**

Wonford Rd, Exeter
Devon, EX2 4UG
Phone: 01392 276591

Nuffield Hospitals

At the Exeter Nuffield Hospital, consultants of all specialties undertake minor surgery. A diagnostic X-ray department, physiotherapy, health screening, pharmacy and pathology services are provided.

price guide	£
Hip replacement	8345-9595
Cataract removal	1995-2895
Number of beds	46
ALS staff	3
heart services	-
Cancer services	☺ ✓

Gloucester · **Winfield Hospital**

Tewkesbury Road, Longford
Gloucester, GL2 9WH

Community Hospitals

Winfield Hospital offers a range of medical and surgical services including a well-regarded sports injury clinic. Patients have notably praised the hospital's peaceful environment and apparent calm of the staff.

price guide	£
Hip replacement	-
Cataract removal	-
Number of beds	-
ALS staff	-
heart services	-
Cancer services	-

Plymouth · **Plymouth Nuffield Hospital**

Derriford Rd, Plymouth
Devon, PL6 8BG
Phone: 01752 775861

Nuffield Nursing Homes Trust
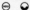

Insurers: Bupa*, PPP*, Norwich*, Standard Life, Royal Sun Alliance*, WPA

The Plymouth Nuffield Hospital is known for plastic and cosmetic surgery, as well as for providing a range of cancer treatments. The hospital offers Fixed Price surgery.

price guide	£
Hip replacement	2280
Cataract removal	8428
Number of beds	41
ALS staff	2
heart services	-
Cancer services	☺ ✓

Poole · **BMI The Harbour Hospital**

St Mary's Rd, Poole
Dorset, BH15 2BH
Phone: 01202 244200

The Harbour Hospital specialises in
oncology and three of its registered
nurses have oncology qualifications.
Consultants are drawn from local
hospitals within the Poole Hospitals
NHS Trust.

General Healthcare Group Ltd

Insurers: Bupa*, PPP*, Norwich*,
Royal Sun Alliance*, WPA

price guide	£
Hip replacement	8114
Cataract removal	-
Number of beds	40
ALS staff	1
heart services	-
Cancer services	

Salisbury · **New Hall Hospital**

Bodenham, Salisbury
Wiltshire, SP5 4EY
Phone: 01722 422 333

New Hall Hospital, located close to
Salisbury city centre, has recently
undergone an extensive £2 m
redevelopment programme. The
redeveloped hospital was opened by
the Earl of Radnor in July 1999.

Capio Healthcare UK

Insurers: Bupa*, PPP*, Norwich,
Standard Life, Royal Sun Alliance, WPA

price guide	£
Hip replacement	7225-10615
Cataract removal	2086-2583
Number of beds	-
ALS staff	1
heart services	-
Cancer services	

Swindon · **BMI The Ridgeway Hospital**

Moormead Rd, Wroughton, Swindon
Wiltshire, SN4 9DD
Phone: 01793 814848

The Ridgeway has a 12-bed day care
unit and a physiotherapy department
with a gymnasium and hydrotherapy
pool. In 1999 it took patients from the
Swindon and Marlborough NHS Trust,
helping to cut waiting lists at the
Princess Margaret Hospital.

General Healthcare Group Ltd

Insurers: Bupa*, PPP*, Norwich,
Standard Life, Royal Sun Alliance, WPA

price guide	£
Hip replacement	7805-8000
Cataract removal	2815-3295
Number of beds	50
ALS staff	1
heart services	-
Cancer services	

Taunton · **Somerset Nuffield Hospital**

Staplegrove Elm, Taunton
Somerset, TA2 6AN
Phone: 01823 286991

The Somerset Nuffield Hospital was extended in 1992 to provide additional beds, a new operating theatre suite, outpatient facilities, physiotherapy and sports injuries, pathology, pharmacy and imaging departments.

Nuffield Nursing Homes Trust

Insurers: Bupa, PPP, Norwich, Standard Life

price guide	£
Hip replacement	5900-7900
Cataract removal	1950-2600

Number of beds	44
ALS staff	3
heart services	-
Cancer services	

Torquay · **Mount Stuart Hospital**

St Vincent's Road, Torquay
Devon, TQ1 4UP

Mount Stuart Hospital has 2 operating theatres, 8 consulting rooms, physiotherapy, diagnostic services including mammography and full colour doppler ultrasound. Fixed Cost Care is available.

Community Hospitals

price guide	£
Hip replacement	-
Cataract removal	-

Number of beds	-
ALS staff	-
heart services	-
Cancer services	-

Truro · **Duchy Hospital**

Penventinnie Lane, Treliske, Truro
Cornwall, TR1 3UP
Phone: 01872 226100

The Duchy Hospital is located next to Torbay District General Hospital, which has the nearest intensive care facilities. Development is under way to increase bed capacity, create a dedicted endoscopy unit and increase the outpatient accommodation.

Community Hospitals Group

Insurers: Bupa*, PPP*, Norwich, Standard Life, Royal Sun Alliance, WPA

price guide	£
Hip replacement	2199
Cataract removal	7399

Number of beds	-
ALS staff	2
heart services	-
Cancer services	

Trent

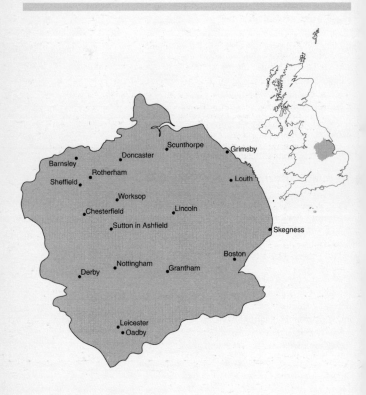

NHS

Barnsley	Barnsley District General Hospital
Boston	Pilgrim Hospital
Chesterfield	Chesterfield and North Derbyshire Royal Hospital
Derby	Derby City General Hospital
Derby	Derbyshire Royal Infirmary
Doncaster	Doncaster Royal Infirmary and Montagu Hospital
Grantham	Grantham and District Hospital
Grimsby	Diana, Princess of Wales Hospital
Leicester	Glenfield Hospital
Leicester	Leicester General
Leicester	Leicester Royal Infirmary
Lincoln	Lincoln County Hospital
Louth	Louth County Hospital
Nottingham	Nottingham City Hospital
Nottingham	Queen's Medical Centre
Rotherham	Rotherham District General Hospital
Scunthorpe	Scunthorpe General Hospital
Sheffield	Northern General Hospital
Sheffield	Royal Hallamshire Hospital
Skegness	Skegness and District Hospital
Sutton in Ashfield	King's Mill Hospital
Worksop	Bassetlaw District General Hospital

Private

Chesterfield	BMI Chatsworth Suite
Derby	East Midlands Nuffield Hospital
Doncaster	Park Hill Hospital
Humberside	St Hugh's Hospital
Leicester	BUPA Hospital Leicester
Leicester	Leicester Nuffield Hospital
Lincoln	Lincoln Nuffield Hospital
Nottingham	Nottingham Nuffield Hospital
Nottingham	BMI The Park Hospital
Sheffield	Claremont Hospital
Sheffield	Thornbury Hospital

Barnsley · **Barnsley District General Hospital**

Gawber Road, Barnsley
South Yorkshire, S75 2EP
Phone: 01226 730000

Trust: Barnsley District General
Hospital NHS Trust

Barnsley District General is a large hospital. Last year the hospital spent over £4.5 m improving equipment and facilities including a cancer helpdesk to ensure that patients with suspected cancer are seen within 8 days. The hospital's death rate for emergency fractured hip admissions is low but for emergency stroke admissions it is high. Inpatient waiting times are higher than average.

Number of beds		526
⊕ ⊕ ⊕ ⊗ ⊕ ⊕		
		regional
Overall mortality	105	102
Vacancy rates	10	4
Doctors per 100 beds	33	33
Nurses per 100 beds	125	117
Cancelled operations	0.3	9
Complaints	3	3
Complaints clear up	42	48
waiting times		
Inpatient	87	77
Outpatient	77	81

Boston · **Pilgrim Hospital**

Sibsey Road, Boston
Lincolnshire, PE21 9QS
Phone: 01205 364801

Trust: United Lincolnshire Hospitals
NHS Trust

The Pilgrim Hospital is one of a number of hospitals run by United Lincolnshire hospitals NHS Trust. The Trust has an average overall mortality rate and a lower than average death rate for patients admitted with broken hips. However, waiting times in A&E are above average. The A&E department has separate waiting and treatment areas for children and paediatric surgery is also performed but a paediatrician is not on site 24 hours a day. The hospital will undergo a £1m extension to improve dermatology and ENT outpatient services in 2002.

Number of beds		681
⊕ ⊕ ⊕ ⊗ ⊕ ⊕		
		regional
Overall mortality	105	102
Vacancy rates	3	4
Doctors per 100 beds	31	33
Nurses per 100 beds	112	117
Cancelled operations	3	9
Complaints	2.8	3
Complaints clear up	28	48
waiting times		
Inpatient	74	77
Outpatient	83	81

Chesterfield · **Chesterfield & North Derbyshire**

Calow, Chesterfield
Derbyshire, S44 5BL
Phone: 01246 277271

Trust: Chesterfield & North Derbyshire
**   Royal Hospital NHS**

Chesterfield and North Derbyshire Royal is a large acute hospital. Last year, the hospital spent £1.8m on cancer care development and a rapid-access chest pain clinic opens this year. Death rates for emergency admissions for fractured hips and strokes are high and stroke patients do not receive a CT scan within the recommended 48 hours of admission. A&E has separate treatment and waiting areas for children and two-thirds of patients in A&E are dealt with within 4 hours.

Number of beds		572
➊ ➕ ⏀ ✖ Ⓖ ⊚		
		regional
Overall mortality	102	102
Vacancy rates	1	4
Doctors per 100 beds	36	33
Nurses per 100 beds	119	117
Cancelled operations	2	9
Complaints	3.3	3
Complaints clear up	84	48
waiting times		
Inpatient	75	77
Outpatient	99	81

Derby · **Derby City General Hospital**

Uttoxeter Road, Derby
Derbyshire, DE22 3NE
Phone: 01332 340131

Trust: Southern Derbyshire Acute
**   Hospitals NHS Trust**

Derby City Hospital is a medium-sized district general serving Derby and the surrounding areas. There is no A&E and emergency services are provided by Derby Royal Infirmary. New plans have recently been announced to radically reshape Derby hospital services. The current hospital site will house a single-site 'super hospital' providing most acute services for the area. Derby City has a coronary care unit and a renal unit.

Number of beds		514
⏀ ➕ ✖ Ⓖ		
		regional
Overall mortality	105	102
Vacancy rates	3	4
Doctors per 100 beds	35	33
Nurses per 100 beds	125	117
Cancelled operations	-	9
Complaints	1.6	3
Complaints clear up	68	48
waiting times		
Inpatient	76	77
Outpatient	79	81

Derby · **Derbyshire Royal Infirmary**

London Road, Derby
Derbyshire, DE1 2QY
Phone: 01332 347141

Trust: Southern Derbyshire Acute
   Hospitals NHS Trust

This hospital has a lower than expected death rate for patients requiring emergency treatment for a broken hip. However, the death rate for emergency stroke admissions is higher than expected despite the fact that the hospital has dedicated stroke facilities and all suspected stroke patients receive a CT scan within 48 hours of admission. By 2007/8 Derbyshire Royal Infirmary will have a community facility, providing therapy and rehabilitation, outpatient clinics and treatment units.

Number of beds		606
⊕ ⊕ ⊗ ⊗ ☎ ◉		
		regional
Overall mortality	105	102
Vacancy rates	3	4
Doctors per 100 beds	35	33
Nurses per 100 beds	125	117
Cancelled operations	-	9
Complaints	1.6	3
Complaints clear up	68	48
waiting times		
Inpatient	76	77
Outpatient	79	81

Doncaster · **Doncaster Royal Infirmary & Montagu**

Armthrope Road, Doncaster
South Yorkshire, DN2 5LT
Phone: 01302 366 666

Trust: Doncaster & Bassetlaw Hospitals
   NHS Trust

Doncaster Royal Infirmary & Montagu Hospital is a large district general hospital. The death rate for emergency stroke patients is higher than average. The hospital does not have a dedicated stroke unit and does not ensure that suspected stroke patients receive a CT scan within 48 hours. However, the hospital recently opened a new CT suite, enabling scans to go direct to consultant neurosurgeons at Sheffield's Royal Hallamshire Hospital. Other death rates are in line with national averages.

Number of beds		718
⊕ ⊕ ⊗ ⊗ ☎ ◉		
		regional
Overall mortality	108	102
Vacancy rates	1	4
Doctors per 100 beds	40	33
Nurses per 100 beds	126	117
Cancelled operations	-	9
Complaints	0	3
Complaints clear up	0	48
waiting times		
Inpatient	88	77
Outpatient	88	81

Grantham · **Grantham & District Hospital**

101 Manthorpe Road, Grantham
Lincolnshire, NG31 8DG

Trust: United Lincolnshire Hospitals
NHS Trust

Grantham and District Hospital is a small hospital which has recently received NHS cash injections enabling it to open an additional critical care bed and to extend and modernise the A&E department. There are separate treatment and waiting areas for children in A&E, and heart attack patients receive thrombolytic drugs within an average of 30 minutes of arrival. The death rate for patients admitted as emergencies with a broken hip are lower than expected.

Number of beds		198
➕ ⊕ 🅰 ❌ 🆑		
		regional
Overall mortality	105	102
Vacancy rates	3	4
Doctors per 100 beds	31	33
Nurses per 100 beds	112	117
Cancelled operations	2	9
Complaints	2.8	3
Complaints clear up	28	48
waiting times		
Inpatient	74	77
Outpatient	83	81

Grimsby · **Diana, Princess of Wales Hospital**

Scartho Road, Grimsby
South Humberside, DN33 2BA
Phone: 01472 874 111

Trust: Northern Lincolnshire and Goole
Hospitals NHS Trust

Diana, Princess of Wales Hospital serves Cleethorpes and Immingham, plus a large rural population. Over £3 m has been spent on service improvements including a children's waiting area in A&E. All A&E patients are dealt with within 4 hours and the hospital meets one of 2 key targets for treating heart disease by performing over 500 catheterisations a year and by ensuring heart attack patients receive thrombolysis within 30 minutes of arrival in A&E. However, not all suspected stroke patients are given a CT scan within 48 hours.

Number of beds		657
➕ ⊕ 🅰 ⊕ ❌ 🆑 🅰		
		regional
Overall mortality	99	102
Vacancy rates	4.4	4
Doctors per 100 beds	31	33
Nurses per 100 beds	122	117
Cancelled operations	0.8	9
Complaints	0	3
Complaints clear up	0	48
waiting times		
Inpatient	75	77
Outpatient	85	81

Leicester · **Glenfield Hospital**

Groby Road, Leicester
Leicestershire, LE3 9QP
Phone: 0116 287 1471

Trust: University Hospitals of Leicester
NHS Trust

Glenfield Hospital is a centre for treatment of heart disease and is an NHS beacon site for its rapid-access chest pain clinic, although the hospital as a whole has no A&E unit. Heart bypass surgery is performed at the hospital, which has an average death rate for this procedure. The hospital is also one of the leading sites carrying out extra corporeal membrane oxygenation (EMO), used to support patients with damaged lungs. There is also a renal unit here. The overall mortality rate for the Trust is lower than average.

Number of beds		482
		regional
Overall mortality	97	102
Vacancy rates	0	4
Doctors per 100 beds	48	43
Nurses per 100 beds	127	132
Cancelled operations	3	9
Complaints	3	3
Complaints clear up	56	48
waiting times		
Inpatient	77	77
Outpatient	72	81

Leicester · **Leicester General Hospital**

Gwendolen Road, Leicester
Leicestershire, LE5 4PW
Phone: 0116 249 0490

Trust: University Hospitals of Leicester
NHS Trust

Leicester General Hospital's acute stroke and rehabilitation wards have recently been refurbished and modernised. The Trust that runs this hospital has below average overall death rates and waiting times are in line with other hospitals. It has no A&E department and this is provided by the Leicester Royal infirmary. There is a renal unit here also.

Number of beds		701
		regional
Overall mortality	97	102
Vacancy rates	0	4
Doctors per 100 beds	48	43
Nurses per 100 beds	127	132
Cancelled operations	3	9
Complaints	3	3
Complaints clear up	56	48
waiting times		
Inpatient	77	77
Outpatient	72	81

Leicester · **Leicester Royal Infirmary**

Leicester
Leicestershire, LE1 5WW
Phone: 0116 254 1414

Trust: University Hospitals of Leicester
NHS Trust

Leicester Royal Infirmary has an A&E department as well as acute facilities. The overall mortality rate is below average, but the number of deaths following emergency broken hip admissions is above average. Coronary angiography is not available. The A&E department has separate child waiting and treatment areas and there is a paediatrician on site 24 hours a day.

Number of beds		1061
⊕ ⊕ ⊘ ⊕ ⊗ ⊕ ⊚		
		regional
Overall mortality	97	102
Vacancy rates	0	4
Doctors per 100 beds	48	43
Nurses per 100 beds	127	132
Cancelled operations	3	9
Complaints	3	3
Complaints clear up	56	48
waiting times		
Inpatient	77	77
Outpatient	72	81

Lincoln · **Lincoln County Hospital**

Greetwell Road, Lincoln
Lincolnshire, LN2 5QY
Phone: 01522 512512

Trust: United Lincolnshire Hospitals
NHS Trust

This hospital has a £10 m radiotherapy and oncology unit with a CT scanner and 32 beds. It has recently opened a new 6-bed CCU. However, CT scans for suspected stroke patients are not yet provided within the maximum recommended time of 48 hours from admission. Services for heart patients include angiography and the hospital meets the Government target of performing at least 500 catheterisations per year.

Number of beds		774
⊕ ⊕ ⊘ ⊗ ⊕ ⊚		
		regional
Overall mortality	105	102
Vacancy rates	3	4
Doctors per 100 beds	31	33
Nurses per 100 beds	112	117
Cancelled operations	1	9
Complaints	2.8	3
Complaints clear up	28	48
waiting times		
Inpatient	74	77
Outpatient	83	81

Louth · **Louth County Hospital**

High Holme Road, Louth
Lincolnshire, LN11 0EU
Phone: 01507 600100

Trust: United Lincolnshire Hospitals
  NHS Trust

Louth County Hospital is a small acute hospital, which opened a rapid-access chest pain clinic last year. The Trust has below average mortality rates for patients admitted as emergencies with broken hips. Heart attack patients are given thrombolysis within an average of 30 minutes of arrival at A&E. The hospital does not offer a coronary angiography service and there are no MRI or CT scanning facilities.

Number of beds		124
➕		
		regional
Overall mortality	105	102
Vacancy rates	3	4
Doctors per 100 beds	31	33
Nurses per 100 beds	112	117
Cancelled operations	-	9
Complaints	2.8	3
Complaints clear up	28	48
waiting times		
Inpatient	74	77
Outpatient	83	81

Nottingham · **Nottingham City Hospital**

Hucknall Road, Nottingham
Nottinghamshire, NG5 1PB
Phone: 0115 969 1169

Trust: Nottingham City Hospital NHS
  Trust

Nottingham City Hospital is a major teaching hospital and provides routine hospital care for almost 300,000 people each year. The hospital has a dedicated stroke unit and below average death rates for emergency stroke admissions. It does not yet meet the Government target of performing CT scans on all suspected stroke patients within 48 hours of being admitted. Single-sex wards are provided and stomach, breast and lung cancers are all treated at the hospital. Government targets on coronary angiographies are also met.

Number of beds		1100
⚕ ✖ 🆑 ⬤		
		regional
Overall mortality	91	102
Vacancy rates	4	4
Doctors per 100 beds	29	43
Nurses per 100 beds	127	132
Cancelled operations	2	9
Complaints	2.9	3
Complaints clear up	45	48
waiting times		
Inpatient	71	77
Outpatient	86	81

Nottingham · **Queen's Medical Centre**

Queen's Medical Centre, Nottingham
Nottinghamshire, NG7 2UH
Phone: 0115 924 9924

Trust: Queen's Medical Centre
University Hospital NHS Trust

The Queen's Medical Centre has embarked on a £6.2 m A&E modernisation programme. It has a combined stroke unit but does not offer all suspected stroke patients a CT scan within 48 hours of admission. Death rates for emergency stroke patients are higher than average. The major cancers are treated here (apart from breast cancer) and multidisciplinary teams are in place for each. The hospital performs coronary angiography but does not administer thrombolysis within 30 minutes of emergency admission.

Number of beds		1400
⊕ ⊕ ⊕ ⊕ ⊗ 🖶 ⊚		
		regional
Overall mortality	109	102
Vacancy rates	2	4
Doctors per 100 beds	46	43
Nurses per 100 beds	144	132
Cancelled operations	0.9	9
Complaints	3	3
Complaints clear up	37	48
waiting times		
Inpatient	80	77
Outpatient	75	81

Rotherham · **Rotherham District General Hospital**

Moorgate Road
Rotherham, S60 2UD
Phone: 01709 820000

Trust: Rotherham General Hospitals
NHS Trust

Rotherham General provides a range of acute services and is a centre for ophthalmology. Death rates are average and waiting times are better than average. Thrombolysis is not currently administered to heart attack patients within the target average of 30 minutes of being admitted. The hospital has a stroke unit and CT scanning facilities.

Number of beds		850
⊕ ⊕ ⊗ 🖶		
		regional
Overall mortality	108	102
Vacancy rates	7	4
Doctors per 100 beds	28	33
Nurses per 100 beds	105	117
Cancelled operations	-	9
Complaints	4.4	3
Complaints clear up	39	48
waiting times		
Inpatient	90	77
Outpatient	84	81

Scunthorpe · **Scunthorpe General Hospital**

Cliff Gardens, Scunthorpe
North Lincolnshire, DN15 7BH
Phone: 01724 282282

Trust: Northern Lincolnshire and Goole
  Hospitals NHS Trust

Scunthorpe General Hospital has introduced a number of one-stop clinics as part of a major drive to create rapid access to specialist consultants. It has an efficient A&E department with most patients dealt with within the recommended maximum time of 4 hours. The hospital does not perform coronary angiography. The overall mortality rate is average, although the death rate for emergency patients with broken hips is low, and the death rate for emergency stroke patients is relatively high.

Number of beds		513
✚ ⊕ ⊛ ⊕ ✖ ⊕		
		regional
Overall mortality	99	102
Vacancy rates	4.1	4
Doctors per 100 beds	31	29
Nurses per 100 beds	120	110
Cancelled operations	0.3	9
Complaints	0	3
Complaints clear up	0	48
waiting times		
Inpatient	75	77
Outpatient	85	81

Sheffield · **Northern General Hospital**

Herries Road, Sheffield
Yorkshire, S5 7AU
Phone: 0114 243 4343

Trust: Sheffield Teaching Hospital NHS
  Trust

The Northern General Hospital, Sheffield, is an important teaching hospital. It is a centre for heart surgery and has an average mortality rate for people undergoing heart bypass operations. It has managed to reduce its cardiology waiting times from 6 months to 4 weeks by moving its echocardiography service to a new, state-of-the-art department. It has an efficient A&E department, in which three-quarters of patients are dealt with within 4 hours. The hospital offers multidisciplinary teams for all major cancers.

Number of beds		1200
✚ ⊛ ✖ ⊕ ⊙		
		regional
Overall mortality	95	102
Vacancy rates	0	4
Doctors per 100 beds	35	43
Nurses per 100 beds	124	132
Cancelled operations	-	9
Complaints	0	3
Complaints clear up	0	48
waiting times		
Inpatient	73	77
Outpatient	76	81

Sheffield · **Royal Hallamshire Hospital**

Glossop Road, Sheffield
Yorkshire, S10 2JF
Phone: 0114 271 1900

Trust: Sheffield Teaching Hospital NHS
Trust

The hospital has opened a £27 m women's unit bringing the city's obstetric, gynaecology and neonatal services under one roof. There is no A&E department and cancellations for elective surgery are higher than most other hospitals. The Trust's overall mortality rate is low. MRI and CT scanning facilities are available.

		regional
Number of beds		740
Overall mortality	85	102
Vacancy rates	3	4
Doctors per 100 beds	51	43
Nurses per 100 beds	148	132
Cancelled operations	4	9
Complaints	0	3
Complaints clear up	0	48
waiting times		
Inpatient	73	77
Outpatient	76	81

Skegness · **Skegness & District Hospital**

Dorothy Avenue, Skegness
Lincolnshire, PE25 2BS
Phone: 01754 762401

Trust: United Lincolnshire Hospitals
NHS Trust

Skegness & District Hospital is a small acute facility forming part of the United Lincolnshire Hospitals NHS Trust. The Trust has below average death rates for emergency broken hip admissions and average death rates for stroke admissions.

		regional
Number of beds		40
Overall mortality	105	102
Vacancy rates	3	4
Doctors per 100 beds	31	33
Nurses per 100 beds	112	117
Cancelled operations	-	9
Complaints	2.8	3
Complaints clear up	28	48
waiting times		
Inpatient	74	77
Outpatient	83	81

Sutton in Ashfield · **King's Mill Hospital**

**Mansfield Road, Sutton in Ashfield
Nottinghamshire, NG17 4JL
Phone: 01623 622515**

**Trust: Sherwood Forest Hospitals NHS
Trust**

King's Mill Hospital provides a full range of surgical and medical specialties to a population of around 329,000 in Mansfield and surrounding areas. Death rates are average or low with a low death rate for emergency fractured hip admissions. There is an A&E department and, on average, heart attack patients receive thrombolytic drugs within the target 30 minutes of arrival at the hospital's A&E department as recommended by the Government. Outpatient waiting times are longer than average.

Number of beds		635
➕ ⊕ ⚕ ✖ ⚕		
		regional
Overall mortality	104	102
Vacancy rates	7	4
Doctors per 100 beds	35	33
Nurses per 100 beds	115	117
Cancelled operations	4	9
Complaints	2.6	3
Complaints clear up	22	48
waiting times		
Inpatient	74	77
Outpatient	70	81

Worksop · **Bassetlaw District General Hospital**

**Kilton Hill, Worksop
Nottinghamshire, S81 0BD
Phone: 01909 500990**

**Trust: Doncaster & Bassetlaw Hospitals
NHS Trust**

Bassetlaw Hospital saw many developments last year including the addition of a new day surgery unit, critical care units and a bone scanner. The A&E department has separate children's waiting and treatment areas. Most A&E patients are dealt with within 4 hours and all suspected stroke patients receive a CT scan within the recommended 48 hours of admission. However, thrombolytic drugs are not given to heart attack patients within 30 minutes of their arrival in A&E.

Number of beds		376
➕ ⊕ ⚕ ✖ ⚕		
		regional
Overall mortality	102	102
Vacancy rates	9	4
Doctors per 100 beds	28	29
Nurses per 100 beds	100	110
Cancelled operations	-	9
Complaints	0	3
Complaints clear up	0	48
waiting times		
Inpatient	88	77
Outpatient	88	81

Chesterfield · **BMI Chatsworth Suite**

Chesterfield Royal Hospital,
Chesterfield, Derbyshire, S44 5BL
Phone: 01246 544 400

BMI Chatsworth Suite is the private
patient facility on the site of the
Chesterfield and North Derbyshire
Royal Hospital, so benefits from the
services offered by a district general
hospital as well as offering specialties
including dermatology and
oral/maxillo-facial surgery.

General Healthcare Group Ltd

Insurers: Bupa*, PPP*, Norwich*,
Standard Life, Royal Sun Alliance*, WPA

price guide	£
Hip replacement	6801-8434
Cataract removal	1936-1936

Number of beds	18
ALS staff	2
heart services	-
Cancer services	◑ ✔

Derby · **East Midlands Nuffield Hospital**

Rykneld Rd, Littleover, Derby
Derbyshire, DE23 7SN
Phone: 01332 517891

The East Midlands Nuffield Hospital is
currently expanding its facilities to
include a third operating theatre, a 6-
bay recovery unit, and an 8-bay day
care unit.

Nuffield Nursing Homes Trust

Insurers: Bupa*, PPP*, Norwich*,
Standard Life*, Royal Sun Alliance*, WPA

price guide	£
Hip replacement	7452-9752
Cataract removal	2762-2912

Number of beds	32
ALS staff	1
heart services	-
Cancer services	◑

Doncaster · **Park Hill Hospital**

Thorne Rd, Doncaster
South Yorkshire, DN2 5TH
Phone: 01302 730 300

Services offered at Park Hill Hospital
include a wide range of cardiac
services, hip replacement and cataract
removal.

Caplo Healthcare UK

Insurers: Bupa*, PPP*, Norwich*,
Standard Life*, Royal Sun Alliance*, WPA*

price guide	£
Hip replacement	7180
Cataract removal	1861

Number of beds	22
ALS staff	0
heart services	
Cancer services	-

Humberside · **St Hugh's Hospital**

Peaks Lane, Grimsby South
Humberside, NE Lincolnshire, DN32 9RP
Phone: 01472 251100

St Hugh's has a High Dependency
Unit. The nearest Intensive Care Unit is
at Diana, Princess of Wales NHS
Hospital, just over a mile away.

The Hospital Management Trust

Insurers: Bupa*, PPP*, Norwich*,
Standard Life*, Royal Sun Alliance*, WPA*

price guide	£
Hip replacement	6268-6886
Cataract removal	1975-2025

Number of beds	30
ALS staff	0
heart services	-
Cancer services	

Leicester · **BUPA Hospital Leicester**

Gartree Road, Oadby
Leicester, LE2 2FF
Phone: 0116 272 0888

The hospital has undergone recent
development, adding a fourth
operating theatre, improved
chemotherapy facilities, and a re-
equipped Intensive Care Unit. It now
also includes an ambulatory care and
day care unit.

BUPA Hospitals

Insurers: Bupa, PPP, Norwich, Standard Life,
Royal Sun Alliance, WPA

price guide	£
Hip replacement	7425-7425
Cataract removal	2330-2565

Number of beds	76
ALS staff	2
heart services	
Cancer services	

Leicester · **Leicester Nuffield Hospital**

Scraptoft Lane, Leicester
Leicestershire, LE5 1HY
Phone: 0116 2769401

In addition to the usual surgical and
medical services, the Leicester Nuffield
Hospital runs an eating disorders clinic
and a PMS clinic.

Nuffield Nursing Homes Trust

Insurers: Bupa*, PPP, Norwich*,
Standard Life*, Royal Sun Alliance*, WPA

price guide	£
Hip replacement	7400-10500
Cataract removal	1999-2085

Number of beds	46
ALS staff	10
heart services	
Cancer services	-

Lincoln · **Lincoln Nuffield Hospital**

Nettleham Rd, Lincoln
Lincolnshire, LN2 1QU
Phone: 01522 578 000

The Lincoln Nuffield Hospital's specialist capabilities include general surgery, diagnostics, physiotherapy and health screening. It also takes medical and surgical emergencies on a 24-hour basis.

Nuffield Nursing Homes Trust

Insurers: Bupa*, PPP*, Norwich*, Standard Life*, Royal Sun Alliance*, WPA

price guide	£
Hip replacement	7284-8082
Cataract removal	2262-2270

Number of beds	40
ALS staff	1
heart services	-
Cancer services	

Nottingham · **Nottingham Nuffield Hospital**

748 Mansfield Rd, Woodthrope
Nottingham, NG5 3FZ
Phone: 0115 9209209

The Nottingham Nuffield Hospital is nearing the completion of a £3.5 m refurbishment which includes an upgraded X-ray facility, outpatient facilities, as well as a new endosocopy suite.

Nuffield Nursing Homes Trust

Insurers: Norwich, Standard Life, Royal Sun Alliance, WPA

price guide	£
Hip replacement	6432-6632
Cataract removal	1800-2000

Number of beds	38
ALS staff	2
heart services	-
Cancer services	-

Nottingham · **BMI The Park Hospital**

Sherwood Lodge Drive, Arnold,
Nottingham, NG5 8RX
Phone: 0115 9670670

The Park Hospital caters for most surgical specialties. The hospital has a well-equipped and staffed Intensive Therapy Unit, a day case chemotherapy suite and provides a full range of fertility treatments.

General Healthcare Group

Insurers: Bupa*, PPP*, Norwich*, Standard Life*, Royal Sun Alliance*, WPA*

price guide	£
Hip replacement	6600
Cataract removal	1850

Number of beds	93
ALS staff	6
heart services	
Cancer services	

Sheffield · **Claremont Hospital**

401 Sandygate Rd, Sheffield
South Yorks, S10 5UB
Phone: 0114 263 0330

Founded in 1953, the Claremont
Hospital employs over 200 of the
region's consultants, providing a
variety of services including brain,
plastic and maxillofacial surgery.

The Hospital Management Trust

Insurers: Bupa, Norwich, Standard Life,
Royal Sun Alliance, WPA

price guide	£
Hip replacement	7107
Cataract removal	1500

Number of beds	60
ALS staff	2
heart services	-
Cancer services	⊘

Sheffield · **Thornbury Hospital**

312 Fulwood Rd, Sheffield
South Yorkshire, S10 3BR
Phone: 0114 2661133

The Thornbury Hospital has a
pathology lab on site. Services offered
include a sexual health clinic, hip and
knee services and a breast clinic.
Consultants are drawn from local NHS
hospitals.

General Healthcare Group Ltd

Insurers: Bupa*, PPP*, Norwich,
Royal Sun Alliance, WPA

price guide	£
Hip replacement	8135-8500
Cataract removal	1590-2060

Number of beds	77
ALS staff	2
heart services	⊘ ⊛
Cancer services	⊘ ✓

West Midlands

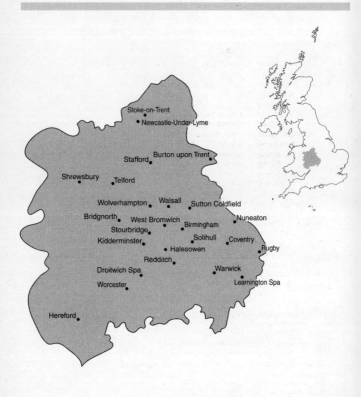

NHS

Birmingham	Birmingham Heartlands Hospital
Birmingham	City Hospital
Birmingham	Queen Elizabeth Hospital
Birmingham	Selly Oak Hospital
Burton-upon-Trent	Queen's Hospital (Burton)
Coventry	Coventry & Warwickshire Hospital
Coventry	Walsgrave Hospital
Hereford	County Hospital
Hereford	General Hospital
Kidderminster	Kidderminster Hospital
Nuneaton	George Eliot Hospital
Redditch	Alexandra Hospital
Rugby	Hospital of St Cross
Shrewsbury	Royal Shrewsbury Hospital
Solihull	Solihull Hospital
Stafford	Staffordshire General Hospital
Stoke-on-Trent	North Staffordshire Hospital
Stourbridge	Russells Hall, Wordsley, Corbett & Guest Hospitals
Sutton Coldfield	Good Hope District General Hospital
Telford	Princess Royal Hospital
Walsall	Manor Hospital
Warwick	Warwick Hospital
West Bromwich	Sandwell General Hospital
Wolverhampton	New Cross Hospital
Worcester	Worcester Royal Infirmary

Private

Birmingham	Birmingham Nuffield Hospital
Birmingham	BMI The Priory Hospital
Droitwich Spa	BMI Droitwich Spa Hospital
Halesowen	West Midlands Hospital
Hereford	Wye Valley Nuffield Hospital
Leamington Spa	Warwickshire Nuffield Hospital
Newcastle-under-Lyme	North Staffordshire Nuffield Hospital
Nuneaton	BMI Nuneaton Private Hospital
Shrewsbury	Shropshire Nuffield Hospital
Solihull	BUPA Parkway Hospital
Stafford	Rowley Hall Hospital
Sutton Coldfield	BUPA Hospital Little Aston
Tettenhall	Wolverhampton Nuffield Hospital
Worcester	BUPA South Bank Hospital

Birmingham · **Birmingham Heartlands Hospital**

Bordesley Green East
Birmingham, B9 5SS
Phone: 0121 424 2000

Trust: Birmingham Heartlands and
      Solihull NHS Trust

This large hospital has a purpose-built helipad for the County Air Ambulance. In the past year, a new block has become fully operational which houses the infectious diseases and elderly medicine wards. The A&E has separate children's waiting and treatment areas. Emergency stroke admission death rates are low and all suspected stoke patients will receive a CT scan within 24 hours of admission. The hospital also meets Government targets by providing thrombolysis within 30 minutes of admission and performing 500 cardiac catheterisations a year.

Number of beds		976
✚ ⊕ ♿ ✖ 🕮 ◉		
		regional
Overall mortality	93	103
Vacancy rates	0	3
Doctors per 100 beds	34	37
Nurses per 100 beds	117	124
Cancelled operations	5.7	3
Complaints	3.4	3
Complaints clear up	32	43
waiting times		
Inpatient	77	78
Outpatient	82	75

Birmingham · **City Hospital**

Dudley Road
Birmingham, B18 7QH
Phone: 0121 554 3801

Trust: City Hospital NHS Trust

City Hospital is a large acute hospital in Birmingham City Centre. It has recently expanded and upgraded its Critical Care Unit and plans a new Ambulatory Care Centre. The hospital also has the West Midlands' first Sickle Cell and Thalassaemia Centre. City's A&E department has separate children's waiting and treatment areas. Only 58 per cent of A&E patients are dealt with within 4 hours, but all stroke patients receive a CT scan within 24 hours of admission and heart attack patients are given thrombolysis within 30 minutes of arriving in the hospital.

Number of beds		700
✚ ⊕ ♿ ✖ 🕮 ◉		
		regional
Overall mortality	105	103
Vacancy rates	7	3
Doctors per 100 beds	60	37
Nurses per 100 beds	144	124
Cancelled operations	2	3
Complaints	2.9	3
Complaints clear up	41	43
waiting times		
Inpatient	92	78
Outpatient	83	75

Birmingham · **Queen Elizabeth Hospital**

Edgbaston,
Birmingham, B15 2TH
Phone: 0121 472 1311

Trust: University Hospital Birmingham
NHS Trust

The Queen Elizabeth Hospital has the largest critical care unit in Europe, combining ITU and HDU facilities. Coronary angiography is performed to the Government recommended standard of 500 cardiac catheterisations per year. It also delivers thrombolysis to heart attack patients within the target average of 30 minutes of arrival. The hospital performs heart bypass surgery, for which death rates are average. The hospital also has a dedicated stroke unit.

Number of beds		553
❶ ⚕ ❌ 🅰 ◉		
		regional
Overall mortality	99	103
Vacancy rates	2	3
Doctors per 100 beds	45	45
Nurses per 100 beds	134	134
Cancelled operations	2	3
Complaints	3	3
Complaints clear up	33	43
waiting times		
Inpatient	71	78
Outpatient	89	75

Birmingham · **Selly Oak Hospital**

Raddlebarn Road
Birmingham, B29 6JD
Phone: 0121 627 1627

Trust: University Hospital Birmingham
NHS Trust

Selly Oak Hospital, Birmingham, opened a new £1m ambulatory care unit in December 2000, allowing the Trust to undertake more day case and cataract operations. Thrombolysis is offered to heart attack patients within the target average of 30 minutes of arrival and meets a key Government target for coronary angiography, performing 500 cardiac catheterisations each year. Patients are accommodated on single-sex wards. Overall mortality rates are average.

Number of beds		454
❶ ⊕ ⚕ ❌ 🅰 ◉		
		regional
Overall mortality	99	103
Vacancy rates	2	3
Doctors per 100 beds	45	45
Nurses per 100 beds	134	134
Cancelled operations	2	3
Complaints	3	3
Complaints clear up	33	43
waiting times		
Inpatient	71	78
Outpatient	89	75

Burton upon Trent · **Queen's Hospital**

Belvedere Road, Burton upon Trent
Straffordshire, DE13 0RB
Phone: 01283 566 333

Trust: Burton Hospitals NHS Trust

Queen's Hospital serves around 200,000 people in Burton upon Trent and parts of South Staffordshire, Leicestershire and Derbyshire. Although the hosptital does not have a stroke unit or administer a CT scan to all suspected stroke patients within the recommended 48 hours of admission, the death rate for emergency stroke admissions is low. There is a coronary care unit and the hospital meets Government targets in one out of two key areas for heart disease therapy.

Number of beds		480
⊕ ⊕ ⊛ ⊗ ⊕ ⊙		
		regional
Overall mortality	102	103
Vacancy rates	0	3
Doctors per 100 beds	35	35
Nurses per 100 beds	120	112
Cancelled operations	-	3
Complaints	3.8	3
Complaints clear up	56	43
waiting times		
Inpatient	73	78
Outpatient	84	75

Coventry · **Coventry and Warwickshire Hospital**

Stoney Stanton Road
Coventry, CV1 4FH
Phone: 02476 224 055

Trust: University Hospitals Coventry
and Warwickshire NHS Trust

Coventry and Warwickshire Hospital is a small acute facility run by the University Hospitals of Coventry and Warwickshire NHS Trust which also runs the Walsgrave hospital and the Hospital of St Cross in Rugby. The hospital has an A&E department with separate children's facilities. There is no MRI scanner but there is a CT scanner operational 24 hours a day. The Trust's death rate for emergency hip fracture admissions is low. However, deaths following emergency stroke admissions are more frequent than expected. There is no stroke unit at this hospital.

Number of beds		146
⊕ ⊕ ⊛ ⊗ ⊕		
		regional
Overall mortality	107	103
Vacancy rates	5	3
Doctors per 100 beds	35	37
Nurses per 100 beds	120	124
Cancelled operations	3	3
Complaints	2.2	3
Complaints clear up	20	43
waiting times		
Inpatient	80	78
Outpatient	66	75

Coventry · **Walsgrave Hospital**

Clifford Bridge Road
Coventry, CV2 2DX
Phone: 024 7660 2020

Trust: University Hospitals Coventry and Warwickshire NHS Trust

The Walsgrave Hospital, Coventry, is to be rebuilt as part of a £200 m development plan. The hospital has low death rates for emergency stroke operations. The hopsital performs heart bypass surgery but its death rate for this is high. The hospital also performs angiography and meets the government target of 500 catheterisations per year. It also ensures that heart attack patients receive thrombolysis within 30 minutes. The hospital has multidisciplinary teams for cancer treatment.

Number of beds		942
⚕ ✖ 🚑 ◕		
		regional
Overall mortality	107	103
Vacancy rates	5	3
Doctors per 100 beds	35	37
Nurses per 100 beds	120	124
Cancelled operations	3	3
Complaints	2.2	3
Complaints clear up	20	43
waiting times		
Inpatient	80	78
Outpatient	66	75

Hereford · **County Hospital**

Hereford, HR1 2ER
Phone: 01432 355 444

Trust: Hereford Hospitals NHS Trust

County Hospital Hereford is a medium-sized district general serving Herefordshire and the Powys area of Wales. The overall mortality rate and the death rate for emergency fractured hip admissions are low. Over 95 per cent of A&E patients are dealt with within 4 hours, but not all heart attack patients receive thrombolysis within the recommended average time of 30 minutes of A&E arrival nor does the hospital perform the recommended 500 cardiac catheterisations a year.

Number of beds		340
➕ ⊕ ⚕ ✖ 🚑 ◕		
		regional
Overall mortality	86	103
Vacancy rates	4	3
Doctors per 100 beds	38	35
Nurses per 100 beds	125	112
Cancelled operations	3	3
Complaints	2.5	3
Complaints clear up	61	43
waiting times		
Inpatient	70	78
Outpatient	76	75

Hereford · **General Hospital**

Nelson Street
Hereford, HR1 2NZ
Phone: 01432 355 444

Trust: Hereford Hospitals NHS Trust

Hereford General Hospital is a small hospital, which together with the larger County Hospital in Hereford, is managed by the Hereford NHS Trust. The A&E department is due to be closed but emergency services will continue to be provided by the County Hospital.

Number of beds		118
✚ ⚕		
		regional
Overall mortality	86	103
Vacancy rates	4	3
Doctors per 100 beds	38	35
Nurses per 100 beds	125	112
Cancelled operations	-	3
Complaints	2.5	3
Complaints clear up	61	43
waiting times		
Inpatient	70	78
Outpatient	76	75

Kidderminster · **Kidderminster Hospital**

Bewdley Road, Kidderminster
Worcestershire, DY11 6RJ
Phone: 01562 823 424

Trust: Worcestershire Acute Hospitals
NHS Trust

Kidderminster Hospital is an outpatient only unit with 18 day-case beds. The hospital has been the subject of a campaign to prevent the closure of services on the site. It does not have an A&E department but does provide a range of acute services and has MRI and CT scanners. The hospital provides a diagnostic facility for breast and lung cancer but surgery is performed at Worcester or Redditch.

Number of beds		-
⚛ ◉		
		regional
Overall mortality	105	103
Vacancy rates	3	3
Doctors per 100 beds	38	37
Nurses per 100 beds	125	124
Cancelled operations	1	3
Complaints	3	3
Complaints clear up	40	43
waiting times		
Inpatient	71	78
Outpatient	77	75

Nuneaton · **George Eliot Hospital**

College Street, Nuneaton
Warwickshire, CV10 7DJ
Phone: 02476 351351

Trust: George Eliot Hospital NHS Trust

Specialist services at George Eliot Hospital include cancer therapy and diabetes and asthma centres. All A&E patients are seen within 4 hours and all suspected stroke patients receive a CT scan within 24 hours. However, death rates at the hospital are higher than average, including death rates for emergency stroke patients and patients with broken hips. The recently modernised A&E has separate children's waiting and treatment areas.

Number of beds		413

		regional
Overall mortality	115	103
Vacancy rates	0	3
Doctors per 100 beds	32	35
Nurses per 100 beds	98	112
Cancelled operations	1	3
Complaints	3.2	3
Complaints clear up	73	43
waiting times		
Inpatient	74	78
Outpatient	75	75

Redditch · **Alexandra Hospital**

Woodrow Drive, Redditch
Worcestershire, B98 7UB
Phone: 01527 503030

Trust: Worcestershire Acute Hospitals NHS Trust

This small hospital is part of Wocestershire Acute Hospitals NHS Trust, which is in line with national averages for overall mortality and staffing levels. There is no stroke unit at this hospital and emergency stroke admission death rate for the Trust is high. The A&E department has recently been updated to include a children's waiting area and most patients admitted to A&E are dealt with within 4 hours. Multi-disciplinary teams are in place to treat most major cancers.

Number of beds		312

		regional
Overall mortality	105	103
Vacancy rates	3	3
Doctors per 100 beds	38	37
Nurses per 100 beds	125	124
Cancelled operations	1	3
Complaints	3	3
Complaints clear up	40	43
waiting times		
Inpatient	71	78
Outpatient	77	75

Rugby · **Hospital of St Cross**

Barby Road, Rugby
Warwickshire, CV22 5PX
Phone: 01788 572831

Trust: University Hospitals Coventry
and Warwickshire NHS Trust

The Hospital of St Cross is a small acute facility serving Rugby. It recently opened a new renal dialysis unit and has a cancer unit providing treatment for breast, lung, colorectal and stomach cancers, with multidisciplinary teams in place for each. The death rate following emergency hip fracture admission is below average. However, the death rate following emergency admission for stroke is higher than average.

Number of beds		138
✪ ⊕ ♫ ✖		
		regional
Overall mortality	107	103
Vacancy rates	5	3
Doctors per 100 beds	35	37
Nurses per 100 beds	120	124
Cancelled operations	3	3
Complaints	2.2	3
Complaints clear up	20	43
waiting times		
Inpatient	80	78
Outpatient	66	75

Shrewsbury · **Royal Shrewsbury Hospital**

Mytton Oak Road, Shrewsbury
Shropshire, SY3 8XQ
Phone: 01743 261 000

Trust: Royal Shrewsbury Hospital NHS
Trust

The overall mortality rate at the Royal Shrewsbury is lower than average, as is the death rate for emergency stroke admissions. Nine out of the patients awaiting treatment in A&E are dealt with within the recommended maximum time of 4 hours. The hospital does not yet meet the government target of 500 cardiac catheterisations a year, but provides a CT scan to all suspected stroke patients within 48 hours. Wards are single-sex.

Number of beds		488
✪ ⊕ ♫ ✖ ⊕		
		regional
Overall mortality	90	103
Vacancy rates	0	3
Doctors per 100 beds	37	28
Nurses per 100 beds	128	111
Cancelled operations	2	3
Complaints	2.7	3
Complaints clear up	68	43
waiting times		
Inpatient	79	78
Outpatient	71	75

Solihull · **Solihull Hospital**

Lade Lane, Solihull
West Midlands, B91 2JL
Phone: 0121 424 2000

Trust: Birmingham Heartlands and
Solihull NHS Trust

Solihull Hospital, part of the Birmingham Heartlands and Solihull NHS Trust, has high death rates for emergency broken hip admissions but a low death rate for emergency stroke patients. Almost all patients awaiting treatment in A&E are dealt with within the recommended maximum of 4 hours. Solihull has dedicated units for acute stroke care and stroke rehabilitation.

Number of beds		976
➕ 🔆 ❌ GP 🌣		
		regional
Overall mortality	93	103
Vacancy rates	0	3
Doctors per 100 beds	34	37
Nurses per 100 beds	117	124
Cancelled operations	3.2	3
Complaints	3.4	3
Complaints clear up	32	43
waiting times		
Inpatient	77	78
Outpatient	82	75

Stafford · **Staffordshire General Hospital**

Weston Road
Stafford, ST16 3SA
Phone: 01785 257 731

Trust: Mid Staffordshire General
Hospitals NHS Trust

Serving a population of around 320,000, the Staffordshire General Hospital provides a range of services including A&E and cancer treatment. The hospital has multidisciplinary teams for treating lung, breast, stomach and colorectal cancers. It provides thrombolysis within 30 minutes emergency admission for heart attack. It has a CCU and a designated stroke unit, but does not yet offer coronary angiography. The hospital meets Government targets to provide single-sex wards.

Number of beds		547
➕ ⊕ 🔆 ❌ 🚑 🌣		
		regional
Overall mortality	107	103
Vacancy rates	3	3
Doctors per 100 beds	19	28
Nurses per 100 beds	102	111
Cancelled operations	1	3
Complaints	3.7	3
Complaints clear up	57	43
waiting times		
Inpatient	72	78
Outpatient	69	75

Stoke-on-Trent · **North Staffordshire Infirmary**

Royal Infirmary, Princes Road
Stoke-on-Trent, ST4 7LN
Phone: 01782 715 444

Trust: North Staffordshire Hospital NHS
  Trust

North Staffordshire Royal Infirmary houses the acute services for Stoke-on-Trent, Newcastle-under-Lyme and Staffordshire Moorlands. All suspected stroke patients are given a CT scan within 48 hours of being admitted. Coronary angiography is performed and the recommended figure of 500 catheterisations a year is met. However, heart attack patients are not given thrombolytic drugs within an average of 30 minutes of arrival. Death rates are average, including for heart bypass surgery, which is performed at the hospital.

Number of beds		1386
⊕ ⊕ ⊕ ⊕ ⊗ ☎ ◉		
		regional
Overall mortality	105	103
Vacancy rates	4	3
Doctors per 100 beds	38	37
Nurses per 100 beds	140	124
Cancelled operations	-	3
Complaints	2.4	3
Complaints clear up	32	43
waiting times		
Inpatient	79	78
Outpatient	61	75

Stoke-on-Trent · **North Staffordshire City General**

Newcastle Road, Stoke-on-Trent
Staffordshire, ST4 6QG
Phone: 01782 715444

Trust: North Staffordshire Hospital NHS
  Trust

The North Staffordshire Hospital operates from both the Royal Infirmary (above) and the City General site which houses the maternity department. The two sites are operated as one hospital and the data presented are the same for each.

Number of beds		830
⊕ ⊕ ☎ ◉		
		regional
Overall mortality	105	103
Vacancy rates	4	3
Doctors per 100 beds	38	37
Nurses per 100 beds	140	124
Cancelled operations	-	3
Complaints	2.4	3
Complaints clear up	32	43
waiting times		
Inpatient	79	78
Outpatient	61	75

Stourbridge · **Dudley Group of Hospitals**

Wordsley Hospital, Stourbridge
West Midlands, DY8 5QX
Phone: 01384 456 111

Trust: Dudley Group of Hospitals NHS
Trust (The)

The Dudley Group of hospitals comprising Russells Hall, Wordsley, Corbett and Guest Hospitals meet government targets on coronary heart disease in two key areas. They provide over 500 cardiac catheterisations each year and heart attack patients receive thrombolysis with an average of 30 minutes of entering the hospital. Waiting times in A&E are longer than average, with 50 per cent of patients dealt with within the recommended time of 4 hours. However, inpatient and outpatient waiting times better than average.

Number of beds		830
⊕ ⊕ ⊕ ⊗ ☎ ◉		
		regional
Overall mortality	103	103
Vacancy rates	2	3
Doctors per 100 beds	33	37
Nurses per 100 beds	103	124
Cancelled operations	2	3
Complaints	2.8	3
Complaints clear up	30	43
waiting times		
Inpatient	84	78
Outpatient	81	75

Sutton Coldfield · **Good Hope District General**

Rectory Road, Sutton Coldfield
West Midlands, B75 7RR
Phone: 0121 378 2211

Trust: Good Hope Hospital NHS Trust

Good Hope Hospital provides a wide range of services to North Birmingham and South Staffordshire. It received two NHS Beacon awards for cancer services and waiting times. Despite having a dedicated stroke unit, the death rate following emergency stroke admission is high. However, overall the mortality rate for the hospital is in line with expectations. For heart patients, the hospital has a Coronary Care Unit and performs coronary angiography although it does not yet meet the government target of performing at least 500 catheterisations per year.

Number of beds		566
⊕ ⊕ ⊕ ⊗ ☎ ◉		
		regional
Overall mortality	105	103
Vacancy rates	2	3
Doctors per 100 beds	32	28
Nurses per 100 beds	117	111
Cancelled operations	2	3
Complaints	2.9	3
Complaints clear up	22	43
waiting times		
Inpatient	75	78
Outpatient	87	75

Telford · **Princess Royal Hospital**

Apley Castle, Telford
Shropshire, TF1 6TF
Phone: 01952 641 222

Trust: Princess Royal Hospital NHS
Trust

The Princess Royal Hospital plans to upgrade its A&E department with a £600,000 grant from the government's modernisation programme. Paediatric surgery is performed and the A&E department has separate child treatment and waiting areas. The hospital has a lower than average overall mortality rate and ensures that all patients in A&E are dealt with within 4 hours. Heart attack patients do not receive thrombolysis within the target average of 30 minutes of arrival.

Number of beds		330
➊ ⊕ ⚕ ✖ ☎ ☻		
		regional
Overall mortality	90	103
Vacancy rates	5	3
Doctors per 100 beds	30	35
Nurses per 100 beds	100	112
Cancelled operations	-	3
Complaints	3.1	3
Complaints clear up	41	43
waiting times		
Inpatient	88	78
Outpatient	61	75

Walsall · **Manor Hospital**

Walsall, WS2 9PS
Phone: 01922 721172

Trust: Walsall Hospitals NHS Trust

Manor Hospital, Walsall, provides a full range of acute services including A&E, outpatients and intensive care to Walsall, Wolverhampton and Sutton Coldfield. The hospital achieves a key Government standard for coronary angiography, and heart attack patients are given thrombolytic drugs within the target 30 minutes of arrival. Waiting times are better than average. However, the overall mortality rate at the hospital is higher than would be expected.

Number of beds		776
➊ ⊕ ⚕ ✖ ☎ ☻		
		regional
Overall mortality	120	103
Vacancy rates	4	3
Doctors per 100 beds	25	28
Nurses per 100 beds	97	111
Cancelled operations	1	3
Complaints	2.6	3
Complaints clear up	98	43
waiting times		
Inpatient	90	78
Outpatient	76	75

Warwick · **Warwick Hospital**

Lakin Road, Warwick
Warwickshire, CV34 5BW
Phone: 01926 495 321

Trust: South Warwickshire General
Hospitals NHS Trust

Warwick Hospital recently opened a
£3.6 m medical unit and is currently
nearing the completion of a new A&E
department which has separate child
waiting and treatment areas. It has
low cancellation rates for operations.
Death rates are broadly in line with
similar hospitals. Thrombolysis is
administered to heart attack patients
within 30 minutes of arrival.

Number of beds		418
✛ ⊕ ♺ ✗ ☎		
		regional
Overall mortality	108	103
Vacancy rates	0	3
Doctors per 100 beds	35	35
Nurses per 100 beds	103	112
Cancelled operations	0.3	3
Complaints	-	3
Complaints clear up	69	43
waiting times		
Inpatient	80	78
Outpatient	72	75

West Bromwich · **Sandwell General Hospital**

Lyndon, West Bromwich
West Midlands, B71 4HU
Phone: 0121 553 1831

Trust: Sandwell Healthcare NHS Trust

Sandwell General Hospital has higher
than average death rates, particularly
for emergency stroke admissions. It
has a CCU and carries out the
recommended 500 coronary
angiography catheterisations each
year. It provides heart attack patients
with thrombolysis within the target
average of 30 minutes of arrival. Eight
out of 10 patients awaiting treatment
in A&E are currently dealt with within
4 hours and there are multidisciplinary
teams for treating lung, breast,
colorectal and stomach cancers.

Number of beds		557
✛ ⊕ ♺ ✗ ☎ ◑		
		regional
Overall mortality	118	103
Vacancy rates	0	3
Doctors per 100 beds	29	37
Nurses per 100 beds	111	124
Cancelled operations	1	3
Complaints	3.2	3
Complaints clear up	52	43
waiting times		
Inpatient	90	78
Outpatient	71	75

Wolverhampton · **New Cross Hospital**

Wednesfield Road, Wolverhampton
West Midlands, WV10 0QP
Phone: 01902 307 999

Trust: Royal Wolverhampton Hospitals
Trust

During 2001, New Cross Hospital invested £10 million in patient services, improving areas such as coronary heart disease and renal care. The hospital treats breast, lung, stomach and colorectal cancers and multidisciplinary teams are in place for each. Government guidelines on performing CT scans on suspected stroke patients within 48 hours of admission are met, while on average, thrombolysis is given to heart attack patients in less than the target 30 minutes from arrival. Death rates for the hospital are average or low.

Number of beds		853
✚ ✚ ✪ ✖ 🚑		
		regional
Overall mortality	101	103
Vacancy rates	7	3
Doctors per 100 beds	36	37
Nurses per 100 beds	128	124
Cancelled operations	0.4	3
Complaints	2.9	3
Complaints clear up	20	43
waiting times		
Inpatient	82	78
Outpatient	76	75

Worcester · **Worcester Royal Infirmary**

Ronkswood Branch, Worcester
Worcestershire, WR5 1HN
Phone: 01905 763333

Trust: Worcestershire Acute Hospitals
NHS Trust

Worcestershire Royal Infirmary has recently opened a new medical assessment unit providing rapid access for emergency stroke patients. The hospital's death rate for emergency operations for stroke patients is high. The A&E department deals with most cases within 4 hours. Heart attack patients are given thrombolytic drugs within 30 minutes. However, the Government target to provide 500 cardiac catheterisations per year is not yet met by the hospital's angiography service nor are stroke patients given a CT scan within 48 hours.

Number of beds		513
✚ ✪ ✖ 🚑 ◉		
		regional
Overall mortality	105	103
Vacancy rates	3	3
Doctors per 100 beds	38	37
Nurses per 100 beds	125	124
Cancelled operations	1	3
Complaints	3	3
Complaints clear up	40	43
waiting times		
Inpatient	71	78
Outpatient	77	75

Birmingham · **Birmingham Nuffield Hospital**

22 Somerset Road, Edgbaston
Birmingham, B15 2QQ
Phone: 0121 4562000

In addition to the surgical and medical procedures offered, Birmingham Nuffield Hospital also incorporates Edgbaston Health Centre, providing inpatient and outpatient physiotherapy services and hydrotherapy pools.

Nuffield Hospitals

Insurers: Bupa*, Norwich*, Standard Life, Royal Sun Alliance*, WPA

price guide	£
Hip replacement	7940-9720
Cataract removal	1999-2500

Number of beds	57
ALS staff	0
heart services	–
Cancer services	

Birmingham · **BMI The Priory Hospital**

Priory Rd, Edgbaston,
Birmingham, B5 7UG
Phone: 0121 4402323

The Priory Hospital is the only private hospital in the West Midlands with an Intensive Therapy Unit (ITU). The hospital provides most major specialities and has a fertility clinic.

General Healthcare Group

Insurers: Bupa*, PPP*, Norwich, Standard Life, Royal Sun Alliance, WPA

price guide	£
Hip replacement	7100-8500
Cataract removal	1985-2110

Number of beds	114
ALS staff	0
heart services	
Cancer services	

Droitwich Spa · **BMI Droitwich Spa Hospital**

St Andrew's Road, Droitwich Spa
Worcestershire, WR9 8DN
Phone: 01905 794 793

Droitwich Spa Hospital takes advantage of its situation by a natural spa, operating a unique brine baths facility for treating sports injuries, back pain and joint problems. The hospital also offers a wide range of more traditional services including a fertility clinic, breast screening and keyhole surgery.

General Healthcare Group Ltd

Insurers: Bupa, PPP, Norwich, Royal Sun Alliance, WPA

price guide	£
Hip replacement	6500-7500
Cataract removal	2000-2500

Number of beds	43
ALS staff	2
heart services	
Cancer services	

Halesowen · **West Midlands Hospital**

Colman Hill, Halesowen
West Midlands, B63 2AH
Phone: 01384 560 123

West Midlands Hospital offers a range
of treatments from general surgery to
cosmetic surgery. The hospital has a
High Dependency Unit, but the
nearest intensive care facility is at the
Russells Hall NHS hospital.

Capio Healthcare UK

Insurers: Bupa*, PPP*, Norwich,
Standard Life, Royal Sun Alliance, WPA

price guide	£
Hip replacement	7128
Cataract removal	1897

Number of beds	14
ALS staff	1
heart services	-
Cancer services	

Hereford · **Wye Valley Nuffield Hospital**

Venns Lane, Hereford
Herefordshire, HR1 1DF
Phone: 01432 355131

The Wye Valley Nuffield Hospital
recently extended outpatient facilities
to include new suites for
physiotherapy, ophthalmology, ENT
and Health screening. The radiology
department has also been upgraded.

Nuffield Nursing Homes Trust

Insurers: Bupa, PPP, Norwich, Standard Life,
Royal Sun Alliance, WPA

price guide	£
Hip replacement	7300-8000
Cataract removal	1699-1850

Number of beds	23
ALS staff	1
heart services	-
Cancer services	-

Leamington Spa · **Warwickshire Nuffield Hospital**

The Chase, Leamington Spa,
Warwickshire, CV32 6RW
Phone: 01926 427971

The Warwickshire Nuffield Hospital
recently completed an £8m
refurbishment adding a third
operating theatre, 11 new consulting
rooms and improved diagnostic
facilities including a static MRI scanner.

Nuffield Hospitals

Insurers: Bupa*, PPP*, Norwich*,
Standard Life*, Royal Sun Alliance*, WPA

price guide	£
Hip replacement	6500-7500
Cataract removal	2100-2600

Number of beds	43
ALS staff	2
heart services	-
Cancer services	

Newcastle · **North Staffordshire Nuffield Hospital**

Clayton Rd, Newcastle
Staffordshire, ST5 4DB
Phone: 01782 625431

The North Staffordshire Nuffield Hospital is located 1.5 miles south of Newcastle-under-Lyme town centre. Major surgery is undertaken in all specialities and fixed cost surgery is available.

Nuffield Nursing Homes Trust

Insurers: Bupa*, PPP*, Norwich*, Standard Life*, Royal Sun Alliance*, WPA

price guide	£
Hip replacement	7655-9255
Cataract removal	1950-2050

Number of beds	32
ALS staff	1
heart services	-
Cancer services	

Nuneaton · **BMI Nuneaton Private Hospital**

132 Coventry Road, Nuneaton
Warwickshire, CV10 7AD
Phone: 02476 357500

Nuneaton hospital provides a range of services to its patients including surgery for breast and colorectal cancer. The hospital has a bone density scanning facility.

General Healthcare Group

Insurers: Bupa*, PPP*, Norwich*, Standard Life*, Royal Sun Alliance*, WPA*

price guide	£
Hip replacement	6900-8000
Cataract removal	2100-2500

Number of beds	24
ALS staff	1
heart services	-
Cancer services	-

Shrewsbury · **Shropshire Nuffield Hospital**

Longden Rd, Shrewsbury
Shropshire, SY3 9DP
Phone: 01743 282500

The purpose-built Shropshire Nuffield has diagnostic services which include a radiology department with a colour doppler ultrasound machine, mammography and a mobile MRI scanner that visits regularly.

Nuffield Hospitals

Insurers: Bupa*, PPP*, Norwich*, Standard Life*, Royal Sun Alliance*, WPA

price guide	£
Hip replacement	8140-8640
Cataract removal	2100-2600

Number of beds	34
ALS staff	1
heart services	-
Cancer services	

Solihull · **BUPA Parkway Hospital**

1 Damson Parkway, Solihull
West Midlands, B91 2PP
Phone: 0121 704 1451

The hospital provides a general medical service and paramedical support services on site. A multidisciplinary team approach to breast care and back pain has recently been launched.

BUPA Hospitals

Insurers: Bupa, PPP, Norwich, Standard Life, Royal Sun Alliance, WPA

price guide	£
Hip replacement	8522
Cataract removal	1850-2690

Number of beds	51
ALS staff	2
heart services	-
Cancer services	

Stafford · **Rowley Hall Hospital**

Rowley Park, Stafford
Staffordshire, ST17 9DQ
Phone: 01785 223203
Fax: 01785 249532

Rowley Hall hospital offers a range of medical and surgical services including cataract removal and hip replacement. The hospital also has access to a mobile diagnostic imaging service.

Community Hospitals Group

Insurers: Bupa*, PPP*, Norwich*, Standard Life*, Royal Sun Alliance*, WPA*

price guide	£
Hip replacement	6575
Cataract removal	1975

Number of beds	20
ALS staff	0
heart services	-
Cancer services	-

Sutton Coldfield · **BUPA Hospital Little Aston**

Little Aston Hall Drive, Sutton Coldfield,
West Midlands, B74 3UP
Phone: 0121 353 2444

This purpose-built hospital offers a comprehensive range of medical and surgical services both for insured patients and those wishing to pay for their own care.

BUPA Hospitals

Insurers: Bupa, PPP, Norwich, Standard Life, Royal Sun Alliance, WPA

price guide	£
Hip replacement	7360-7360
Cataract removal	2546-2546

Number of beds	69
ALS staff	2
heart services	-
Cancer services	

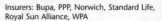

Tettenhall · **Wolverhampton Nuffield Hospital**

Wood Rd, Tettenhall
Wolverhampton, WV6 8LE
Phone: 01902 754177

In 1999 Wolverhampton Nuffield
treated 150 NHS patients sent from
Royal Wolverhampton Hospitals NHS
Trust in an attempt to wating times for
treatment.

Nuffield Nursing Homes Trust

Insurers: Bupa*, PPP*, Norwich*,
Standard Life*, Royal Sun Alliance*, WPA

price guide	£
Hip replacement	8100-9200
Cataract removal	1999-2274

Number of beds	41
ALS staff	2
heart services	–
Cancer services	

Worcester · **BUPA South Bank Hospital**

139 Bath Road
Worcester, WR5 3YB
Phone: 01905 350003

In addition to the usual medical and
surgical specialties, the hospital offers
alternative treatments including
acupuncture and aromatherapy. Other
services include clinics for back pain,
impotence and incontinence.

BUPA Hospitals

Insurers: Bupa, PPP, Norwich, Standard Life,
Royal Sun Alliance, WPA

price guide	£
Hip replacement	7829-9929
Cataract removal	2490-2677

Number of beds	41
ALS staff	2
heart services	–
Cancer services	

Scotland

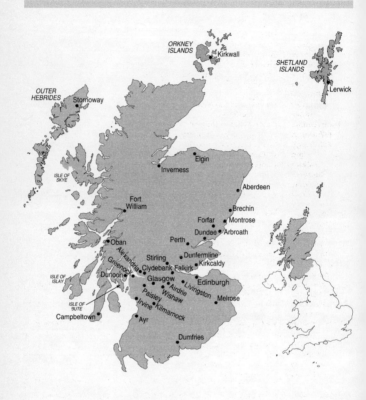

ORKNEY
ISLANDS
Kirkwall

SHETLAND
ISLANDS

Lerwick

OUTER
HEBRIDES
Stornoway

ISLE OF
SKYE

Elgin
Inverness

Aberdeen

Fort
William

Brechin

Forfar   Montrose

Dundee Arbroath

Perth

Oban

Dunfermline

Stirling

Alexandria

Clydebank Falkirk

Kirkcaldy

Greenock

Dunoon

ISLE OF
ISLAY

Glasgow

Edinburgh

Airdrie

Livingston

Paisley

Wishaw

Melrose

ISLE OF
BUTE

Irvine

Kilmarnock

Campbeltown

Ayr

Dumfries

NHS

Aberdeen	Aberdeen Royal Infirmary
Aberdeen	Woodend Hospital
Airdrie	Monklands Hospital
Alexandria	Vale of Leven District General Hospital
Ayr	Ayr Hospital
Brechin	Stracathro Hospital
Dumfries	Dumfries and Galloway Royal Infirmary
Dundee	Ninewells Hospital
Dunfermline	Queen Margaret Hospital
Edinburgh	Royal Infirmary of Edinburgh
Edinburgh	Western General Hospital
Elgin	Dr Gray's Hospital
Falkirk	Falkirk Royal Infirmary
Glasgow	Gartnavel General Hospital
Glasgow	Glasgow Royal Infirmary
Glasgow	Hairmyres Hospital
Glasgow	Southern General Hospital
Glasgow	Stobhill Hospital
Glasgow	Victoria Infirmary
Glasgow	Western Infirmary
Greenock	Inverclyde Royal Hospital
Inverness	Raigmore Hospital
Kilmarnock	Crosshouse Hospital
Kirkcaldy	Victoria Hospital
Kirkwall	Balfour Hospital
Lerwick	Gilbert Bain Hospital
Livingston	St John's Hospital at Howden
Melrose	Borders General Hospital
Oban	Lorn and Islands District General Hospital
Paisley	Royal Alexandra Hospital
Perth	Perth Royal Infirmary
Stirling	Stirling Royal Infirmary
Stornoway	Western Isles Hospital
Wishaw	Wishaw Hospital

Private

Aberdeen	Albyn Hospital
Ayr	Abbey Carrick Glen Hospital
Clydebank	HCI International Medical Centre
Dundee	Fernbrae Hospital
Edinburgh	BUPA Murrayfield Hospital
Glasgow	Glasgow Nuffield Hospital
Glasgow	BMI Ross Hall Hospital
Stirling	Abbey Kings Park Hospital

Aberdeen · **Aberdeen Royal Infirmary**

Foresthill
Aberdeen, AB25 2ZN
Phone: 01224 681818

Trust: Grampian University Hospitals
   NHS Trust

Aberdeen Royal Infirmary is a large district hospital providing services to Aberdeen and the surrounding Grampian area. The hospital has one of the lowest overall mortality rates in Scotland and is well below average. The hospital is equipped with an A&E department and ITU and has MRI and CT scanning facilities. Coronary angiography is performed at the hospital; however, not at the recommended rate of 500 cardiac catheterisations per year.

Number of beds		1200
Overall mortality	82	low

		national
Doctors per 100 beds	43	37
Nurses per 100 beds	125	130
Complaints	5	5
Complaints clear up	46	60

waiting times		
Inpatient	91	93
Outpatient	65	74

Aberdeen · **Woodend Hospital**

Eday Road
Aberdeen, AB15 6XS
Phone: 01224 663 131

Trust: Grampian University Hospitals
   NHS Trust

Woodend Hospital is a medium-sized facility forming part of Grampian University Hospitals NHS Trust. The Trust has higher than average staffing levels for doctors but figures are slightly lower than average for nurses. However, it has MRI facilities and a CT scanner available 24 hours a day. The hospital does not have an A&E unit; this service is provided nearby at Aberdeen Royal Infirmary.

Number of beds		422
Overall mortality	-	-

		national
Doctors per 100 beds	43	37
Nurses per 100 beds	125	130
Complaints	5	5
Complaints clear up	46	60

waiting times		
Inpatient	91	93
Outpatient	65	74

Airdrie · **Monklands Hospital**

Monkscourt Avenue, Airdrie
Lanarkshire, ML6 0JS
Phone: 01236 748748

Trust: Lanarkshire Acute Hospitals NHS
Trust

Monklands Hospital, part of the
Lanarkshire Acute Hospitals NHS Trust,
is a district general hospital that
provides services for communicable
diseases, renal medicine, ENT and oral
surgery to the population of
Lanarkshire. The Trust has an average
ratio of doctors and nurses to beds.
However, its outpatient waiting times
are slightly longer than average.
Monklands has an Intensive Care Unit
and CT and X-ray facilities are
available 24 hours a day.

Number of beds		498
✚ ⚕ ✖ ☎		
Overall mortality	102	average

		national
Doctors per 100 beds	38	37
Nurses per 100 beds	137	130
Complaints	4	5
Complaints clear up	80	60

waiting times		
Inpatient	95	93
Outpatient	69	74

Alexandria · **Vale of Leven District General Hospital**

Main Street, Alexandria
Dunbartonshire, G83 0UA
Phone: 01389 754121

Trust: Argyll & Clyde Acute Hospitals
NHS Trust

Vale of Leven District General Hospital
is part of the Argyll & Clyde Acute
Hospitals NHS Trust. Although the
Trust has lower than average staffing
levels, A&E services are efficient, with
the majority of patients being treated
within the recommended time of 2.5
hours. The hospital does not have a
dedicated stroke unit and wards are
not all single-sex.

Number of beds		276
✚ ⚕ ✖		
Overall mortality	103	average

		national
Doctors per 100 beds	28	37
Nurses per 100 beds	100	130
Complaints	4	5
Complaints clear up	70	60

waiting times		
Inpatient	91	93
Outpatient	78	74

Ayr · **Ayr Hospital**

Dallmellington Road, Ayr
Ayrshire, KA6 6DX
Phone: 01292 610555

Trust: Ayrshire and Arran Acute
Hospitals NHS Trust

The Ayr Hospital was opened 10 years ago and is part of the Ayrshire and Arran Acute Hospitals NHS Trust. The overall death rate for the hospital is higher than average. Services for heart patients include coronary angiography and the hospital performs the recommended 500 cardiac catheterisations a year. Patients can expect average waiting times in A&E across the Trust.

Number of beds		348
➊ ➌ ➍ ➎ ➏ ➐		
Overall mortality	112	high

		national
Doctors per 100 beds	29	37
Nurses per 100 beds	122	130
Complaints	4	5
Complaints clear up	70	60

waiting times		
Inpatient	93	93
Outpatient	72	74

Brechin · **Stracathro Hospital**

Brechin
Angus, DD9 7QA
Phone: 01356 647291

Trust: Tayside University Hospitals NHS
Trust

Stracathro Hospital, part of the Tayside University Hospitals NHS Trust, is based in Brechin. The Trust is well staffed with above average doctors and nurses. It has an efficient complaint clearance procedure. The hospital meets Government guidelines by providing CT scans to emergency stroke patients within 48 hours of being admitted and complies with the recommendations on single-sex wards.

Number of beds		148
➊ ➋ ➌		
Overall mortality	107	average

		national
Doctors per 100 beds	54	37
Nurses per 100 beds	164	130
Complaints	6	5
Complaints clear up	64	60

waiting times		
Inpatient	91	93
Outpatient	72	74

Dumfries · **Dumfries and Galloway Royal Infirmary**

Bankend Road
Dumfries, DG1 4AP
Phone: 01387 246246

Trust: Dumfries & Galloway Acute &
Maternity Hospitals NHS Trust

The Dumfries and Galloway Royal is part of the Dumfries and Galloway Acute and Maternity Trust and provides a wide range of acute services and outreach clinics. A&E services are run efficiently within the Trust, with both walking wounded and trolley waits dealt with more quickly than the national average. Staffing levels at the Trust are above average, with a particularly high number of nurses per 100 beds.

Number of beds		363
➕ ⊕ ⚕ ✖ 🚑		
Overall mortality	96	average

		national
Doctors per 100 beds	38	37
Nurses per 100 beds	148	130
Complaints	6	5
Complaints clear up	67	60

waiting times		
Inpatient	97	93
Outpatient	79	74

Dundee · **Ninewells Hospital**

Dundee, DD4 9NN
Phone: 01382 660111

Trust: Tayside University Hospitals NHS
Trust

The Ninewells Hospital, Dundee, is a teaching hospital that is part of the University of Dundee. The Tayside University Hospitals NHS Trust, which operates the hospital, has a higher ratio of doctors and nurses to beds than most Scottish NHS Trusts. The overall mortality rate at Ninewells is average. Complaints are slightly above average, as is the time taken to deal with them. A high percentage of A&E walking wounded are dealt with within 2.5 hours.

Number of beds		823
➕ ⚕ ⊕ ✖ 🚑 ◉		
Overall mortality	98	average

		national
Doctors per 100 beds	54	37
Nurses per 100 beds	164	130
Complaints	6	5
Complaints clear up	64	60

waiting times		
Inpatient	91	93
Outpatient	72	74

Dunfermline · **Queen Margaret Hospital**

Whitefield Road, Dunfermline
Fife, KY12 0SU
Phone: 01383 623623

Trust: Fife Acute Hospitals NHS Trust

Queen Margaret's Hospital, part of the Fife Acute Hospitals NHS Trust, provides the trauma service for the whole of Fife, as well as urology, ophthalmology and dermatology services. The Trust has a below average number of doctors per 100 beds and an above average mortality rate. It provides a fast A&E service to walking wounded patients, treating or discharging them within the recommended 2.5 hours. However, A&E trolley cases are not always seen within 2 hours.

Number of beds		356
➕ 🔄 ✖️ 🔂		
Overall mortality	130	high

		national
Doctors per 100 beds	33	37
Nurses per 100 beds	136	130
Complaints	4	5
Complaints clear up	61	60

waiting times		
Inpatient	86	93
Outpatient	65	74

Edinburgh · **Royal Infirmary of Edinburgh**

Lauriston Place
Edinburgh, EH3 9YW
Phone: 0131 5361000

Trust: Lothian University Hospitals NHS Trust

The Royal Infirmary of Edinburgh, part of the Lothian University Hospitals NHS Trust, is a major teaching hospital that provides a range of general and specialist services for the population of Edinburgh. The trust is well staffed and complaints are cleared quickly. The overall mortality rate is average. Waiting times in A&E for both walking wounded and trolley cases are the longest in the country.

Number of beds		737
➕ 🔄 ✖️ 🔂 🔵		
Overall mortality	97	average

		national
Doctors per 100 beds	50	37
Nurses per 100 beds	143	130
Complaints	6	5
Complaints clear up	63	60

waiting times		
Inpatient	93	93
Outpatient	75	74

Edinburgh · **Western General Hospital**

Crewe Road
Edinburgh, EH3 9EF
Phone: 0131 5371000

Trust: Lothian University Hospitals NHS Trust

Western General Hospital, part of the Lothian University Hospitals NHS Trust, does not offer full A&E facilities but has a minor injuries unit. The Trust's staffing levels are above average for both doctors and nurses and the hospital has one of the lowest mortality rates in the country. There is a dedicated stroke unit. There are no separate waiting and treatment areas for children in A&E. Western General provides coronary angiographies and performs the recommended number of 500 catheterisations per year.

Number of beds		571
Overall mortality	77	low

		national
Doctors per 100 beds	50	37
Nurses per 100 beds	143	130
Complaints	6	5
Complaints clear up	63	60

waiting times		
Inpatient	93	93
Outpatient	75	74

Elgin · **Dr Gray's Hospital**

Elgin, IV30 1SN
Phone: 01343 543 131

Trust: Grampian University Hospitals NHS Trust

Dr Gray's Hospital is a small acute hospital based in Elgin and part of the Grampian University Hospitals NHS Trust. The Trust has more doctors per bed than average but fewer nurses. Across the Trust, those seeking inpatient appointments are seen quickly but outpatient waiting times are slightly longer than average. A&E services are efficient, with the majority of walking wounded being treated or discharged within 2.5 hours.

Number of beds		197
Overall mortality	103	average

		national
Doctors per 100 beds	43	37
Nurses per 100 beds	125	130
Complaints	5	5
Complaints clear up	46	60

waiting times		
Inpatient	91	93
Outpatient	65	74

Falkirk · **Falkirk Royal Infirmary**

Major's Loan, Falkirk
FK1 5QE
Phone: 01324 624000

Trust: Forth Valley Acute Hospitals NHS Trust

At Falkirk Royal Infirmary death rates are average although waiting times in A&E are longer than average. Beds are available in the day surgery unit for routine minor surgery and by arrangement in the surgical unit for medically compromised patients and more major cases. There is an Intensive Care Unit with 5 beds and a High Dependency Unit with 4 beds. The outpatient department in the hospital has treatment areas with surgeries and offices. Within the same unit are orthodontics, community dentistry and an endoscopy suite.

Number of beds		412
➊ ⚕ ✖ ⊕ ◉		
Overall mortality	98	average

		national
Doctors per 100 beds	31	37
Nurses per 100 beds	120	130
Complaints	4	5
Complaints clear up	54	60

waiting times		
Inpatient	90	93
Outpatient	68	74

Glasgow · **Gartnavel General Hospital**

1053 Great Western Road
Glasgow, G12 0NY
Phone: 0141 211 3000

Trust: North Glasgow University Hospitals NHS

Gartnavel General Hospital is managed with the Western Infirmary and the two operate effectively as one hospital managed by the North Glasgow University Hospitals NHS Trust. It provides a broad range of medical and surgical sub-specialties, supported by an 8-theatre inpatient operating department. The Trust has an above average number of doctors, but fewer than average nurses. The overall mortality rate is lower than average. The hospital has no A&E department.

Number of beds		465
⚕ ✖ ⊕		
Overall mortality	94	low

		national
Doctors per 100 beds	47	37
Nurses per 100 beds	117	130
Complaints	4	5
Complaints clear up	40	60

waiting times		
Inpatient	94	93
Outpatient	73	74

Glasgow · **Glasgow Royal Infirmary**

84 Castle Street
Glasgow, G4 0SF
Phone: 0141 211 4000

Trust: North Glasgow University
Hospitals NHS

Glasgow Royal Infirmary, part of the North Glasgow University Hospitals NHS Trust, provides a broad range of regional and national acute clinical services. The mortality rate for the hospital is average. The number of inpatients seen within the recommended 6-month waiting time is just above average. There is an A&E department.

Number of beds		765
➕ ⚕ ✖ ☎ ◉		
Overall mortality	97	average

		national
Doctors per 100 beds	47	37
Nurses per 100 beds	117	130
Complaints	4	5
Complaints clear up	40	60

waiting times		
Inpatient	94	93
Outpatient	73	74

Glasgow · **Hairmyres Hospital**

Eaglesham Road, East Kilbride
Glasgow, G75 8RG
Phone: 01355 220292

Trust: Lanarkshire Acute Hospitals NHS
Trust

Hairmyres Hospital is based in East Kilbride and is part of Lanarkshire Acute Hospitals NHS Trust. The Trust has average staffing levels but A&E times for trolley waits and walking wounded are longer than average. Cardiology services have improved following construction of a new £67.5 m facility. There is a coronary angiography service that performs the recommended number of 500 cardiac catheterisations per year. CT scans are carried out within the recommended 48 hours. Children are referred elsewhere for surgery.

Number of beds		447
➕ ⚕ ☎		
Overall mortality	101	average

		national
Doctors per 100 beds	38	37
Nurses per 100 beds	137	130
Complaints	4	5
Complaints clear up	80	60

waiting times		
Inpatient	95	93
Outpatient	69	74

Glasgow · **Southern General Hospital**

1345 Govan Road
Glasgow, G51 4TF
Phone: 0141 201 1100

Trust: South Glasgow University
Hospitals NHS Trust

Southern General Hospital provides a range of medical and surgical services including urology, dermatology and ophthalmology, to the south west of Glasgow.

The hospital forms part of the South Glasgow University Hospitals NHS Trust, which has a notably low rate of nurses per bed. The number of outpatients seen within 13 weeks is lower than average, as is the number of A&E patients seen within target times for both the walking wounded and trolley cases. The hospital death rate is average.

Number of beds		576
Overall mortality	100	average

		national
Doctors per 100 beds	34	37
Nurses per 100 beds	111	130
Complaints	5	5
Complaints clear up	50	60

waiting times		
Inpatient	92	93
Outpatient	65	74

Glasgow · **Stobhill Hospital**

Balornock Road
Glasgow, G21 3UW
Phone: 0141 201 3000

Trust: North Glasgow University
Hospitals NHS

Stobhill Hospital, part of the North Glasgow University Hospitals NHS Trust, provides a range of acute medical and surgical services to over 200,000 people living in North Glasgow. The Trust has more doctors per 100 beds than average, but fewer than average numbers of nurses. The death rate for the hospital is average. The number of emergency patients dealt with in A&E within target times is below average for both walking wounded patients and trolley cases. The hospital has a CT scanner but it is not operational 24 hours a day.

Number of beds		476
Overall mortality	97	average

		national
Doctors per 100 beds	47	37
Nurses per 100 beds	117	130
Complaints	4	5
Complaints clear up	40	60

waiting times		
Inpatient	94	93
Outpatient	73	74

Glasgow · **Victoria Infirmary**

Langside
Glasgow, G42 9TT
Phone: 0141 201 6000

Trust: South Glasgow University
 Hospitals NHS Trust

Victoria Infirmary, part of the South Glasgow University Hospitals NHS Trust, provides a wide range of medical and surgical services. The Trust has low staffing levels compared to other Trusts and the hospital has a higher than average death rate. But A&E deals with trolley cases and walking wounded quicker than average. The hospital has a CT scanner but cannot guarantee that a suspected stroke patient will receive a CT scan within 48 hours.

Number of beds		485
➕ ❖ ⒞⒯		
Overall mortality	115	high

		national
Doctors per 100 beds	34	37
Nurses per 100 beds	111	130
Complaints	5	5
Complaints clear up	50	60

waiting times		
Inpatient	92	93
Outpatient	65	74

Glasgow · **Western Infirmary**

Dumbarton Road
Glasgow, G11 6NT
Phone: 0141 211 2000

Trust: North Glasgow University
 Hospitals NHS

The Western Infirmary, which operates as one hospital with the Gartnavel, houses most of the acute emergency services for the west of Glasgow. The North Glasgow University Hospitals NHS Trust has higher than average staffing levels for doctors but fewer nurses than average. Inpatient and outpatient waiting times are average, but A&E waiting times are longer than average. The hospital does perform coronary angiography but does not yet meet the recommended 500 cardiac catheterisations per year.

Number of beds		493
➕ ❖ ❌ ⒞⒯ ◉		
Overall mortality	94	average

		national
Doctors per 100 beds	47	37
Nurses per 100 beds	117	130
Complaints	4	5
Complaints clear up	40	60

waiting times		
Inpatient	94	93
Outpatient	73	74

Greenock · **Inverclyde Royal Hospital**

**Larkfield Road, Greenock
Renfrewshire, PA16 0XN
Phone: 01475 633777**

**Trust: Argyll & Clyde Acute Hospitals
NHS Trust**

The hospital is run by Argyll & Clyde Acute Hospitals Trust, which is also responsible for the Vale of Leven District General Hospital. Despite low staffing levels, the Trust's A&E waiting times compare favourably to other hospitals and the overall mortality rate is lower than other hospitals. The coronary angiography service does not yet carry out the recommended number of 500 cardiac catheterisations per year. Wards are single-sex. The hospital provides round-the-clock access to a paediatrician but there is no paediatric ITU.

Number of beds		386
✚ ⊕ ♫ ✖ ⚙		
Overall mortality	99	average

		national
Doctors per 100 beds	28	37
Nurses per 100 beds	100	130
Complaints	4	5
Complaints clear up	70	60

waiting times		
Inpatient	91	93
Outpatient	78	74

Inverness · **Raigmore Hospital**

**Old Perth Road
Inverness, IV2 3UJ
Phone: 01463 704000**

**Trust: Highland Acute Hospitals NHS
Trust**

Raigmore Hospital provides acute services to the sparsely populated Highland area of Scotland. Cancer services for the Highland Acute Hospitals NHS Trust are centred at Raigmore. The hospital offers radiotherapy, chemotherapy and scanning facilities. Work has begun on installing a new Linear Accelerator. The hospital is a clinical teaching centre and the University of Aberdeen's second undergraduate medical teaching site. The University of Stirling's department of nursing and midwifery is also located on site.

Number of beds		643
✚ ♫ ✖ ⚙		
Overall mortality	-	-

		national
Doctors per 100 beds	34	37
Nurses per 100 beds	114	130
Complaints	3	5
Complaints clear up	72	60

waiting times		
Inpatient	96	93
Outpatient	81	74

Kilmarnock · **Crosshouse Hospital**

Crosshouse
Kilmarnock, KA2 0BE
Phone: 01563 521133

Trust: Ayrshire and Arran Acute Hospitals NHS Trust

The Crosshouse Hospital is part of the Ayrshire and Arran Acute Hospitals NHS Trust. The number of doctors and nurses per 100 beds in the Trust is below the national average and the mortality rate is higher than average. Both inpatient and outpatient waiting times are average. Patients attending A&E are largely dealt with within target waiting times, particularly trolley waits. The Trust receives a below average number of complaints and aims to deal with any that are received quickly.

Number of beds		540
✚ ⊕ ⚕ ✖ 🆒 ◉		
Overall mortality	120	high

		national
Doctors per 100 beds	29	37
Nurses per 100 beds	122	130
Complaints	4	5
Complaints clear up	70	60

waiting times		
Inpatient	93	93
Outpatient	72	74

Kirkcaldy · **Victoria Hospital**

Hayfield Road, Kirkcaldy
Fife, KY2 5AH
Phone: 01592 643355

Trust: Fife Acute Hospitals NHS Trust

Victoria Hospital, part of Fife Acute Hospitals NHS Trust, provides a wide range of acute services including paediatrics and ear, nose and throat surgery. The Trust has average staffing levels. Inpatient and outpatient waiting times are slightly longer than other hospitals but in the A&E department most "walking wounded" patients are seen within the recommended time of 2.5 hours. The hospital has MRI and CT scanning facilities.

Number of beds		328
✚ ⊕ ⚕ ✖ 🆒 ◉		
Overall mortality	-	-

		national
Doctors per 100 beds	33	37
Nurses per 100 beds	136	130
Complaints	4	5
Complaints clear up	61	60

waiting times		
Inpatient	86	93
Outpatient	65	74

Kirkwall · **Balfour Hospital**

New Scapa Road, Kirkwall
Orkney, KW15 1BH

Trust: Orkney Health Board

Balfour is the only hospital serving the island of Orkney. It is staffed by 17 doctors who provide a range of services including a maternity department and an A&E unit. There is little problem waiting for services in A&E – 100 per cent of both trolley cases and walking wounded are dealt with within target times. For more specialist services patients are transferred to the mainland.

Number of beds		93
✗		
Overall mortality	-	-

		national
Doctors per 100 beds	17	37
Nurses per 100 beds	-	130
Complaints	-	5
Complaints clear up	-	60

waiting times		
Inpatient	96	93
Outpatient	91	74

Lerwick · **Gilbert Bain Hospital**

Lerwick
Shetland, ZE1 0TB
Phone: 01595 743000

Trust: Shetland Health Board

Gilbert Bain Hospital is a small acute facility serving the island of Shetland with a small team of doctors providing emergency cover and other services. Waiting times are shorter than average, particularly outpatient waiting times. In A&E, however, 50 per cent of trolley cases wait longer than the target 2 hours to be dealt with.

Number of beds		68
✚ ✗		
Overall mortality	112	average

		national
Doctors per 100 beds	16	37
Nurses per 100 beds	-	130
Complaints	-	5
Complaints clear up	-	60

waiting times		
Inpatient	99	93
Outpatient	98	74

Livingston · **St John's Hospital at Howden**

Howden Road West, Livingston
West Lothian, EH54 6PP
Phone: 01506 419666

West Lothian Healthcare NHS Trust

St John's Hospital is part of the West Lothian Healthcare NHS Trust. The Trust is well staffed, particularly in the area of nurses, and it has an efficient complaint clearance procedure. Emergency stroke patients will receive a CT scan within 48 hours of being admitted and the hospital has a rehabilitation stroke unit.

Number of beds		560
➊ ➋ ➌ ➍		
Overall mortality	104	average

		national
Doctors per 100 beds	46	37
Nurses per 100 beds	206	130
Complaints	5	5
Complaints clear up	78	60

waiting times		
Inpatient	94	93
Outpatient	74	74

Melrose · **Borders General Hospital**

Melrose
Roxburghshire, TD6 9BS
Phone: 01896 826000

Trust: Borders General Hospital NHS Trust

Borders General Hospital in Melrose provides acute health care services and has inpatient, day case and outpatient facilities for most medical specialties. The hospital has below average death rates. Across the Trust, around half of all A&E trolley cases will be dealt with within 2 hours but a large majority of walking wounded will be seen within 2.5 hours. A higher number of outpatients and inpatients are seen within target waiting times than the national average.

Number of beds		328
➊ ➋ ➌ ➍		
Overall mortality	92	low

		national
Doctors per 100 beds	33	37
Nurses per 100 beds	132	130
Complaints	7	5
Complaints clear up	60	60

waiting times		
Inpatient	97	93
Outpatient	84	74

Oban · **Lorn and Islands District General Hospital**

Glengallon Road, Oban
Argyll, PA34 4HH
Phone: 01631 567500

Trust: Argyll & Clyde Acute Hospitals
NHS Trust

Lorn and the Islands Hospital, part of the Argyll and Clyde Acute Hospitals NHS Trust, is a new general hospital that provides services to the population of North Argyll and the Islands. The Trust has lower than average staffing levels but both inpatient and outpatient waits are average as are the percentage of complaints dealt with within 4 weeks. Stroke patients receive CT scans within the recommended 48 hours. The A&E department can only deal with 2 major traumas at any one time.

Number of beds		132
✪ ✪ ⒸⓉ		
Overall mortality	90	average

		national
Doctors per 100 beds	28	37
Nurses per 100 beds	100	130
Complaints	4	5
Complaints clear up	70	60

waiting times		
Inpatient	91	93
Outpatient	78	74

Paisley · **Royal Alexandra Hospital**

Corsebar Road, Paisley
Renfrewshire, PA2 9PN
Phone: 0141 8879111

Trust: Argyll & Clyde Acute Hospitals
NHS Trust

The Royal Alexandra Hospital, Paisley, part of the Argyll and Clyde Acute Hospitals NHS Trust, is a 600-bed hospital. The number of admitted or transferred patients dealt with in A&E within 2 hours is above average, despite lower than average staffing levels. It also manages to resolve an above average rate of complaints within 20 days. There are separate waiting and treatment areas for children in A&E.

Number of beds		600
✪ ⊕ ⚡ ✪ ⒸⓉ		
Overall mortality	98	average

		national
Doctors per 100 beds	28	37
Nurses per 100 beds	100	130
Complaints	4	5
Complaints clear up	70	60

waiting times		
Inpatient	91	93
Outpatient	78	74

Perth · **Perth Royal Infirmary**

Taymount Terrace
Perth, PH1 1NX
Phone: 01738 623311

Trust: Tayside University Hospitals NHS
Trust

Perth Royal Infirmary forms part of the Tayside University Hospitals NHS Trust. The Trust is well staffed with above average numbers of doctors and nurses. It clears complaints efficiently and has a well-organised A&E department with both emergency and walking wounded patients seen within the respective 2- and 2.5-hour time recommendations. However, inpatient and outpatient waiting times are slightly longer than average.

Number of beds		284
➕ ♿ ✖ 🚊 ◉		
Overall mortality	99	average

		national
Doctors per 100 beds	54	37
Nurses per 100 beds	164	130
Complaints	6	5
Complaints clear up	64	60

waiting times		
Inpatient	91	93
Outpatient	72	74

Stirling · **Stirling Royal Infirmary**

Livilands
Stirling, FK8 2AU
Phone: 01786 434000

Trust: Forth Valley Acute Hospitals NHS
Trust

Stirling Royal Infirmary is a district general hospital providing a range of acute services. It is part of the Forth Valley Acute Hospitals NHS Trust, which has lower than average numbers of doctors and nurses. However, the number of emergency patients dealt with in A&E within 2 hours is above average, as is the amount of "walking wounded" treated and discharged within 2.5 hours. Emergency stroke patients will receive a CT scan within 48 hours of being admitted.

Number of beds		475
➕ ⊕ ♿ ✖ 🚊 ◉		
Overall mortality	94	average

		national
Doctors per 100 beds	31	37
Nurses per 100 beds	120	130
Complaints	4	5
Complaints clear up	54	60

waiting times		
Inpatient	90	93
Outpatient	68	74

Stornoway · **Western Isles Hospital**

Macaulay Road, Stornoway
Isle of Lewis, HS1 2AF
Phone: 01851 704704

Trust: Western Isles Health Board

The Western Isles Hospital opened in 1992 as a new facility replacing the County and Lewis Hospitals in Stornoway. The hospital is managed by Western Isles Health Board. Inpatient and outpatient waiting times are shorter than average and 8 out of 10 trolley cases in A&E are seen within the recommended 2 hours. Almost all walking wounded patients are seen within the recommended 2.5 hours.

Number of beds		212
✚		
Overall mortality	92	average

		national
Doctors per 100 beds	14	37
Nurses per 100 beds	-	130
Complaints	-	5
Complaints clear up	-	60

waiting times		
Inpatient	97	93
Outpatient	92	74

Wishaw · **Wishaw Hospital**

Netherton Street, Wishaw
lanarkshire, ML2 0EF
Phone: 01698 361100

Trust: Lanarkshire Hospitals Acute NHS Trust

Wishaw Hospital has replaced the old Law Hospital and the migration to the new site was completed this year. As a result we do not have any figures for this hospital. The old Law hospital was one of four in Scotland with a higher than average mortality rate. This state-of-the-art new hospital has a low rise design with the main facilities on only three floors. The nursing stations make use of new technology with features such as videophones and pneumatic tubes for sending samples.

Number of beds		-
Overall mortality	-	-

		national
Doctors per 100 beds	-	37
Nurses per 100 beds	-	130
Complaints	-	5
Complaints clear up	-	60

waiting times		
Inpatient	-	93
Outpatient	-	74

Aberdeen · **Albyn Hospital**

21-24 Albyn Place, Aberdeen
AB10 1RW
01244 595993

This hospital draws on consultants from Aberdeen Royal Infirmary and provides a range of medical and surgical services. It has more nursing staff trained in Advance Life Support than most hospitals; however, there is no ITU, only high dependency beds.

Healthcare Scotland

Insurers: BUPA*, PPP*, Norwich Union, Standard Life, Royal Sun Alliance, WPA

price guide	£
Hip replacement	7762
Cataract removal	1960

Number of beds	44
ALS staff	5
heart services	-
Cancer services	

Ayr · **Abbey Carrick Glen Hospital**

Dalmellington Road, Ayr
Ayrshire, KA6 6PG
Phone: 01292 288882

Abbey Carrick Glen hospital has 22 beds and provides a range of medical, surgical and diagnostic services. Complementary therapy is offered at the hospital as is cancer treatment.

Abbey Hospitals Ltd

Insurers: BUPA*, PPP*, Norwich*, Standard Life*, Royal Sun Alliance*, WPA*

price guide	£
Hip replacement	6500
Cataract removal	2350-2500

Number of beds	22
ALS staff	3
heart services	-
Cancer services	

Clydebank · **HCI International Medical Centre**

Beardmore Street, Clydebank
Dunbartonshire, G81 4HX
Phone: 0141 951 5000

HCI International Medical Centre is an independent tertiary care medical complex based in Glasgow. In addition to its clinical services, HCI also offers dialysis, radiotherapy, reconstructive surgery and paediatric surgery.

HCI

Insurers: Norwich, Standard Life, Royal Sun Alliance, WPA

price guide	£
Hip replacement	5950
Cataract removal	2355-2726

Number of beds	52
ALS staff	0
heart services	
Cancer services	

Dundee · **Fernbrae Hospital**

329 Perth Rd
Dundee, DD2 1LJ
Phone: 01382 667203

Fernbrae Hospital provides a large
range of services including "tailor
made" health screening. In February
2000 the hospital was the first in
Scotland to install a computerised and
digital processing system in its X-ray
department.

Healthcare Scotland

Insurers: BUPA*, PPP*, Norwich,
Standard Life, Royal Sun Alliance, WPA

price guide	£
Hip replacement	6000-8000
Cataract removal	1880-2000

Number of beds	26
ALS staff	2
heart services	-
Cancer services	-

Edinburgh · **BUPA Murrayfield Hospital**

122 Corstorphine Road
Edinburgh, EH12 6UD
Phone: 0131 334 0363

Providing the usual medical and
surgical services, the hospital also
offers recompression treatment for
sufferers of carbon monoxide
poisoning to speed toxin removal from
the blood.

BUPA Hospitals

Insurers: BUPA, PPP, Norwich, Standard Life,
Royal Sun Alliance, WPA

price guide	£
Hip replacement	7360-7360
Cataract removal	2380-2380

Number of beds	69
ALS staff	2
heart services	-
Cancer services	

Glasgow · **Glasgow Nuffield Hospital**

Beaconfield Rd,
Glasgow, G12 0PJ
Phone: 0141 334 9441

The Glasgow Nuffield Hospital has a
comprehensive diagnostic service. It's
second site, Nuffield House, is an
outpatient centre offering a fully
integrated service for all musculo-
skeletal problems.

Nuffield Hospitals

Insurers: BUPA*, PPP, Norwich*,
Standard Life*, Royal Sun Alliance*, WPA

price guide	£
Hip replacement	6725-6975
Cataract removal	2345-2800

Number of beds	33
ALS staff	2
heart services	-
Cancer services	

Glasgow · **BMI Ross Hall Hospital**

221 Crookston Rd
Glasgow, G52 3NQ
Phone: 0141 8103151

The hospital is one of the largest private hospitals in Scotland and offers services ranging from general surgery to more specialised procedures such as neurosurgery, vascular surgery and laser surgery.

BMI Healthcare

Insurers: BUPA, PPP, Norwich, Standard Life, Royal Sun Alliance, WPA

price guide	£
Hip replacement	6000
Cataract removal	2295-2750

Number of beds	101
ALS staff	0
heart services	
Cancer services	

Stirling · **Abbey Kings Park Hospital**

Polmaise Road
Stirling, FK7 9PU
Phone: 01786 451669

Abbey Kings Park Hospital provides medical services to Stirling and it's neighbouring regions in Scotland. A wide range of specialities are available, including: dental surgery, ear nose and throat, general medicine, general surgery, gynaecology, ophthalmology and orthopaedics.

Abbey Hospitals Limited

Insurers: BUPA*, PPP*, Norwich*, Standard Life*, Royal Sun Alliance*, WPA*

price guide	£
Hip replacement	6600
Cataract removal	2500-2600

Number of beds	24
ALS staff	4
heart services	-
Cancer services	

Wales

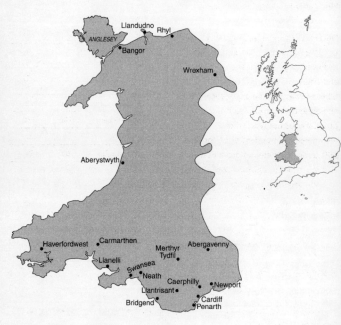

NHS

Abergavenny	Nevil Hall Hospital
Bangor	Ysbyty Gwynedd
Bridgend	Princess of Wales Hospital
Caerphilly	Caerphilly District Miners' Hospital
Cardiff	University Hospital of Wales
Carmarthen	West Wales General Hospital
Ceredigion	Bronglais General Hospital
Haverfordwest	Withybush General Hospital
Llandudno	Llandudno General Hospital
Llanelli	Prince Philip Hospital
Llantrisant	Royal Glamorgan Hospital
Merthyr Tydfil	Prince Charles Hospital
Neath	Neath General Hospital
Newport	Royal Gwent Hospital
Penarth	Llandough Hospital
Rhyl	Glan Clwyd District General Hospital
Swansea	Morriston Hospital
Swansea	Singleton Hospital
Wrexham	Wrexham Maelor Hospital

Private

Bancyfelin	BMI Werndale Hospital
Cardiff	BUPA Hospital Cardiff
Wrexham	BUPA Yale Hospital

Abergavenny · **Nevill Hall Hospital**

Brecon Road, Moumouthshire
Abergavenny, Gwent, NP7 7EG
Phone: 01873 732732

Trust: Gwent Healthcare NHS Trust

Nevill Hall Hospital performs thrombolysis within 30 minutes of a heart attack patient arriving in A&E and suspected stroke victims receive a CT scan within 48 hours. Coronary angiography is performed but the hospital does not reach the recommended standard of performing 500 cardiac catheterisations a year. Children's facilities at the hospital have recently undergone a £273,000 extension, providing more space for clinics and consulting.

Number of beds		423

		national
Doctors per 100 beds	24	24
Nurses per 100 beds	106	110
Complaints	4	6
Complaints clear up	65	71

waiting times		
Inpatient	62	66
Outpatient	44	49

Bangor · **Ysbyty Gwynedd**

Penrhosgarnedd, Bangor
Gwynedd, LL57 2PW
Phone: 01248 384 384

Trust: North West Wales NHS Trust

Ysbyty Gwynedd hospital is part of North West Wales NHS Trust, which has one of the lowest numbers of doctors and nurses per 100 beds in Wales. Waiting times are significantly shorter for the Trust than other trusts in Wales. Emergency stroke patients all receive a CT scan within 48 hours of arriving in the hospital.

Number of beds		512

		national
Doctors per 100 beds	18	24
Nurses per 100 beds	100	110
Complaints	7	6
Complaints clear up	69	71

waiting times		
Inpatient	88	66
Outpatient	55	49

Bridgend · **Princess of Wales Hospital**

Coitoi Road, Bridgend
Glamorgan, CF31 1RQ
Phone: 01656 752 752

Trust: Bro Morgannwg NHS Trust

The Princess of Wales Hospital's surgical material testing laboratory is a leader in its specialisation and is particularly well known for its research into the use of maggots in wound healing. The hospital does not give thrombolytic drugs to heart attack patients within an average 30 minutes of arrival. However, it does carry out CT scans on stroke patients within 48 hours.

Number of beds		529

⊕ ⊕ ✢ ✖ ⏇

		national
Doctors per 100 beds	17	24
Nurses per 100 beds	108	110
Complaints	4	6
Complaints clear up	66	71

waiting times		
Inpatient	75	66
Outpatient	60	49

Caerphilly · **Caerphilly District Miners' Hospital**

St Martin's Road, Caerphilly
Caerphilly County Borough, CF83 2WW
Phone: 02920 801215

Trust: Gwent Healthcare NHS Trust

Although the hospital has a stroke unit, it does not offer all stroke patients a CT scan within 48 hours. In the last year, day case activity at the hospital has risen by 21 per cent which can help to free up beds and bring down waiting lists. An 8-bed medical assessment unit has recently opened at the hospital to handle the increasing number of medical admissions. There is a separate treatment area for children in the A&E although no separate waiting area.

Number of beds		109

⊕ ✖

		national
Doctors per 100 beds	24	24
Nurses per 100 beds	106	110
Complaints	4	6
Complaints clear up	65	71

waiting times		
Inpatient	62	66
Outpatient	44	49

Cardiff · **University Hospital of Wales**

Heath Park
Cardiff, CF14 4XW
Phone: 029 2074 7747

Trust: Cardiff and Vale NHS Trust

The hospital is the main teaching hospital in Wales and is the leading centre for regional referrals. It is part of Cardiff and Vale NHS Trust, which has one of the highest numbers of doctors and nurses per 100 beds in Wales. During 2002, all emergency surgery and children's services in the Trust will transfer to the site. The high complaints rate reflects issues with waiting lists that are caused, in part, by the hospital's status as a tertiary referral centre.

Number of beds		929

		national
Doctors per 100 beds	36	24
Nurses per 100 beds	123	110
Complaints	13	6
Complaints clear up	75	71

waiting times		
Inpatient	51	66
Outpatient	32	49

Carmarthen · **West Wales General Hospital**

Glangwili
Carmarthen, SA31 2AF
Phone: 01267 235151

Trust: Carmarthenshire NHS Trust

There are plans to replace the A&E department at the West Wales hospital in order to reduce the current strain the unit is under. It currently fails to perform thrombolysis within 30 minutes of a heart attack patient arriving. Carmarthenshire NHS Trust, which manages the hospital, has also recently launched a major international recruitment drive, taking on 102 nurses from the Philippines as well as locally qualified nurses.

Number of beds		388

		national
Doctors per 100 beds	27	24
Nurses per 100 beds	106	110
Complaints	5	6
Complaints clear up	56	71

waiting times		
Inpatient	59	66
Outpatient	47	49

Ceredigion · **Bronglais General Hospital**

Aberystwyth, Ceredigion
Dyfed, SY23 1ER
Phone: 01970 623 131

Trust: Ceredigion and Mid Wales NHS Trust

Bronglais General is managed by Ceredigion and Mid Wales NHS Trust, which has one of the highest numbers of nurses per 100 beds in Wales. The hospital does not meet the recommended standard of administering thrombolysis within 30 minutes of a patient arriving at the hospital. However, it is one of relatively few hospitals in Wales to offer all stroke patients a CT scan within 24 hours. The intensive care unit at the hospital has recently been upgraded and a new dialysis unit opened.

Number of beds		181

⊕ ⊕ ⊕ ⊕ ⊗ ⊙

		national
Doctors per 100 beds	26	24
Nurses per 100 beds	123	110
Complaints	4	6
Complaints clear up	90	71

waiting times		
Inpatient	67	66
Outpatient	56	49

Haverfordwest · **Withybush General Hospital**

Fishguard Road, Haverfordwest
Pembrokeshire, SA61 2PZ
Phone: 01437 764 545

Trust: Pembrokeshire and Derwen NHS Trust

The hospital is part of Pembrokeshire and Derwen NHS Trust, which has one of the highest numbers of nurses per 100 beds in Wales. Stroke patients receive a CT scan within 48 hours, and heart attack victims receive thrombolysis within 30 minutes. The hospital performs surgery on children under general anaesthetic but does not meet Royal College of Surgeons guidelines requiring a paediatrician to be on site 24 hours a day. There is a separate treatment area for children in A&E but no separate waiting area.

Number of beds		332

⊕ ⊕ ⊗ ⊙

		national
Doctors per 100 beds	21	24
Nurses per 100 beds	123	110
Complaints	7	6
Complaints clear up	78	71

waiting times		
Inpatient	63	66
Outpatient	58	49

Llandudno · **Llandudno General Hospital**

Llandudno
Gwynedd, LL30 1LB
Phone: 01492 860066

Trust: North West Wales NHS Trust

Llandudno General Hospital is part of North West Wales NHS Trust, which has one of the lowest numbers of doctors and nurses per 100 beds in Wales. Catering services at the site have recently undergone a £400,000 upgrade. There is an A&E department but diagnostic services are relatively limited, with no CT scanner. However, X-ray services are available around the clock. There is a separate treatment area for children in A&E but no separate waiting area.

Number of beds		111

		national
Doctors per 100 beds	18	24
Nurses per 100 beds	100	110
Complaints	7	6
Complaints clear up	69	71

waiting times		
Inpatient	88	66
Outpatient	55	49

Llanelli · **Prince Philip Hospital**

Bryngwynmawr, Dafen
Llanelli, SA14 8QF
Phone: 01554 756 567

Trust: Carmarthenshire NHS Trust

The Prince Phillip Hospital has recently received a £13.7 m investment to cover the cost of services being transferred to the site following the closure of Bryntirion Hospital. A 9-bed orthopaedic ward has been opened at the hospital together with a breast care centre funded largely by public donations. It does not provide thrombolysis to heart attack patients within an average of 30 minutes of arrival. The A&E has a separate waiting area for children, but no separate treatment area.

Number of beds		239

		national
Doctors per 100 beds	27	24
Nurses per 100 beds	106	110
Complaints	5	6
Complaints clear up	56	71

waiting times		
Inpatient	59	66
Outpatient	47	49

Llantrisant · **Royal Glamorgan Hospital**

Ynys Maerdy, Llantrisant
Mid Glamorgan, CF72 8XR
Phone: 01443 443443

Trust: Pontypridd and Rhondda NHS
  Trust

The Royal Glamorgan Hospital was opened by the Prince of Wales in March 1999. The hospital performs thrombolysis within 30 minutes of arrival in A&E. It also meets Royal College of Surgeons guidelines on children's surgery, with a paediatrician on site 24 hours a day. However, the Trust has one of the lowest numbers of nurses per 100 beds in Wales.

Number of beds		503

		national
Doctors per 100 beds	22	24
Nurses per 100 beds	96	110
Complaints	6	6
Complaints clear up	57	71

waiting times		
Inpatient	64	66
Outpatient	50	49

Merthyr Tydfil · **Prince Charles Hospital**

Merthyr Tydfil,
Mid Glamorgan, CF47 9DT
Phone: 01685 721721

Trust: North Glamorgan NHS Trust

North Glamorgan NHS Trust, which manages Prince Charles Hospital, has a lower than average number of nurses per 100 beds for Wales. The hospital performs thrombolysis within 30 minutes of a heart attack victim arriving in A&E or CCU and meets Royal College of Surgeons guidelines of having a paediatrician on site 24 hours a day.

Number of beds		440

		national
Doctors per 100 beds	21	24
Nurses per 100 beds	99	110
Complaints	4	6
Complaints clear up	71	71

waiting times		
Inpatient	63	66
Outpatient	45	49

Neath · **Neath General Hospital**

Briton Ferry Rd
Neath, SA11 2LQ
Phone: 01639 641161

Trust: Bro Morgannwg NHS Trust

Neath General Hospital is part of Bro Morgannwg NHS Trust, which has a lower than average number of doctors per 100 beds for Wales. The hospital offers CT scans to stroke victims within 48 hours but does not offer thrombolysis within 30 minutes of heart attack patients arriving in A&E or CCU. During 2002, a new 270-bed hospital is due to open to replace services currently offered on both the Neath and Talbot sites.

Number of beds		230

➕ ✖ 🆖

		national
Doctors per 100 beds	17	24
Nurses per 100 beds	108	110
Complaints	4	6
Complaints clear up	66	71

waiting times		
Inpatient	75	66
Outpatient	60	49

Newport · **Royal Gwent Hospital**

Cardiff Road, Newport
Gwent, NP20 2UB
Phone: 01633 234234

Trust: Gwent Healthcare NHS Trust

The Royal Gwent Hospital's location in the heart of Newport means that little space is available on the site, although outpatient facilities have been improved. New ophthalmology facilities have also opened on the site. In heart services, the hospital performs thrombolysis within the recommended 30 minutes. The hospital performs coronary angiography but not perform 500 catheterisations a year as recommended.

Number of beds		774

➕ ⊕ 〽 ✖ 🆖 ◉

		national
Doctors per 100 beds	24	24
Nurses per 100 beds	106	110
Complaints	4	6
Complaints clear up	65	71

waiting times		
Inpatient	62	66
Outpatient	44	49

Penarth · **Llandough Hospital**

Penlan Road, Llandough
Penarth Vale of Glamorgan, CF64 2XX
Phone: 029 20711711

Trust: Cardiff and Vale NHS Trust

The hospital is part of Cardiff and Vale NHS Trust, which has more doctors and nurses per 100 beds than any other Welsh Trust. It does not have an A&E unit, and emergency services are provided at University Hospital of Wales in Cardiff. However, from spring 2002 Llandough will become the Trust's main centre for booked general surgery. A new chemotherapy unit will also open, and discussions are under way for a new day care and diagnostic centre, mainly for orthopaedic patients.

Number of beds		500

		national
Doctors per 100 beds	36	24
Nurses per 100 beds	123	110
Complaints	13	6
Complaints clear up	75	71

waiting times		
Inpatient	51	66
Outpatient	32	49

Rhyl · **Glan Clwyd District General Hospital**

Bodelwyddan, Rhyl
Clwyd, LL18 5UJ
Phone: 01745 583910

Trust: Conwy and Denbighshire NHS Trust

Glan Clwyd District General is one of relatively few hospitals in Wales to offer a paediatric Intensive Care Unit and also to provide a CT scan for all stroke patients within 24 hours. However, it does not meet the recommended standard of carrying out thrombolysis within 30 minutes of a heart attack victim arriving in A&E or CCU. Conwy and Denbighshire NHS Trust, which manages the hospital, plans to build a 32-bed admissions ward in order to relieve pressure on beds.

Number of beds		683

		national
Doctors per 100 beds	1	24
Nurses per 100 beds	114	110
Complaints	6	6
Complaints clear up	74	71

waiting times		
Inpatient	83	66
Outpatient	57	49

Swansea · **Morriston Hospital**

Morriston
Swansea, SA6 6NL
Phone: 01792 702222

Trust: Swansea NHS Trust

Morriston Hospital houses the regional burns and plastic surgery units. The hospital meets two key standards in cardiac services, providing thrombolysis within 30 minutes and ensuring that its angiography service performs the recommended number of 500 cardiac catheterisations each year. Although the hospital performs surgery on children, a paediatrician is not on site 24 hours a day. A 4-bed HDU has recently been added to the hospital, and A&E and ITU services at the hospital will be redeveloped.

Number of beds		723

		national
Doctors per 100 beds	28	24
Nurses per 100 beds	111	110
Complaints	3	6
Complaints clear up	90	71

waiting times		
Inpatient	60	66
Outpatient	43	49

Swansea · **Singleton Hospital**

Sketty Road
Swansea, SA2 8QA
Phone: 01792 205666

Trust: Swansea NHS Trust

Singleton hospital overlooks Swansea Bay and is located next to the University of Swansea's campus. A dedicated cancer unit is based at the hospital, and there has been an expansion of the chemotherapy day unit. The A&E department is currently being upgraded, and the main outpatients entry has been renovated. All suspected stroke admissions receive a CT scan within 48 hours of admission.

Number of beds		550

		national
Doctors per 100 beds	28	24
Nurses per 100 beds	111	110
Complaints	3	6
Complaints clear up	90	71

waiting times		
Inpatient	60	66
Outpatient	43	49

Croesnewydd Road, Wrexham
Clwyd, LL13 7TD
Phone: 01978 291100

Trust: North East Wales NHS Trust

The hospital is located on the western side of Wrexham. In the past 8 years, £40 m has been invested in order to place most of the patient services at Wrexham Maelor Hospital into one building. An integrated Child Health Unit, which includes health and social services for paediatric outpatients and children with special needs, has been built, and the hospital has a paediatric ITU. The unit fails to provide thrombolysis within 30 minutes of a heart attack patient arriving in A&E or CCU. The hospital has a comparatively high number of complaints.

Number of beds		595

⊕ ⊕ ⊕ ⊗ ☎

		national
Doctors per 100 beds	21	24
Nurses per 100 beds	112	110
Complaints	14	6
Complaints clear up	56	71

waiting times		
Inpatient	72	66
Outpatient	49	49

Bancyfelin · **BMI Werndale Hospital**

Bancyfelin
Carmathenshire, SA33 5NE
Phone: 01267 211500

BMI Werndale has an operating theatre, day care unit and intensive care unit as part of its facilities. It provides a wide range of procedures using the latest technology and has a large nursing team and resident medical officers.

General Healthcare Group Ltd

Insurers: Bupa*, PPP*, Norwich, Standard Life, Royal Sun Alliance, WPA

price guide	£
Hip replacement	7500
Cataract removal	1968

Number of beds	28
ALS staff	1
heart services	⊘
Cancer services	⊕ ⊕ ⊘

Cardiff · **BUPA Hospital Cardiff**

Croescadarn Road, Pentwyn
Cardiff, CF23 8XL
Phone: 029 2073 5515

BUPA Hospital Cardiff offers treatment in most main specialities. The hospital runs a successful fertility clinic and has a scheme to assist women who cannot afford infertility treatment.

BUPA Hospitals

Insurers: Bupa, PPP, Norwich, Standard Life, Royal Sun Alliance, WPA

price guide	£
Hip replacement	6900-8148
Cataract removal	2300-2525

Number of beds	62
ALS staff	2
heart services	-
Cancer services	⊕ ⊘

Wrexham · **BUPA Yale Hospital**

Wrexham Technology Park
Wrexham, LL13 7YP
Phone: 01978 291306

BUPA Hospital Yale offers a wide range of medical services and facilities including an ultra-modern operating theatre with an optimum sterile environment allowing the hospital to undertake deep wound and joint replacement surgery.

BUPA Hospitals

Insurers: Bupa, PPP, Norwich, Standard Life, Royal Sun Alliance, WPA

price guide	£
Hip replacement	7425-7425
Cataract removal	2085-2085

Number of beds	25
ALS staff	1
heart services	-
Cancer services	⊕

Northern Ireland

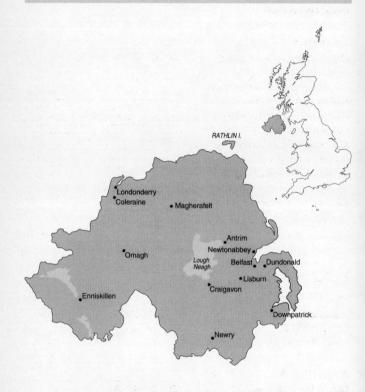

RATHLIN I.

Londonderry
Coleraine
Magherafelt
Antrim
Newtonabbey
Omagh
Lough Neagh
Belfast
Dundonald
Lisburn
Craigavon
Enniskillen
Downpatrick
Newry

	NHS
Antrim	Antrim Hospital
Belfast	Belfast City Hospital
Belfast	Mater Hospital
Belfast	The Royal Hospitals
Coleraine	Causeway Hospital
Craigavon	Craigavon Area Hospital
Downpatrick	Downe Hospital
Dundonald	Ulster Hospital
Enniskillen	Erne Hospital
Lisburn	Lagan Valley Hospital
Londonderry	Altnagelvin Area Hospital
Magherafelt	Mid-Ulster Hospital
Newry	Daisy Hill Hospital
Newtonabbey	Whiteabbey Hospital
Omagh	Tyrone & Fermanagh Hospital

Antrim · **Antrim Hospital**

45 Bush Road, Antrim
Co. Antrim, BT41 2RL
Phone: 028 94424000

Trust: United Hospitals Group HSS
Trust

Antrim Hospital is a medium-sized District General managed by the United Hospitals Group HSS Trust. A full range of services for children are available including operations on children under general anaesthetic and a paediatrician on site 24 hours. The A&E department also has separate children's areas for waiting and treatment. The hospital cannot guarantee that a suspected stroke patient will receive a CT scan within 48 hours of admission.

Number of beds		370

⊕ ⊕ ⚕ ⊗ ☏

		national
Doctors per 100 beds	33	40
Nurses per 100 beds	98	105
Complaints	4	8
Complaints clear up	67	72

waiting times

Inpatient	67	66
Outpatient	53	55

Belfast · **Belfast City Hospital**

Lisburn Road, Belfast
Belfast, BT9 7AB
Phone: 028 90329241

Trust: Belfast City Hospital HSS Trust

Belfast City Hospital is situated within Queen's University in south Belfast and is part of the Belfast City Hospital HSS Trust. The Trust has an above average number of doctors and nurses per 100 beds. Inpatient waiting times are notably longer than average but the majority of patients seeking outpatient appointments will be seen within 13 weeks. Stroke patients in need of a CT scan are likely to receive one within 48 hours of being admitted to the hospital. Single-sex wards are provided.

Number of beds		900

⊕ ⚕ ⊗ ☏

		national
Doctors per 100 beds	48	40
Nurses per 100 beds	140	105
Complaints	4	8
Complaints clear up	60	72

waiting times

Inpatient	51	66
Outpatient	72	54

Belfast · **Mater Hospital**

47-51 Crumlin Road
Belfast, BT14 6AB
Phone: 028 90741211

Trust: Mater Hospital HSS Trust

Mater Hospital, part of the Mater Hospital HSS Trust, is undergoing redevelopment with the construction of a new hospital building. The Trust has an above average number of doctors, but has fewer than average nurses. It has an efficient complaint clearance procedure and inpatients are seen within the recommended waiting times. The hospital provides CT scans to stroke patients within 24 hours of being admitted.

Number of beds		240

⊕ ⊕ ⋀ ⊗ ⊕

		national
Doctors per 100 beds	50	40
Nurses per 100 beds	94	105
Complaints	8	8
Complaints clear up	81	72

waiting times		
Inpatient	78	66
Outpatient	56	54

Belfast · **The Royal Hospitals**

Grosvenor Road,
Belfast 0, BT12 6BA
Phone: 028 90240503

Trust: Royal Group of Hospitals HSS Trust

This large district general hospital serving Belfast has a high number of doctors and nurses per 100 beds and a full range of facilities including a CT scanner and X-ray service available 24 hours a day. Suspected stroke patients are given a CT scan within 24 hours of admission. However, waiting times for both inpatients and outpatients are longer than average for Northern Ireland.

Number of beds		750

⊕ ⊕ ⋀ ⊕ ⊗ ⊕ ◉

		national
Doctors per 100 beds	61	40
Nurses per 100 beds	138	105
Complaints	6	8
Complaints clear up	54	72

waiting times		
Inpatient	51	66
Outpatient	43	54

Coleraine · **Causeway Hospital**

Newbridge Road, Coleraine
Londonderry, BT52 1TT
Phone: 028 70327032

Trust: Causeway HSS

The new, state-of-the-art Causeway Hospital opened during 2001, providing the acute services previously provided by the Route and Coleraine Hospitals. The hospital meets recommended guidelines on delivering thrombolysis and also in the volumes of coronary angiography performed. The hospital performs surgery on children under general anaesthetic but does not meet Royal College of Surgeons guidelines requiring a paediatrician to be on site 24 hours a day.

Number of beds		235

		national
Doctors per 100 beds	39	40
Nurses per 100 beds	101	105
Complaints	15	8
Complaints clear up	76	72

waiting times		
Inpatient	69	66
Outpatient	61	54

Craigavon · **Craigavon Area Hospital**

68 Lurgan Road, Portadown
Craigavon, Co Armagh, BT63 5QQ
Phone: 02838 334444

Trust: Craigavon Area Hospital Group
 HSS Trust

Craigavon Area Hospital is one of the main acute services units in Northern Ireland and is part of the Craigavon Area Hospital Group HSS. The hospital provides coronary angiographies but does not yet perform 500 a year as is recommended. Staffing levels are above average but patients wait longer than average for an inpatient appointment. Outpatient waiting times are similar to other Trusts.

Number of beds		414

		national
Doctors per 100 beds	47	40
Nurses per 100 beds	121	105
Complaints	3	8
Complaints clear up	88	72

waiting times		
Inpatient	54	66
Outpatient	52	54

Downpatrick · **Downe Hospital**

9A Pound Lane, Downpatrick
Co Down, BT30 6JA
Phone: 028 44613311

Trust: Down Lisburn HSS Trust

The 94-bed Downe Hospital is situated in Downpatrick and is part of the Down Lisburn HSS Trust. The Trust has fewer doctors and nurses per 100 beds than the national average. The high complaints figure reflects the fact that the Trust treats all verbal complaints as written complaints. This may lead to the lower than average complaints clear-up figure. The inpatient waiting times are shorter on average than other Trusts although patients will wait slightly longer on average for an outpatient appointment.

Number of beds		94
● ✖		

		national
Doctors per 100 beds	29	40
Nurses per 100 beds	67	105
Complaints	17	8
Complaints clear up	59	72

waiting times		
Inpatient	86	66
Outpatient	48	54

Dundonald · **Ulster Hospital**

Upper Newtownards Road, Dundonald
Belfast, BT16 0RH
Phone: 028 9048 4511

Trust: Ulster Community and Hospitals
HSS Trust

The Ulster Hospital is based in Dundonald and is part of the Ulster Community and Hospitals HSS Trust. The Trust has an average number of nurses and doctors to 100 beds. It has an average number of complaints but deals with them quickly. Inpatient and outpatient waiting times in the Trust are significantly longer than average. The hospital provides coronary angiographies but it has yet to meet the recommended caseload of 500 cardiac catheterisations a year.

Number of beds		576
● ⊕ ✹ ☺		

		national
Doctors per 100 beds	40	40
Nurses per 100 beds	261	105
Complaints	8	8
Complaints clear up	78	72

waiting times		
Inpatient	59	66
Outpatient	44	54

Enniskillen · **Erne Hospital**

Cornagrade Road, Enniskillen
Co Fermanagh, BT74 6AY
Phone: 028 66 324711

Trust: Sperrin Lakeland HSS Trust

Erne Hospital is a small acute facility serving Enniskillen. Sperrin Lakeland HSS Trust, which manages the hospital, has lower than average staffing levels for doctors per 100 beds. Waiting times for both inpatients and outpatients are shorter than average for Northern Ireland. There is no ITU at the hospital but there is a CT scanner and X-ray services are available 24 hours a day.

Number of beds		230

		national
Doctors per 100 beds	25	40
Nurses per 100 beds	102	105
Complaints	4	8
Complaints clear up	76	72

waiting times		
Inpatient	85	66
Outpatient	58	54

Lisburn · **Lagan Valley Hospital**

39 Hillsborough Road, Lisburn
Co Antrim, BT28 1JP
Phone: 028 92665141

Trust: Down Lisburn HSS Trust

Lagan Valley Hospital is a small district general. Down Lisburn HSS Trust, which manages the hospital, has a lower than average number of doctors per 100 beds. The hospital encourages complaints which is why this figure is relatively high. Verbal complaints are treated as written complaints. The Trust has a mixed record for waiting times with shorter than average inpatient waits but longer that average outpatient waits.

Number of beds		287

		national
Doctors per 100 beds	29	40
Nurses per 100 beds	67	105
Complaints	17	8
Complaints clear up	59	72

waiting times		
Inpatient	86	66
Outpatient	48	54

Londonderry · **Altnagelvin Area Hospital**

Gleshane Road, Londonderry
Londonderry, BT47 6SB
Phone: 028 71345171

Trust: Altnagelvin Group HSS Trust

Altnagelvin Hospital in Londonderry is the largest acute hospital in Northern Ireland outside Belfast and part of theAltnagelvin Group HSS Trust. The hospital does not meet recommendations for ensuring stroke patients undergo a CT scan within 48 hours of being admitted. Staffing levels across the Trust are average but outpatient waiting times are longer than average.

Number of beds		542

$\oplus$ $\oplus$ $\otimes$ $\oplus$

		national
Doctors per 100 beds	39	36
Nurses per 100 beds	104	105
Complaints	3	8
Complaints clear up	81	72

waiting times		
Inpatient	75	66
Outpatient	45	54

Magherafelt · **Mid-Ulster Hospital**

59 Hospital Road, Magherafelt
Co Londonderry, BT45 5EX
Phone: 028 7963 1031

Trust: United Hospitals Group HSS Trust

United Hospitals Group HSS Trust manages Mid-Ulster Hospital, a small acute facility serving the Londonderry area. Single-sex wards are available throughout the hospital. There is an A&E department and paediatric surgery is performed under general anaesthetic; however, there is no paediatrician available 24 hours at the hospital.

Number of beds		152

$\oplus$ $\otimes$

		national
Doctors per 100 beds	33	40
Nurses per 100 beds	98	105
Complaints	4	8
Complaints clear up	67	72

waiting times		
Inpatient	67	66
Outpatient	53	54

Newry · **Daisy Hill Hospital**

5 Hospital Road, Newry
County Down, BT35 8DR
Phone: 02830 835 000

Trust: Newry and Mourne HSS Trust

The Daisy Hill Hospital is part of the Newry and Mourne HSS Trust. It has dedicated acute, rehabilitation and combined stroke units and provides stroke patients a CT scan within 24 hours of admission to hospital. Staffing levels are slightly lower than average but inpatient and outpatient waiting times are lower than average.

Number of beds		301

⊕ ⊗ ☎

		national
Doctors per 100 beds	31	40
Nurses per 100 beds	87	105
Complaints	6	8
Complaints clear up	67	72

waiting times		
Inpatient	77	66
Outpatient	57	54

Newtownabbey · **Whiteabbey Hospital**

Doagh Road, Newtownabbey
Co Antrim, BT37 9RH
Phone: 02890 865181

Trust: United Hospitals Group HSS Trust

Whiteabbey Hospital is a small acute facility that is managed by United Hospitals Group HSS Trust. There is an A&E department in which 96 per cent of patients are dealt with within the target waiting time of 4 hours. Children admitted to casualty are treated in a separate area; however, paediatric surgery is not performed at the hospital.

Number of beds		160

⊕ ⊗

		national
Doctors per 100 beds	33	40
Nurses per 100 beds	98	105
Complaints	4	8
Complaints clear up	67	72

waiting times		
Inpatient	67	66
Out patient	53	54

Omagh · **Tyrone County Hospital**

Hospital Road, Omagh
Co Tyrone, BT79 0AP
Phone: 02882 245211

Trust: Sperrin Lakeland HSS Trust

Tyrone County Hospital is a small acute facility managed by the Sperrin Lakeland HSS Trust. Around 115,000 people in mostly rural areas around Omagh are served by the Trust. According to recent figures there are fewer than average doctors per 100 beds at the hospital but inpatient waiting times are shorter than average. Services and facilities include a renal unit and day procedure unit. Mental health care and services for the elderly are provided at the nearby Tyrone and Fermanagh Hospital.

Number of beds		-

		national
Doctors per 100 beds	25	40
Nurses per 100 beds	102	105
Complaints	4	8
Complaints clear up	76	72

waiting times		
Inpatient	85	66
Outpatient	58	54

Methodology

Establishing scope of research and data collection

The scope of the guide was established in consultation with the Department of Health and patient representative organisations which were invited to propose areas they felt of most concern to patients. Focus groups of patients were held around the country at which patients expressed their concerns and talked about the types of information they would like to have access to. This was used to produce a questionnaire which was sent to every hospital in the country. The questionnaires were adapted slightly for Scotland to reflect minor differences in accepted clinical standards.

MORTALITY FIGURES
English Overall Hospital Mortality Figures

In their initial study (Jarman et al, 1999), Imperial College of Science, Technology & Medicine looked at four years of Hospital Episode Statistics (HES) data, from 1991–2 to 1994–5. The exercise was repeated for HES data for the five years 1995–6 to 1999–2000. These mortality rates were published in January 2001. The mortality rates published here used HES data from 1995–6 to 2000–2001, with the five years 1995–6 to 1999–2000 used for standardisation. Community, specialty institutions and small hospitals (under 10,000 admissions during the five years) were excluded, leaving 174 hospital trusts which were in place on 1 April 2001 (about 90 per cent of hospital activity in England for those years). Hospital data was also excluded for any year for which that hospital had poor quality data (usually because data was missing, they were informed of poor data quality, or other quality checks indicated poor quality – details of these omissions are available). A total of 3 per cent (26 of the 870 available years) of the data was excluded. They included discharge records only, that is episodes which ended in discharge (alive or dead) from the hospital rather than transfer to the care of another consultant within the hospital. They eliminated from the analyses all transfers between hospitals (2 per cent of admissions and 3 per cent of discharges in the first four years).

Discharges were included in the analysis if the primary diagnosis was one of 81 primary diagnoses which accounted for 82 per cent of all hospital deaths in England. For the first four years (from 1991–2 to 1994–5) HES uses ICD9 and for the next five years it uses ICD10. A list of equivalent diagnoses between these two data sets was made: in eight of the diagnoses there was not a very close equivalent and the closest corresponding diagnoses were used. This enabled comparisons to be made across all nine years for most of the data analysed – these comparisons are not part of the current publication but allowed Imperial College to show consistency in the data over this period.

Hospital standardised mortality ratios (HSMRs) were calculated, using indirect standardisation, as the ratio of the actual number of deaths to the expected number of deaths multiplied by 100. Death rates were calculated for the six years 1995–2001 for all Trusts in England stratified by age (using the HES age groups), sex, emergency or non-emergency, and length of stay (0–7, 8–14,15–28 and 29–365 days) for each of the 81 primary diagnoses leading to 82 per cent of all deaths. These were used to calculate the expected deaths for each hospital by multiplying the number of hospital inpatient admissions in each stratum by the England death rates for that stratum and adding across all the strata.

In addition to standardising for primary diagnosis, several measures of co-morbidity were based on discharge diagnoses for each hospital: the number of bodily systems affected by disease, the percentage of patient admissions with one of the 15 most serious primary diagnoses (responsible for 50 per cent of all deaths), and the percentage both of cases and of deaths with co-morbidities (that is, sub-diagnoses) in each of the 85 diagnoses that led to over 80 per cent of all deaths. Sub-diagnoses were ranked by their univariable correlation with HSMRs and created a measure of co-morbidity by combining the top two or three co-morbidity diagnoses. Each of these measures was used in their regression model as independent estimates of the severity of illness treated. However, they had already standardised within each of the diagnoses in calculating the hospital standardised mortality ratios, and when regression analyses were carried out using a wide range of possible explanatory variables (Jarman et al, 1999), it was found that additional measures of case-mix and co-morbidities were not very powerful explanatory variables. Measures of local deprivation were also not powerful explanatory variables after the above standardisations had been carried out. They found that the ratio of hospital doctors per bed (total doctors per total beds averaged over the years in question) was by far the most powerful explanatory variable for both the four years (1991–2 to 1994–5) and for the five years 1995–6 to 1999–2000.

They also examined the data for consistency of case-mix. This was done by scaling the proportions of expected deaths for each of the 80 diagnoses for each trust to be the same as the average proportions as the overall figure for England. The numbers of observed deaths were then similarly scaled for each of the 80 diagnoses and the sums of these scaled expected and observed deaths used to calculate HSMRs adjusted to have the same proportions of expected deaths as the England average (for example, diagnoses of malignancies total 22.2 per cent across all trusts).

This was found to make very little difference to the HSMRs, except in the cases of North Middlesex NHS Trust and Bart's and the London NHS Trust, which had unusual levels of malignancy.

Scottish Overall mortality figures

The hospital mortality figures for Scotland are based on the Scottish Mortality Record (SMR) for the years 1996–2000. The figures were calculated using similar methodologies to the figures for England using English data from 1995–2000 for standardisation. However, the variation in case-mix between Scottish hospitals is much greater than for English hospitals, and it was found in a number of cases that the HSMR strongly altered when the case-mix was scaled to the English average. The 14 hospitals affected by this have been excluded from the analysis. The figures published are standardised mortality rates after the case-mix has been scaled to match the average. Those hospitals identified as high or low had a significantly higher than average mortality rate at 99 per cent confidence both when case-mix was scaled and when it was not.

For further details on methodology please refer to the 1999 British Medical Journal (BMJ) article in which the original study, based on 1991 to 1995 data, was published. Note that the latest figures have additionally been standardised for emergency admission and length of stay. Jarman B, Gault S, Alves B, Hider A, Dolan S, Cook A, Hurwitz B, Iezzoni LI. Explaining differences in English hospital death rates using routinely collected data. *BMJ* 1999;318:1515–1520.

Mortality data for fractured neck of femur, stroke and heart bypass.

The mortality rates are based on an analysis of the Hospital Episode Statistics between 1995 and 2001 by Imperial College of Science, Technology and Medicine. Analysis of each of the 80 diagnoses that lead to 80 per cent of deaths in hospital (see above), as well as some of the most common procedures that are associated with a high death rate, allowed them to identify two diagnoses – stroke and fractured neck of femur (broken hip) – as demonstrating the necessary statistical quality for further analyses – sufficiently high numbers of deaths to allow meaningful comparison and reasonably stable rates of mortality year on year. In addition, one procedure, coronary artery bypass graft (CABG) surgery – or heart bypass surgery – was also considered to be statistically robust.

Stroke and neck of femur

Hospital standardised mortality ratios (HSMRs) were calculated as the ratio of actual number of deaths to the expected number of deaths. Standardisation was by age (using the HES age groups), sex and length of stay (0–7, 8–14, 15–28 and 29–365 days). Inter-hospital transfers were removed. Only emergency admissions were studied (only 1 or 2 per cent of admissions were not emergencies). Regression analyses were carried out using the HSMR as the dependent variable and a measure of social deprivation (the underprivileged area score – UPA – using the average value of the electoral ward of residence of the patients admitted to each trust) as the explanatory variable, along with several other possible explanatory variables. The regression model was used to calculate a value for the HSMR allowing for social deprivation. They also considered using secondary diagnoses recorded in HES as a measure of severity. Although some measures based on secondary diagnoses were found to correlate with mortality rates, the relationship was far less strong than that with measures of social deprivation, which is linked to incidence and severity of illness.

Standardisation of the Dr Foster data for Coronary Artery Bypass Graft (CABG)

HSMRs were created by standardising for age, sex and admission method (elective or planned, emergency and transfer from another hospital). Various severity measures were considered, such as the co-morbidities, waiting times, lengths of stay and methods of discharge, but none were found to improve on using the admission method. Transfers have 2.5 times the mortality of planned admissions with emergencies intermediate between these.

They removed all cases with one of a selected list of other operations carried out during the same admission which made the operation more complex than a simple coronary artery bypass graft. The original number of cases was about 130,000 over the six years: 11,000 cases were removed because they involved heart valve surgery (mainly plastic repair of the aortic or mitral valve but included all OPCS4 codes K02 to K39). In addition 2,500 operations were removed, because they involved operations with a high mortality (on average 34 per cent) carried out at the same time as, but not directly related to, the CABG operations. Overall, the excluded cases accounted for about 42 per cent of all deaths amongst the CABG patients despite only representing about 10 per cent of the cases.

Regression analyses were carried out using the standardised CABG SMRs as the dependent variable and a measure of social deprivation and a variety of other factors as the explanatory variable. GPs per 1000 population and the percentage of trusts doing more than 70 per cent of their CABG operations as arterial grafts were the best explanatory variables when SMRs were not standardised for admission method, but when admission method was included in the standardisation GPs per 1000 population was no longer significant. The explanatory variables included the percentage of diagnoses with heart failure, myocardial infarction, and aneurysm as co-morbidities (these were the highest mortality of the relatively common co-morbidities): these were not significant in explaining the variation of SMRs between units. SMR for units doing high (>70 per cent) and low (<70 per cent) percentages of their CABG operations with at least one arterial graft were significantly different (but not allowed for in the standardisation as this was considered to be a factor under the units' control).

OTHER DATA
England
Vacancy Rates: Department of Health, three-month vacancy rates, all consultants, 2001. Consultant posts that trusts are actively trying to fill that have been vacant for three months or more as a percentage of all posts (staff in post plus three-month vacancies) as at 30 September 2001.

Inpatient Waiting Times: NHS Executive 'Green Book', 2001/2002 Q2 (Nov 2001). Percentage of patients waiting less than 6 months for admission.

Outpatient Waiting Times: NHS Executive 'Red Book', 2001/2002 (Nov 2001). Percentage of those GP written referrals seen who waited less than 13 weeks.

Complaints & Complaints clear up: 'Handling complaints: monitoring the NHS complaints procedure'. Department of Health, Financial Year 2000/2001. Number of inpatient complaints per 1000 inpatient episodes. Percentage of complaints answered within 20 working days.

Bed Numbers: NHS Executive 'Blue Book', 2000/2001. Figure used is the number of overnight beds.

Doctor Numbers: Specific data request from the Department of Health, 2001. Figures are from March 2000. Whole time equivalent (wte) figures for all staff, excluding hospital practitioner, clinical assistant, dental staff and other staff.

Nurse Numbers: Manager, midwife, registered sick children's, other level 1, other level 2. We amalgamate whole time equivalent (wte) figures for qualified staff in these categories. Health visitors and district nurses (1 and 2) were excluded.

SCOTLAND

Doctor Numbers: Supplied by ISD. Whole time equivalents for all medical staff (consultant, staff grade, senior registrar, specialist registrar, registrar, SHO, HO, associate specialist, limited specialist, hospital practitioner, GMP). Source: Medical & Dental Staff Census (MEDMAN), Sept 2000.

Nurse Numbers: Supplied by ISD. Whole time equivalents for qualified nursing staff, both hospital and community, excluding health visitors and district nurses level 1 and 2.

Bed Numbers: Scottish Health Statistics. Hospital & Clinical Activity September 2001

Complaints and complaints and clear up. Scottish Health Statistics. NHS Scotland Complaints. April 2001. The complaints index is the total number of complaints divided by the number of inpatient and day case episodes. The episodes figure is the sum of Emergency Inpatients, Elective Inpatients, and Day Cases. Source: ISD Scotland National Statistics, Trends in Acute Activity, November 2001.

Inpatient Waiting Times: ISD Scotland National Statistics. March 2001. Percentage of patients waiting less than 6 months for admission.

Outpatient Waiting Times: ISD Scotland National Statistics November 2001. Percentage of those GP written referrals seen who waited less than 13 weeks.

A&E Trolley Waits (percentage seen within 2 hours). Source : ISD Scotland National Statistics SMR30C (April/May 2001).

A&E Walking Wounded (percentage seen within 2.5 hours). Source : ISD Scotland National Statistics SMR30C (April/May 2001).

WALES

Doctor Numbers: Whole time equivalent medical and dental staff in post as at 30 September 2000 (excluding locums). National Assembly for Wales.

Nurse Numbers: Non Medical Staff Directly Employed by the NHS in Post at 30 September 2000, Nursing, Midwifery and Health Visiting Staff. National Assembly for Wales. We have included whole time equivalents for Nurse Manager, registered sick children's nurse, registered midwife, and other level 1 and 2 nurses.

Complaints: Complaints to the NHS in Wales 2000–2001. We give a complaints index and the percentage of complaints responded to within 4 weeks. The complaints index is the total number of complaints divided by the number of inpatient episodes for each trust for the year to March 2001. Source: National Assembly for Wales.

Inpatient Waiting Times: NHS Wales Hospital Waiting Times, National Assembly for Wales, 2001. Percentage of patients waiting less than 6 months for admission.

Outpatient Waiting Times: NHS Wales Hospital Waiting Times, National Assembly for Wales, 2001. Percentage of those GP written referrals seen, who waited less than 3 months.

Bed Numbers: Average daily available beds 1999–2000. National Assembly for Wales, 2001.

NORTHERN IRELAND

Bed Numbers: Inpatient Activity Data by Hospital Provider 2000–1. Department of Health, Social Services and Public Safety (DHSSPS).

Complaints & Complaints Clear up: Charter for Patients and Clients. Performance Tables for 1999–2000. Department of Health, Social Services and Public Safety (DHSSPS).

Doctor Numbers: General Acute Trust Hospital Staff In Post By Category And Provider. Mixed Activity Trust Hospital, Community And Personal Social Services Staff In Post By Category And Provider. Department of Health, Social Services and Public Safety (DHSSPS). Nurse Numbers: Data request from Department of Health, Social Services and Public Safety (DHSSPS). Source: Human Resource Information System. Numbers of Qualified Nurses. Figures exclude the following: bank or agency staff; community-based staff; hospital-based staff who work in the community, health visitors and district nurses; unqualified staff.

Inpatient Waits: Ordinary Admission Waiting List by Provider and Time Waiting (March 2001) plus Day Case Waiting List by Provider and Time Waiting (March 2001). Department of Health, Social Services and Public Safety (DHSSPS). Percentage of patients waiting less than 6 months for admission.

Outpatient Waits: Outpatient Waiting List by Provider and Time Waiting (March 2001). Department of Health, Social Services and Public Safety (DHSSPS). Percentage of those GP written referrals seen who waited less than 2 months.

REFERENCES

1. Jarman B, Alves B, Hider A, Dolan S, Cook A, Hurwitz B, Iezzoni LI. Explaining differences in English hospital death rates using routinely collected data. *British Medical Journal* **318**, 1515–1520 (1999).

Glossary

Accident and Emergency (A&E) The gateway for patients who require hospital admission due to an acute illness or injury. A&E staff work with other hospital specialties to organise appropriate treatment for the patients who attend. Many patients can be dealt with in the department and can then go home. Some are given a hospital outpatient appointment or are referred to their GP. A minority are admitted to hospital.

Acute condition A condition of short duration that starts quickly and has severe symptoms, for instance, heart failure. It may also refer to a symptom, for example, severe pain. An "acute" abdomen is a serious disorder of the abdomen requiring urgent treatment, usually surgery.

Advanced Life Support Staff Hospital staff who have completed training which qualifies them to deal with life-threatening emergencies in a particular field of care, such as Intensive Care or Coronary Care.

Anaesthetist Doctor with specialist training who administers an anaesthetic to induce unconciousness in a patient before a surgical operation. Anaesthetists are also key members of resuscitation and intensive care teams.

Aneurysm A localised swelling or dilation of an artery due to weakening of its wall. The commonest sites are the aorta (the artery that opens out of the left ventricle of the heart and carries blood to the whole body), the arteries of the legs, and those that pass into the upper arms. Aneurysms are most common amongst the elderly, with men affected more commonly than women.

Angina Pectoris Pain in the centre of the chest often brought on by exercise or anxiety. Pain may be severe and also felt in the arms and the jaw. The condition, which is aggravated by cold weather, occurs when the heart muscle is temporarily starved of oxygen.

People who suffer from angina pectoris may need advice on diet and lifestyle and may also have high blood pressure.

Angiography A diagnostic test for heart disease using injected dye and X-rays. This procedure demonstrates whether there is any narrowing or ballooning of the coronary arteries, changes usually caused by disease or injury.

Angioplasty A method of treating a blocked or narrowed artery by inserting a balloon into the constriction to open it up. The technique is used to treat a narrowed artery in the heart or a limb. About 65 per cent of patients treated benefit, but when symptoms persist or recur the procedure may be repeated.

Beta Blockers Any of a group of drugs used to treat various disorders associated with the circulatory system. These disorders include high blood pressure (hypertension), angina pectoris (chest pains caused by reduced oxygen flow to the heart muscle), irregular heartbeat, and migraine headache.

Cardiac Catheterisation A diagnostic procedure in which a tube is inserted into a blood vessel under local anaesthetic and threaded through to the chambers of the heart to monitor blood flow, blood pressure, blood chemistry, and the output of the heart, and to take a sample of heart tissue. The technique is used to diagnose congenital heart disease and coronary artery disease. As part of the catheterisation procedure, angiography may also be performed.

Cardiology The branch of medical science devoted to the study of diseases of the heart, for instance coronary artery (ischaemic heart) disease and angina. Other areas covered by cardiology including abnormal heart rhythms, heart failure and high blood pressure.

Cardiothoracic surgery A specialist area of surgery involving operating on the heart and lungs only available in a minority of hospitals. Often a patient may see a cardiothoracic surgeon upon being referred by a cardiologist. The most common operation these surgeons perform is heart bypass surgery (coronary artery bypass graft), which improves life expectancy and symptoms in patients with coronary heart disease.

CCU (Coronary Care Unit) This is a unit delivering care to high dependency patients with heart conditions.

Chemotherapy This is an important chemical treatment for cancer, which is used to target germ-cell tumours, some leukaemias and lymphomas and ovarian cancer (following surgery). It is also used in some breast cancers and some childhood cancers. Over 20 substances are in common use, the major classes being alkylating agents, antimetabolites, vinca alkaloids and antitumour antibiotics.

Chronic condition This is a persistent or recurring condition, for example, arthritis. The disease, which may or may not be severe, often starts gradually and changes will be slow.

Colonoscopy Internal examination of the large bowel (colon) using a fibre-optic camera called a colonoscope. This is a long flexible tube with a bright light at the end that allows the doctor to look down at the lining of the bowel. In some cases biopsies (small pieces of tissue) may be taken with tiny forceps and sent to the laboratory.

Colorectal surgery The diagnosis and surgical treatment of diseases of the intestinal tract, colon, rectum, and perianal area (eg for colon cancer).

Consultant Senior doctor or surgeon with several years experience of practise in a chosen area of specialisation.

CT (Computed Tomography) scan A scanning examination technique which gives better images of soft tissue than X-ray and can distinguish soft tissue from cysts or fat. Computed tomography is particularly useful in patients with suspected malignancy and is commonly used for brain scanning and head injury.

Dietician Works with people to promote nutritional wellbeing, prevent food-related problems and treat disease. They may be asked to see patients who are undernourished or who need to watch their diet, for instance patients who have had heart attacks or diabetics.

ECG (Electrocardiogram) This is a record of a patient's heartbeat which is monitored by connecting the patient via electrodes to an instrument known as an electrograph. Any muscle in use produces an electric current, but when an individual is at rest the main muscular current in the body is that produced by the heart.

Elective surgery Non-emergency surgery.

Endoscopy Examination of a body cavity using an endoscope – a tube-shaped (fibre-optic) camera to investigate and treat disorders. It is flexible and equipped with lenses and a light source. An endoscope has a different name according to the part of the body it investigates; for the examination of the stomach it is called a gastroscope.

Fluoroscopy The technique for rendering X-rays visible after they have passed through the body by projecting them on a screen of calcium tungstate. It provides a method of being able to watch, for instance, the beating of the heart, or the movements of the intestine after the administration of a barium meal.

Haemodialysis unit Every renal department has a dialysis unit, which treats people with kidney failure. A dialysis machine is an artificial means of filtering the blood when the kidneys cannot. It removes poisonous waste from the blood and keeps body fluids in balance.

HDU (High Dependency Unit) A hospital unit equipped and staffed to nurse patients who require a high level of technically supported care. Patients are usually moved to the HDU when they have made satisfactory progress in an intensive-care unit (ICU) and no longer require ventilation and one-to-one nursing care. Also, patients who have undergone major surgery are often transferred here from the recovery ward.

Holistic Care A method of medical care in which patients are treated as a whole, taking into account their physical and mental state and social background, rather than just treating the disease alone.

Hospice A hospital that cares only for the terminally ill and dying. The emphasis is on providing quality of life, and special care is taken in providing pain relief by whichever methods are deemed best suited to the person's needs.

Hospital Doctor A doctor (physician), whose career is based in hospital medicine. Consultants are the most senior grade. More junior grades are specialist surgeon registrar, senior house officers and house officers.

HRT (Hormone Replacement Therapy) Prescription of natural or synthetic hormones to people who no longer secrete adequate quantities of natural hormones. This term is most often used to refer to hormonal deficiencies in women going through the menopause and commonly include treatment with the hormones oestrogen and progestogen.

Hypertension Abnormally high blood pressure. Some people's blood pressure may vary with daily activity, rising with anxiety or exercise. In more than 90 per cent of people with high blood pressure the cause is not identified and this "variety" is often described as essential hypertension.

ICU (Intensive Care Unit) A hospital unit where patients who have had severe injuries, heart attacks or major operations can be ventilated, and have specialised monitoring, resuscitation and treatment procedures. Units are staffed with highly trained nurses, technicians and doctors and equipped with electronic monitoring devices that allow continuous assessment of vital body functions such as heart rate and blood pressure.

Immunodeficiency Syndrome Impaired immunity resulting from inherited or acquired abnormalities of the immune system. This leads to increased vulnerability to even minor infections.

Keyhole Surgery Also called "Minimally Invasive Surgery" (MIS), this is surgical intervention that causes patients the least physical trauma. It often includes operations (for example to remove stones from the gall bladder) performed through a very small incision with the aid of a fibre-optic camera, to speed up healing and reduce scarring. Patients are often well enough to return home the same day and resume normal activities.

Laparoscopy A technique for examining the interior of the abdomen, taking a biopsy or performing a minor surgical procedure, with the aid of an endoscope (usually fibre-optic) inserted through a small hole made in the abdominal wall.

Linear Accelerators for Radiotherapy High-energy X-rays that can destroy deep-seated tumours. Many head and neck tumours, gynaecological cancers and localised prostate and bladder cancers are curable with radiotherapy.

Mammography The technique whereby X-rays are used to show the structure of the breast or any abnormalities in it. It can detect tumours that are not palpable.

Mortality Index The relative rates of mortality in hospital trusts after allowing for factors such as difference in types of patients treated. A trust with an average performance has an index of 100. Figures greater than 100 indicate a higher mortality rate than expected for the types of patients treated and vice versa.

MRI (Magnetic Resonance Imaging) scan A sophisticated scanning technique that is used particularly to examine the brain, spine and joints. The MRI scanner comprises a strong electromagnet, a radio-wave emitter and a radio-wave detector. The subject is rotated through different planes to obtain a series of images which are viewed on a computer-controlled monitor screen.

National Service Frameworks (NSFs) A range of measures introduced by the Government to raise quality and decrease variations in service. National Service Frameworks set national standards and define service models for a defined service or care group; put in place strategies to support implementation; establish performance milestones against which progress within an agreed time-scale will be measured. Each NSF is developed with the assistance of an external reference group (ERG) which brings together health professionals, service users and carers, health service managers, partner agencies, and other advocates. ERGs adopt an inclusive process to engage the full range of views. The Department of Health supports the ERGs and manages the overall process.

Neurology This is the branch of medicine that treats brain and nerve disorders. Patients with disorders such as Parkinson's, Alzheimer's disease, or multiple sclerosis may consult a neurologist as their principal care physician.

Nurse Works in all aspects of patient care. There are different levels of seniority of qualified nurses. Some also have specialist training, for instance, sick children's nurses and cancer nurses.

Occupational Therapy Helps people to overcome physical, psychological and social problems arising from illness or disability. Occupational therapists concentrate on maximising what people are able to achieve with their current level of function and try to get them to achieve independence in their daily lives. They will often assess the patient's home environment before the patient leaves hospital and organise the installation of aids around the home such as stair rails.

Oncology The management of malignant disease, or cancer, which requires close liaison between the patient, surgeons, physicians, oncologists, haematologists, paediatricians and other specialists. Treatment often involves surgery, radiotherapy or chemotherapy, or a combination of the three.

Orthopaedics The branch of medicine dealing with skeletal deformity (congenital or acquired), fractures and infections of bones, replacement of arthritic joints and the treatment of bone tumours.

Osteoporosis A disease affecting the bones whereby calcium is lost from the bone mass. Sufferers are prone to bone fractures from relatively minor trauma. By the age of 90 one in two women and one in six men are likely to sustain an osteoporosis-related fracture. Treatment is by hormone replacement therapy or anti-resorptive drugs.

Palliative care Palliative care is the active total care of patients whose disease is not responsive to curative treatment. Care aims to control pain and other symptoms and help with psychological, social and spiritual problems. It aims to achieve the best possible quality of life for patients and their families.

Paramedic Senior member of ambulance crew who is trained in pre-hospital emergency care.

Pathology The science that deals with the causes of, and changes produced in the body by disease. It also refers to blood and tissue testing.

Pharmacist Expert in preparation and dispensing of medicines. Pharmacists also have expertise in the use of drugs and can give advice on related matters. They dispense drugs to patients who are going home and also often give advice to the doctors on the wards.

Physiotherapy Treatment after physical injury such as massage and exercise to restore mobility, muscle function, etc. It is an essential part of the rehabilitation of convalescent or disabled patients. Physiotherapists play a particularly large role in treating orthopaedic patients (who have had operations on their bones or joints) and patients who have suffered strokes or spinal injuries, as well as the elderly. Structured exercises are the mainstay of their treatment.

Primary Health Care Team Provide all services outside the hospital in the form of family health services and community health services. Family health services include the four practitioner services: GPs, dental practitioners, pharmacists and opticians. Community health services include community doctors, dentists, nurses, midwives and health visitors and other allied therapies such as physiotherapy and chiropody.

Psychiatrist Doctor who specialises in the treatment of patients with mental disorders.

Psychologist Helps people with mental problems to solve them through discussion. There are various branches of psychology and approaches to treatments of patients according to which the psychologists practise. Some, for example, may use cognitive therapy, or specialise in child psychology.

Radiographer There are two types of radiographers, diagnostic and therapeutic. Diagnostic radiographers produces images (usually X-rays) for doctors to help with diagnosing disease. Therapeutic radiographers use high-energy radiation to treat cancer and other conditions.

Radiologist Doctor who specialises in the use and interpretation of X-rays and other scans such as ultrasound and MRI scans.

Radiotherapy The use of ionising radiation in the treatment of cancer to kill tumour cells. Radiation is by naturally occurring isotopes or artificially produced X-rays. Beams of radiation may be directed at the tumour from a distance or radioactive material, in the form of needles, wires or pellets, may be implanted in the body. Many head and neck tumours, gynaecological cancers and localised prostate and bladder cancers are curable with radiotherapy.

Rapid Access Chest Pain Clinic Ensures that patients with new chest pains, urgently referred to hospital by a GP, see a specialist within 2 weeks.

Speech and Language Therapist Works with people who have problems with communication, including speech defects, or with chewing or swallowing. For instance, they may help patients who are having difficulty speaking after a stroke.

Surgeon Surgeons use the same system of seniority as doctors but have specialist training and experience in surgical techniques. There are various specialties of surgery, the most common being general surgery.

Triage Nurse In A&E, The triage nurse assesses how urgently a patient needs to be seen by a doctor and prioritises patients according to the seriousness of their injuries or disease.

Thrombolysis in 30 minutes The breakdown of a blood clot by enzymic activity within an optimum (half-hour) period after a heart attack.

Tracheostomy An operation to make an artificial opening through the front of the neck into the windpipe so that air may be directly drawn or passed into the lower air passages. The majority of tracheostomies performed nowadays are for patients in intensive care situations. These patients require airway intervention for prolonged periods to facilitate artificial ventilation, which is performed by means of a mechanical ventilator.

Useful Contacts

HEART DISEASE

British Heart Foundation

14 Fitzhardinge Street

London W1H 6DH

Tel: 020 7935 0185

www.bhf.org.uk

Northern Ireland Chest, Heart and Stroke Association

21 Dublin Road

Belfast BT2 7HB

Tel: 028 9032 0184

Helpline:084 5769 7299

www.nichsa.com

Blood Pressure Association

60 Cranmer Terrace

London SW17 0QS

Tel: 020 8772 4994

www.bpassoc.org.uk

Coronary Prevention Group

2 Taviton Street

London WC1H 0BT

Tel: 020 7927 2125

www.healthnet.org.uk

British Cardiac Patients Association

www.cardiac-bcpa.co.uk

Tel: 020 8289 5591

Helpline: 01223 846845

STROKE

The Stroke Association

Stroke House

Whitecross Street

London EC1Y 8JJ

Tel: 020 7566 0300

Helpline: 0845 303 3100

www.stroke.org.uk

Speakability

1 Royal Street

London SE1 7LL

Tel: 020 7261 9572

Helpline: 080 8808 9572

www.speakability.org.uk

CANCER

CancerBACUP

Tel: 020 8800 1234

3 Bath Place, Rivington Street,

London EC2A 3JR

Helpline: 0808 800 1234

www.cancerbacup.org.uk

Macmillan Cancer Relief

89 Albert Embankment

London SE1 7UG

Tel: 020 7840 7840

Information line: 0845 601 6161

www.macmillan.org.uk

The Cancer Research Campaign
10 Cambridge Terrace
London NW1 4JL
Tel: 020 7224 1333
Hotline: 020 7313 5027 (Monday-Friday 9.15am-5.15pm)
www.crc.org.uk or
www.cancerhelp.org.uk

The Bristol Cancer Centre
Grove House
Cornwallis Grove
Bristol BS8 4PG
Tel: 0117 980 9500
www.bristolcancerhelp.org

CHILDREN
National Children's Bureau
8 Wakley Street
London EC1V 7QE
Tel: 020 7843 6000
www.ncb.org.uk

OLDER PEOPLE
Age Concern England
Astral House
1268 London Road
London SW16 4ER
Tel: 020 8765 7200
www.ageconcern.org.uk

Age Concern Scotland
113 Rose Street
Edinburgh EH2 3DT
Tel: 0131 220 3345

Age Concern Wales
1, Cathedral Road
Cardiff CF11 9SD
Tel: 029 2037 1566

Age Concern Northern Ireland
3 Lower Crescent
Belfast BR7 1NR
Tel: 028 9024 5729

Alzheimer's Society
Gordon House
10 Greencoat Place
London SW1P 1PH
Tel: 020 7306 0808
Helpline: 0845 300 0336
www.alzheimers.org.uk

Carers National Association
20-25 Glasshouse Yard
London EC1A 4JT
Tel: 020 7490 8818
Carer's Line: 0808 808 7777
(Monday-Friday 10am-12pm and 2pm-4pm)

COMPLEMENTARY MEDICINE
ACUPUNCTURE
The British Acupuncture Council
63 Jeddo Road
London W12 9HQ
Tel: 020 8735 0400
www.acupuncture.org.uk

The British Medical Acupuncture Society
12 Marbury House
Higher Whitley, Warrington
Cheshire WA4 4QW
www.medical-acupuncture.co.uk

HOMEOPATHY

The British Homeopathic Association

15 Clerkenwell Close
London EC1R 0AA
Tel: 020 7566 7800
www.trusthomeopathy.org

Society of Homeopaths

4a Artizan Road
Northampton, NN1 4HU
www.homeopathy-soh.org

OSTEOPATHY

General Osteopathic Council

176 Tower Bridge Road
London SE1 3LU
Tel: 020 7357 6655
www.osteopathy.org.uk

British Osteopathic Association

Langham House West
Mill Street, Luton
Bedfordshire, LU1 2NA
Tel: 01582 488 455
www.osteopathy.org

CHIROPRACTIC

General Chiropractic Association

344-354 Gray's Inn Road
London WC1X 8BP
Tel: 020 7713 5155
www.chiropractic-uk.co.uk

British Chiropractic Association

Blagrave House, 17 Blagrave Street
Reading, Berkshire, RG1 1QB
Tel: 0118 950 5950
www.chiropractic-uk.co.uk

OTHER CONTACTS

NHS DIRECT

Tel: 0845 4647
www.nhsdirect.nhs.uk
The NHS Direct Healthcare Guide is
available free from pharmacies.

MEDICENTRES

www.medicentre.co.uk
Full details including location of
Medicentres and a current price list.

SMOKING

The National Quitline

Tel: 0800 169 0169
www.givingupsmoking.co.uk

WAITING TIMES

National Waiting List Helpline

Tel: 020 8983 1133

THE PATIENT'S ASSOCIATION

PO Box 935, Harrow
Middlesex, HA1 3YJ
Tel: 0208 423 911
Helpline: 0845 6084455
www.patients-association.com

HEALTH SERVICE OMBUDSMAN

Millbank Tower, Millbank,
London, SW1P 4QP
Tel: 020 7217 4051
Helpline: 0845 015 4033
www.ombudsman.org.uk

Index of NHS Hospitals

Index of Private Hospitals

Index

coronary care units 77, 78
 private 212, 214
critical care, private hospitals 213-14
CT scan, strokes 105, 111

day-case surgery 37-8
diabetes, heart disease 72
diet
 cancer and 129, 130
 heart disease 72
Disability Living Allowance 184
Disabled Person's Tax Credit 184
discrimination, in hospital 51
doctors, private hospitals 213
drugs
 blood pressure 74
 heart attacks 77-8

ear, nose and throat surgeons 133
echocardiograms 83
electrocardiograms (ECGs) 77, 82
 24-hour monitoring 83
Enduring Power of Attorney 182-3
equipment, private hospitals 213
exercise tolerance tests 82

family history
 cancer 129
 heart disease 72
food, hospitals 48-9

general anaesthetics 40
germs, antibiotic-resistant 47
GPs 2-3
 appointments 3
 choice 6-7
 complaints 7, 10
 history taking 12
 out-of-hours contact 10
 private hospital referrals 208
 private patients 10
 referrals *see* referrals
gynaecologists 133

health service Ombudsman 52-3
heart attacks 76-9
 drugs 77-8
heart bypass surgery 70-1, 84-5
 hospital performance 89

heart disease 70-5
 causes 72
 diagnosis and testing 79, 82-4
 hospital performance 88-99
 operations 84-5
 risk profiling 73
heart failure 87-8
heart valve replacement 85
Hepatitis C 129
high blood pressure, heart disease
 72-4
high dependency units 59
 private 212, 213
hip fracture 185
 mortality 185, 187, 197-201
HIV 129
hormonal manipulation, cancer 138
hospices, cancer care 139
hospitals
 A&E departments 59-64
 admissions 30-1, 36
 cancer care performance 140-51
 children's surgery, performance
 162-70
 choice 15
 complaints 51-3
 emergency admissions, children
 159
 food 48-9
 heart disease, performance 88-99
 hip fracture mortality 197-201
 inpatients 32-3
 length of stay 49
 older people, performance
 187-96
 private *see* private hospitals
 private patients 208-9
 self-discharge 50
 specialist 32
 stroke performance 110-21
 visiting 45, 47
 waiting lists 30-1
 ward cleanliness 47-8
House Officers 39
human papilloma virus 129

Incapacity Benefit 184
Income Support 184
infections, hospital acquired 47

Dr Foster Q&A   **Ⅴermilion**

What is Dr Foster?

Dr Foster is an independent organisation which measures healthcare
standards through ongoing assessments of every major hospital, maternity
unit, care home, consultant, dentist and complementary therapist in the UK.
Information from Government, hospitals and medical professionals is
analysed with the help of leading universities such as Imperial College of
Science, Technology and Medicine, Exeter University and City University. An
ethics committee, made up of some of the most distinguished figures in
healthcare, oversees research and adjudicates on complaints. Supported by
the Government and leading professional healthcare organisations, Dr Foster
brings together world-renowned academics, healthcare experts and media
professionals.

What makes Dr Foster unique?

For the first time ever an independent body of experts has assessed the UK's
health services, ranging from hospitals to maternity services, dentists and
complementary therapists. Their unique content derives from questionnaires,
statistical research and analysis, contributions from industry experts, individual
hospitals, the Department of Health and individual GPs and consultants. These
outstanding guides give you the public an unprecedented opportunity to find
out how and where to get the best possible care and service.

The Doctor Foster Guides

Available now:

0091883792   Dr Foster Good Birth Guide
0091883776   Dr Foster Good Hospital Guide

Forthcoming titles:

0091883784   Dr Foster Good Complementary Therapist Guide
0091883857   Dr Foster Good Care Home Guide
0091883822   Dr Foster Breast Cancer Guide
0091883806   Dr Foster Heart Disease Guide
0091883814   Dr Foster Infertility Guide
0091883830   Dr Foster Good Dentist Guide
0091883849   Dr Foster Good Consultant Guide

How can I order more Dr Foster titles?

To order copies of any of these books direct from Vermilion, an imprint of
the Random House Group Ltd, call The Book Service credit card hotline on
01206 255800.

The Dr Foster guides are also available from all good booksellers.